We all must occasionally deal with major upheavals or emotional distress at some points in our lives. These events can cause a host of unexpected feelings and behaviors from depression and panic attacks to major disruptions in sleep or eating. What is the best way to understand these feelings? What is the best way to fix them? Jeff Wood, in his straightforward book Getting Help, *provides an excellent guide to both the understanding of symptoms as well as options for treatment. This is the kind of book that should be in the waiting room of every physician, lawyer, or even car mechanic. It is an unbiased, scientifically respectable, and readable manual on understanding and treating mental health issues.*

—James W. Pennebaker, Ph.D., professor of psychology at the University of Texas at Austin

This book makes sense of the confusion that often prevents people from getting the best possible help for their emotional and psychological difficulties. Wood helps the reader to understand his or her symptoms, identify the various treatment options available, and assess whether treatment is working. Anyone who is considering trying psychotherapy or medication for a psychological problem should check out this book first.

—Martin M. Antony, Ph.D., ABPP, professor of psychology at Ryerson University in Toronto, Canada, and author of *The Shyness and Social Anxiety Workbook* and more than twenty other books

I liked this book immediately! Clear, concise, comprehensive, and easy to use, it is a valuable resource for the consumer and the mental health clinician alike. The section on what to expect in the process of psychotherapy is especially informative and empowering. A deep bow to Jeff Wood for pulling so much information together so well!

—Jeffrey Brantley, MD, director of the Mindfulness-Based Stress Reduction Program at Duke University's Center for Integrative Medicine and author of *Calming Your Anxious Mind*

Getting Help *takes the mystery out of mental health problems and how to get help for them. In plain language and easy-to-use checklists, Wood explains different psychological problems and disorders, the most effective treatments for them, and the roles different mental health professionals play in their care. I recommend this excellent book to anyone suffering with mental health problems to get the help they need.*

—Kim T. Mueser, Ph.D., professor of psychiatry at the Dartmouth Medical School and coauthor of *The Complete Family Guide to Schizophrenia*

Getting Help *is a one-of-a-kind book. It is an extraordinarily clear guide for those seeking help for emotional difficulties or major psychological disorders. It helps anyone suffering from emotional distress to both understand their particular difficulties and to seek out appropriate professional help.* Getting Help *will assist many, many people to navigate through the mental health maze and find solutions that work.*

— John D. Preston, Psy.D., ABPP, licensed psychologist and author of more than seventeen books, including *The Handbook of Clinical Psychopharmacology for Therapists* and *Clinical Psychopharmacology Made Ridiculously Simple*

GETTING HELP

THE COMPLETE & AUTHORITATIVE GUIDE TO SELF-ASSESSMENT & TREATMENT OF MENTAL HEALTH PROBLEMS

JEFFREY C. WOOD, PSY.D.

New Harbinger Publications, Inc.

Distributed in Canada by Raincoast Books

Copyright © 2007 by   Jeffrey C. Wood
                           New Harbinger Publications, Inc.
                           5674 Shattuck Avenue
                           Oakland, CA 94609
                           www.newharbinger.com

Cover and text design by Amy Shoup
Acquired by Tesilya Hanauer
Edited by Kayla Sussell

Library of Congress Cataloging-in-Publication Data

Wood, Jeffrey C.
   Getting help : the complete & authoritative guide to self-assessment and treatment of mental health problems / Jeffrey C. Wood.
       p. cm.
   Includes bibliographical references.
   ISBN-13: 978-1-57224-475-7
   ISBN-10: 1-57224-475-5
   1. Mental illness--Diagnosis. 2. Self-care, Health. 3. Psychology, Pathological. I. Title.
RC454W6644 2006
616.89'075--dc22
                                        2006035091

09   08   07

10   9   8   7   6   5   4   3   2   1

First printing

To Minnie and Matt—
my two favorite editors
—Jeff

CONTENTS

FOREWORD

If you, or someone you love, is struggling with a problem you don't understand, *Getting Help* could be among the most important books you'll ever read. Whether the problem is emotional, behavioral, or with your thoughts, it's important to define—exactly—what the problem is. Only then can you hope to change it.

Getting Help is unique because it provides a 264-item self-assessment inventory (available nowhere else) that can help you clarify and diagnose what's wrong. This tool will assist you in making sense of puzzling symptoms and recognizing what they mean.

Once you have a tentative diagnosis, *Getting Help* offers something even more important—something no other book does. It tells you exactly what kind of treatment works with a specific problem or diagnosis. For example, there are many different types of medications and psychotherapies. Some work with a broad range of disorders, others work with only a few problems, and a few have no proven effectiveness with any problem. So, that's another reason this book will be important to you—it summarizes all the significant studies about which treatment will be most effective for your problem. You no longer have to wonder what sort of therapy you need, or how to find an appropriate clinician. The answers are here in this book.

Now, let's assume for a moment that you've used *Getting Help* to form a tentative understanding about your problem, and you've read about which treatment is appropriate for this diagnosis. There are a lot of clinicians around who will be only too happy to see you, regardless of whether they really have the tools to help or not. How do you go about interviewing a clinician—either over the phone or during a session—to determine if he or she knows how to treat your problem? *Getting Help* provides you with a series of questions and criteria to evaluate the following issues:

· How skilled a clinician is with the particular treatment you need

· Whether the clinician can offer an appropriate treatment plan

- Whether the relationship feels sufficiently comfortable and helpful to continue

- How to evaluate your progress in meeting your treatment goals

- What to do if you aren't getting better

- How to recognize when it's time to stop

In addition to answering the questions raised above, *Getting Help* identifies all the categories of mental health professionals, and tells you the types of treatment each category of clinician has been trained to offer. It also tells you which types of treatment they may not have the training to provide.

Other important information to be found in *Getting Help* includes:

- How to find a referral

- Your rights as a patient or client

- Ethical guidelines for treatment

- What to do if there is a breach of ethics in your treatment

- The limits of confidentiality

When you are struggling with a mental health problem, knowledge is your most important tool. Getting a clearer understanding of what is wrong and concise information on research-proven treatments can save you time, money, and years of needless suffering. Good effective treatment is out there. You just have to know where and how to find it.

—Matthew McKay, Ph.D.
Author of *Thoughts & Feelings*

ACKNOWLEDGMENTS

A project like *Getting Help* could not have been completed without the additional support and skills of many other people to whom I am indebted. I would like to thank:

The thousands of researchers and mental health care professionals listed in the Reference section whose work made this book possible.

My wife, Minnie Wood, RN, whose love, support, medical knowledge, and editing skills continue to make my life and my work more fulfilling.

Everyone at New Harbinger Publications, especially Matthew McKay, Ph.D., for steering this project from the beginning; Catharine Sutker for her professional guidance and personal encouragement; Tesilya Hanauer for her hard work and personal friendship; and Kayla Sussell for making this a better book in the editing process.

John Preston, Psy.D., for editing the section on medications.

Mike Meyers for naming the book.

Minnie and Robert Cancellaro for their ceaseless love and generosity.

Isadora and Michael Asch, Jamyang and Daniel McQuillen, Judy McKay, Mara and Chad Bronstein, Craig Levine and Scott Gatz, Phil MacEachron and Debbie Kim, Michelle Skeen, Michelle Sokoloff, and Teo Ernst, for providing encouragement and suggestions throughout the two years it took to write *Getting Help*.

Peggy Roth for giving me feedback and encouragement.

And to the Wood family, for their support.

Thank you.

INTRODUCTION

MAKING SENSE OF THIS BOOK

What I know for sure is this: You are built not to shrink down to less, but to blossom into more.

—Oprah Winfrey*

Why I Wrote This Book

I began writing this book after hearing an unfortunate story from my friend and colleague Michelle. She told me about her friend, Kate, who had recently begun seeing a psychotherapist. This took a lot of courage for Kate because she had never been in therapy before, and she was very nervous about it. She had not told anyone in her family or any of her friends that she had started therapy because she was afraid of being labeled "crazy." She told only Michelle because Michelle, like me, is a psychotherapist. Like many other people, Kate sought out psychotherapy only after trying several other ways to solve her problems; but nothing had worked. So, she did what thousands of other people do; she opened a phone book and made an appointment with the first psychotherapist she could find. "After all," Kate (probably) thought, "What's the difference? Isn't all psychotherapy the same?"

Well, since all psychotherapy is not the same, this didn't turn out very well for Kate. As I said, this is an "unfortunate story."

During her first session, Kate found herself sitting in a room with a psychotherapist who just sat there and didn't say anything to her. He didn't even ask her any questions. He said hello, directed Kate to a chair, sat opposite her, and looked at her expectantly. Kate had sought help for a relationship problem, and she knew she

---

* *O Magazine.* February 2003. "This Month's Mission."

wanted someone who would give her some feedback and offer some advice about what to do. But the psychotherapist just sat there.

Kate had no idea what was happening, or what was supposed to happen, so she just started talking. When she paused, she looked at the man sitting across from her expecting him to say something in return, but he just nodded his head and motioned her to continue. Naturally, Kate became very uncomfortable, so she just kept talking. When this first session ended, she had no idea if it had gone well or whether anything beneficial had happened. Remember, she'd never been in psychotherapy before, so she didn't know what to expect.

When she left, she didn't feel any better, but the following week, not knowing what else to do, she returned to the same office and sat through the same process again. After the second session ended, Kate just about gave up. She was very frustrated and felt as though she was getting worse, not better.

"Now I have two people in my life who don't listen to me or respond to anything I say to them," she complained to Michelle. "What's the problem with you psychotherapists, anyway?" Kate asked. "How come you just sit there and don't say anything? How is anyone supposed to get better talking to someone who never talks back?"

Kate's questions were reasonable, and they pointed to three larger questions that most consumers want to know about:

· Does psychotherapy work?

· How does psychotherapy work?

· Is psychotherapy effective for my problems?

Questions like these point to a very real, very understandable lack of knowledge about mental health care that exists within the general public. But it's certainly not the general public's fault that they don't know what happens in psychotherapy. It's my responsibility and the responsibility of other mental health care professionals to educate consumers about these issues. In the twenty-first century, there is 100 percent more advertising for medications than there is for psychotherapy. (Unless you count the television promos for the *Dr. Phil Show*.)

Open any magazine or turn on any television channel and you're guaranteed to see an advertisement for some type of medication. They're everywhere. So, of course, when consumers have mental health problems, most often their first thought is to go to a primary care provider in order to get a prescription for a medication. Usually, their first thought isn't to seek help from a psychotherapist.

Now, don't get me wrong. In some cases, medications for mental health problems are effective treatments. But in most cases, psychotherapy is a necessary additional treatment or, sometimes, even a better treatment, based on the evidence of scientific research.[1-5] But how many people in the general public know that? And how many people in the general public know that, actually, there are many different kinds of psychotherapy? This book alone highlights more than twenty different types of psychotherapy—and many more groups of professionals may be offended because their type of psychotherapy isn't included. But how many consumers are aware of this? Kate sure wasn't.

Michelle, good friend and talented psychologist that she is, told Kate that she was probably getting help from a psychoanalyst.

"What does that mean?" Kate asked.

Michelle went on, telling Kate that *psychoanalysis* is a "nondirective" treatment that uses *free association*, a technique that allows clients to talk in an unguided and open way about whatever comes to mind to uncover unconscious thoughts. "Is that good?" Kate wanted to know.

Michelle went on to explain to Kate some of the basic principles of psychoanalysis. Only after that explanation did Kate make sense of what was happening whenever she visited her psychotherapist. But no one, not even her psychotherapist, had taken the time to explain to her how the process worked.

Imagine walking into your medical doctor's office and, without even speaking to you, she hooks you up to a machine and starts drawing blood. That would certainly make me nervous. So, is it any wonder that some people are nervous and more than a little cautious about beginning psychotherapy? Many people have no idea what's going to happen behind the closed doors or how the process works. Who in their right mind would want to subject themselves to unknown procedures?

And, to top it off, if you already have a mental health problem, such as depression, that's making you feel bad, it's understandable that the idea of coming in for an unknown treatment might make you feel even more nervous or frightened. I've never seen a study about this, but I would bet that most people who come in for psychotherapy do so either because (1) they know someone else who did and they've heard firsthand that it is helpful, or (2) they come in because they are in so much pain that psychotherapy is their last ditch effort to get better. If this is true, it's unfortunate and very sad.

Studies do show that many people with mental health problems wait, on average, as long as several years before seeking help for problems like depression, anxiety, phobias, and post-traumatic stress disorder.[6] Yet, the truth is there are many effective treatments for these and other mental health problems, using psychotherapy, medications, or a combination of the two. But again, most people aren't aware that these treatments exist. So how would you know to ask for one?

Another reason people don't come in for treatment of mental health problems is the *stigma* associated with psychotherapy. That means people are worried they'll be labeled "crazy" or "strange" if they do start psychotherapy. And God forbid anyone they know should find out! It's understandable that people want to keep their personal issues private. But the truth is mental health problems are no different than other health issues. No one wants to live with depression, anxiety, or schizophrenia, just like no one wants to live with constant headaches, backaches, or cancer. These are all painful disorders with which to live.

Furthermore, mental health problems are not a sign of weakness. Millions of people all around the world suffer with these problems, including politicians, movie stars, and mental health care workers themselves. It's time for society to address mental health issues in the same way that we address other illnesses. You would certainly never blame someone for suffering with cancer or heart disease. So why do we, as a society, still stigmatize mental health problems?

I think there are a few answers to that question. First, most people don't know much about mental health problems, so there's a fear of the unknown. Second, most people don't know there are effective treatments for many mental health issues. And third, our collective memories are stocked with horrific, outdated images from old movies about people with mental health problems. Remember the electroshock therapy Jack Nicholson suffered in *One Flew Over the Cuckoo's Nest*? How about Angelina Jolie's treatment in *Girl, Interrupted*? Or have you ever seen pictures of a bearded psychiatrist, smoking his pipe while sitting silently behind his client? Images like these are about as accurate a representation of modern mental health care as a 1965 Ford is of modern transportation.

Many current portrayals of psychotherapy aren't even correct. Despite its popularity (and my personal liking for it), the *Dr. Phil Show* isn't even an accurate portrayal of a typical psychotherapy session. No one gets a lifelong problem solved in fifteen minutes. Dr. Phil McGraw is a psychologist, but he's the first person to say that what he does on television isn't psychotherapy. He points out people's problems to them, and then he steers them in the right direction to get help. But his show is designed for entertainment, so it's confrontational: without that element it wouldn't be dramatic enough to keep an audience's attention. That's why people watch it night after night.

But despite his creative methods, I think Dr. Phil has done a great job of educating the American public about mental health problems. He's also done a great job of shattering the image of the stodgy, old psychotherapist who sits silently behind his clients smoking a pipe. As you can tell by watching his show, many mental health care professionals can become very engaged in their clients' treatment.

But, let's get back to Kate. When we last left her, my friend Michelle had explained to her what was going on during her psychotherapy sessions. Kate was grateful for Michelle's explanations and she returned to that treatment because she finally understood what its goals were. After that, she was able to start benefiting from the treatment and her relationship problem began to improve. The temporary setback she experienced was unfortunate for Kate, but for me, it was the inspiration to write this book. I thought, "Why not create a resource for consumers that outlines how to figure out what their problem is and how to find the best type of help for that problem?"

There have been other attempts to write a book like this, but none of them included all of the elements to be found in *Getting Help*, especially the symptoms checklist, the up-to-date research about the illnesses, the treatment recommendations, and the summaries of many different kinds of treatments. The goal of this book is not to show you how to solve your mental health problem by yourself. The goal is to help you find the best mental health professional for your specific problem who can then provide you with the best treatment plan tailored to your specific needs. In essence, this book is designed to make you a well-educated consumer, and to get you to visit a professional's office.

After you finish reading this book, my goal for you is that you will:

- Feel more hopeful about your life

- Feel more empowered to seek an effective treatment for your problem

- Feel less alone, after reading about how many people share your problem

- Feel less stigmatized about getting treatment for your problem

How to Use This Book

Getting Help isn't designed to be read from cover to cover, although you can certainly do that if you want to be a very educated consumer. It is meant to be used in a step-by-step manner. The book is divided into five main chapters to correspond with the five steps that will help you identify the best treatment for your problems and then help you figure out how to find that treatment.

Start with chapter 1, Making Sense of Your Symptoms. This chapter contains a self-assessment checklist that will help you identify the symptoms that you've been experiencing. The symptoms are organized into groups, which will help you to identify the specific mental health problems with which you might be suffering. The last question of each group is always the same. It asks you to rate the severity of the symptoms you've been experiencing. Then, at the end of the entire checklist, you'll be directed to chapter 2 to find descriptions of the problems that are causing the most distress in your life.

Chapter 2 is called Making Sense of Your Problem. Here, you'll read about the specific problems that you marked as "extremely distressing" and "very distressing" on the symptoms checklist. Each description of a problem contains the same basic information you need to make your research and comparison of the problems easier. Each description contains information about what the disorder is, what some of the related problems are, who is affected by the disorder, what some possible causes might be, and what treatments are recommended.

Be mindful that these descriptions are not official diagnoses. Only a mental health care professional can give you an official diagnosis. These descriptions are designed to give you a better idea about the nature of the problems you're experiencing, so you'll be able to find the best treatment possible. You may even find that several of the descriptions portray how you feel. That's okay. Many people suffer with multiple problems and some problems are closely related.

Chapter 3 is called Making Sense of the Treatments. Here, you'll find descriptions of the recommended psychotherapies and medications available to treat your problem. You'll also find descriptions of some psychotherapies that haven't been recommended for anything specific. These treatments are included in this book because they're popular and because they've been known to work for some people, even if they don't have a wealth of scientific research to support them.

After you've figured out what problem you're suffering with and the type of treatment that you want to find, chapter 4, Making Sense of the Mental Health Care Professionals, will help you determine the type of professional from whom you should seek help. This chapter will help you figure out the differences between psychiatrists, psychologists, master's level counselors, and the rest. For each one, recommendations are made about when you should contact them.

Finally, after you've figured out the treatment and the professional you're looking for, chapter 5, Making Sense of the Process, will walk you through the steps of finding a referral and making that first phone call to a mental health care professional. You'll also be told how to evaluate whether the treatment is working once you've started. Then, you'll get some basic information about the ethics that guide your treatment, and some other information that will help to make your treatment more successful.

Again, the goal of this book is to help you figure out what your mental health problems are. Once you've done that, you can get the most effective treatment possible. With that goal in mind, I've tried to make this book as simple as possible to use. If you want more information, there is a list of additional reading in the appendix, along with some contact information for mental health care organizations in which you might be interested.

CHAPTER 1

MAKING SENSE OF YOUR SYMPTOMS

Your vision will become clear only when you look into your heart....
Who looks outside, dreams; who looks inside, awakens.

—Carl Jung*

How to Use the Symptoms Checklist

The symptoms checklist included in this chapter will help you to identify the mental health problems with which you're suffering. The checklist is divided into twenty-five different groups of questions; each group will help you to identify a particular disorder. Then, at the end of the checklist, you'll be guided to chapter 2, Making Sense of Your Problem, where you can read comprehensive descriptions of your problems, including recommended treatments.

It's very important that you answer the entire checklist before you begin reading the descriptions in chapter 2. You may find a group of questions that more accurately describes your problem later in the checklist rather than at the beginning. This is important because many mental health problems share similar symptoms, but the recommended treatments for those disorders are sometimes very different.

As you read the questions in each group, place a checkmark (✓) next to the ones you're currently experiencing or have experienced in the recent past. Be sure to mark problems even if they apply to you only moderately. There are no right or wrong answers. The purpose of this checklist is to help you find the words to describe how you're feeling and to identify your problem.

---

*   From *C. G. Jung Letters*, volume 1. 1992. Edited by Gerhard Adler and Aniela Jaffe. Princeton, NJ: Princeton University Press.

The last question in each group will ask you to assess how severely those symptoms are affecting your life. Do your best to assign a number between 0 and 4 to the severity of the whole set of symptoms. The ratings all use the following format:

0 = This group of symptoms is not bothering you at all.
1 = This group of symptoms is mildly distressing.
2 = This group of symptoms is moderately distressing.
3 = This group of symptoms is very distressing.
4 = This group of symptoms is extremely distressing.

Then, after you've completed the entire checklist, you'll determine which problems are distressing you the most, and you'll be directed to read more about those disorders in chapter 2 to determine the most effective treatment for your problem.

WOOD SELF-ASSESSMENT CHECKLIST

1. Read each question and decide if it applies to how you feel now or to how you've felt in the recent past.

2. Check (✔) the questions that apply to you—even moderately—in the answer column to the right.

3. For the last question of every group, determine how severely that whole set of symptoms is affecting your life using the 0 to 4 scale below:

    0 = Not bothering you at all
    1 = Mildly distressing
    2 = Moderately distressing
    3 = Very distressing
    4 = Extremely distressing

4. When you've completed the entire checklist, read the directions at the beginning of chapter 2, Making Sense of Your Problem, to find the problems that are the most distressing to you.

1. Do you feel very sad or unhappy, more often than you feel good?   1. _____

2. Are you feeling so unhappy that you don't want to leave your house or do the things you normally like to do?   2. _____

3. Are other people concerned about how unhappy you are?   3. _____

4. Are you having trouble with your sleep: not wanting to get out of bed, sleeping most of the day, or feeling too restless to sleep at all?   4. _____

5. Are you feeling excessively tired or rundown most days?   5. _____

6. Are you having trouble thinking, concentrating, or making decisions?   6. _____

7. Are you feeling excessively restless or nervous?   7. _____

8. Have you experienced an unexpected increase or decrease in your weight?   8. _____

9. Does your life feel meaningless or worthless?   9. _____

10. Do you think that you or other people might be better off if you were dead?   10. _____

11. Do you have suicidal thoughts or have you tried to kill yourself? 11. _____

12. Have all of these feelings been *very intense* for a few weeks or months? 12. _____

13. Do these feelings describe how you generally feel most of the time, for at least a few years? 13. _____

14. Review the questions you checked (✓) in this section. How severely does this group of symptoms distress you and affect your life? (Use the 0 to 4 scale.) **14.** _____

These symptoms are commonly associated with depression. See page 58 for a detailed description.

---

15. Do you ever feel excessively energetic and out of control? (During this time, you may feel excessively happy, high, restless, irritable, or a combination of these feelings.) 15. _____

16. Does this period of excessive energy last about one week and interfere with your life, your work, or your relationships? 16. _____

17. Is the experience just a few days long and only moderately intense, which still allows you to function? 17. _____

18. In addition to feelings of excessive energy, do you also experience periods of excessive sadness or depression? 18. _____

During the periods of excessive energy:

19. Do you feel as though you barely need to sleep at all, and yet you still feel extremely energetic? 19. _____

20. Are you so easily distracted that your attention wanders from one idea to the next faster than you can keep track of them? 20. _____

21. Do you notice that the rate at which you speak is much faster than normal? (Maybe other people have asked you to slow down because they can't understand you.) 21. _____

22. Do you engage in an excessive number of plans and activities, perhaps even impulsive behaviors that you later regret, like shopping sprees, expensive trips, or unsafe sexual activities? 22. _____

23. Do you sometimes think that no one else is as smart, strong, or as powerful as you are? 23. _____

24. During the periods of excessive energy or depression, do you see, hear, smell, taste, or feel things that other people can't? 24. _____

25. Review the questions you checked (✓) in this section. How severely does this group of symptoms distress you and affect your life? (Use the 0 to 4 scale.)

    These symptoms are commonly associated with bipolar disorder/manic depression. *See page 44 for a detailed description.*

25. _____

---

26. Do you have an overwhelming fear of something specific, such as snakes, flying in airplanes, driving over bridges, etc., which is more excessive than what's considered normal worrying?

26. _____

27. Do you have an overwhelming fear of social situations, where you have to meet people or speak in front of them? (This, too, is a much greater fear than normal worrying.)

27. _____

28. When you're in social situations, are you afraid that you might do something that would be horribly embarrassing or are you afraid of being judged by others?

28. _____

29. Does your fear seem irrational or unreasonable to you?

29. _____

30. Do you go out of your way to avoid contact with the feared object, like driving thousands of miles instead of flying; or do you make great efforts to avoid social events where you might be forced to meet people?

30. _____

31. When you're forced to confront a feared situation, does an intense feeling of fear or panic suddenly overwhelm you? (Maybe your heart begins to race, you start to sweat excessively, you find it difficult to speak, you feel nauseous, or you start to shake.)

31. _____

32. Review the questions you checked (✓) in this section. How severely does this group of symptoms distress you and affect your life? (Use the 0 to 4 scale.)

    These symptoms are commonly associated with phobias. *See page 97 for a detailed description.*

32. _____

---

33. Did you ever experience a traumatic event, or witness a traumatic event, in which you or someone else was severely injured, threatened, or killed? (This includes situations such as crimes, wars, rapes, attacks, accidents, etc., and it can be an event that happened a long time ago.)

33. _____

34. Did this event make you feel intensely afraid or hopeless?

34. _____

35. Do you have nightmares about what happened?

35. _____

36. Do you have repetitive, uncontrollable thoughts about what happened?   36. _____

37. Do you have moments when you feel like you're back in the situation reliving it?   37. _____

38. Do you have intense fearful reactions to people, places, or things that remind you about what happened?   38. _____

39. Do you avoid thinking about what happened?   39. _____

40. Do you avoid talking about what happened?   40. _____

41. Do you avoid places associated with the event?   41. _____

42. Since the traumatic event, do you feel as though you've shut down emotionally? Or have others noticed a dramatic change in your emotions?   42. _____

43. Since the traumatic event, do you ever feel like you're suddenly outside your body or not in the room? (Maybe you have episodes of missing time, when you can't remember what happened to you.)   43. _____

44. Do you have trouble remembering certain details about what happened?   44. _____

45. Have you been uninterested in relationships and activities that interested you before the traumatic event occurred?   45. _____

46. Are you having trouble sleeping, either not sleeping at all or not being able to sleep soundly throughout the night?   46. _____

47. Are you having trouble thinking, concentrating, or making decisions?   47. _____

48. Do you feel irritated or easily frustrated most of the time?   48. _____

49. Since the traumatic event, do you feel as if you're constantly looking out for other dangers?   49. _____

50. Review the questions you checked (✓) in this section. How severely does this group of symptoms distress you and affect your life? (Use the 0 to 4 scale.)   **50.** _____

   These symptoms are commonly associated with post-traumatic stress disorder. See page 100 for a detailed description.

---

51. Do you experience sudden attacks of fear or panic that are unpredictable, intense, and overwhelming?   51. _____

52. When these attacks take place, do you also experience physical discomfort that makes you think you are having a heart attack, dying, or going crazy?   52. _____

<u>During these attacks of fear:</u>

53. Does your heart pound intensely?   53. _____

54. Do you get dizzy?   54. _____

55. Does your stomach feel sick?   55. _____

56. Do your hands, feet, or face tingle or go numb?   56. _____

57. Do you start to sweat excessively or get the chills?   57. _____

58. Do you start to shake?   58. _____

59. Are these sudden attacks so intense and frightening that you avoid leaving your house because you're afraid that you might be stranded outside without help?   59. _____

60. Review the questions you checked (✔) in this section. How severely does this group of symptoms distress you and affect your life? (Use the 0 to 4 scale.)   **60.** _____

   These symptoms are commonly associated with panic disorder. *See page 94 for a detailed description.*

---

61. Do you have disturbing thoughts that come up repeatedly and are impossible to stop or control?   61. _____

62. Are you bothered by repetitious fears, such as being contaminated by germs or dirt, being killed, hurting someone else, or being punished by God?   62. _____

63. Are you bothered by repetitious desires, like the desire to keep things in perfect order, to not throw anything away, or to do something strange, like stand up and scream at work?   63. _____

64. Are you bothered by repetitious images in your mind, such as images of pictures, symbols, or pornography?   64. _____

65. Do these intrusive thoughts make you extremely anxious, nervous, or afraid?   65. _____

66. Are you worried that if you continue to think these thoughts something bad will happen?   66. _____

67. Do you do anything after you have the thought, in order to prevent something dangerous or bad from happening? (This includes behaviors like washing your hands repeatedly, praying, checking that the door is locked, arranging objects in a certain order, etc.)   67. _____

68. Have these thoughts and behaviors become regular rituals that you do over and over again?　68. _____

69. Do these thoughts and responses take up much of your time or interfere with your life?　69. _____

70. Do your thoughts and responses seem irrational or unreasonable to you?　70. _____

71. Review the questions you checked (✔) in this section. How severely does this group of symptoms distress you and affect your life? (Use the 0 to 4 scale.)　**71.** _____

    These symptoms are commonly associated with obsessive-compulsive disorder. *See page 90 for a detailed description.*

---

72. Do you worry more than most people about things that might happen in the future?　72. _____

73. Are these worries very time-consuming, very distracting, and do they occur almost every day?　73. _____

74. Is it very hard to control this worrying or to turn it off when you want to?　74. _____

75. Do you have lots of muscle tension, feel stressed-out all the time, or do you often feel physically exhausted?　75. _____

76. Do you feel agitated or easily frustrated most of the time?　76. _____

77. Do you have trouble sleeping, either not sleeping at all or not being able to sleep soundly through an entire night?　77. _____

78. Does your worrying keep you up at night?　78. _____

79. Do you have trouble thinking, concentrating, or making decisions?　79. _____

80. Review the questions you checked (✔) in this section. How severely does this group of symptoms distress you and affect your life? (Use the 0 to 4 scale.)　**80.** _____

    These symptoms are commonly associated with generalized anxiety disorder. *See page 83 for a detailed description.*

---

81. Did you recently experience a very stressful or painful event? (This includes situations such as developing an illness, ending a relationship, moving to a new home, having a child, getting married, retiring, and so forth.)　81. _____

82. Since that situation occurred, have you been feeling very sad, nervous, or anxious?   82. _____

83. Since that situation, have you been having difficulty functioning?   83. _____

84. Do you think your reactions to the situation are excessive, compared to what might be expected?   84. _____

85. Has your recovery from the situation gone beyond the length of time that would be considered reasonable?   85. _____

86. Review the questions you checked (✓) in this section. How severely does this group of symptoms distress you and affect your life? (Use the 0 to 4 scale.)   **86.** _____

These symptoms are commonly associated with adjustment disorder. *See page 29 for a detailed description.*

---

87. Do you have the same types of problems in many of your important relationships? (Maybe your relationships end in the same way or have similar, dissatisfying qualities.)   87. _____

88. Do you pick romantic partners or friends who seem to have the same problems or cause the same types of problems in your relationships?   88. _____

89. Do problems with your current relationships remind you of problems you had with your family while you were growing up?   89. _____

90. Do your friends, family, or romantic partners make you feel bad about yourself all the time? (Maybe they make you feel sad, unlovable, defective, broken, guilty, etc.)   90. _____

91. Do certain relationships trigger certain feelings in you that are so painful that all you care about is stopping the pain?   91. _____

92. Do you handle problems in your relationships the same way, over and over again, even if your methods aren't effective? (Maybe you withdraw, run away, get angry, attack the other person, or become passive and nice, even when you don't want to be.)   92. _____

93. Is it hard to say no to other people or to set limits to protect yourself?   93. _____

94. Do you blow up easily when someone does something wrong?   94. _____

95. Are you pessimistic about your relationships, believing that eventually they'll fall apart as they've always done?   95. _____

96. Review the questions you checked (✔) in this section. How severely does this group of symptoms distress you and affect your life? (Use the 0 to 4 scale.)

    These symptoms are commonly associated with schema-focused relationship problems. See page 104 for a detailed description.

96. _____

---

97. Do you drink alcohol or use drugs on a daily, weekly, or regular basis?

97. _____

98. Do you need to drink or use drugs more than you did in the past in order to get the same feeling or high?

98. _____

99. Are you no longer able to achieve that same feeling, even though you use more alcohol or drugs than you used in the past?

99. _____

100. If you stop drinking or using drugs, or even try lowering your usual amount, do you experience physical pain or emotional distress?

100. _____

101. Are you unable to stop drinking or using drugs, even if you want to?

101. _____

102. Have you been drinking or using drugs for a longer period of time than you thought you would?

102. _____

103. Do you spend lots of time and money getting or using alcohol or drugs?

103. _____

104. Despite family, social, or legal problems associated with your habit, do you continue drinking or using drugs?

104. _____

105. Do you continue to drink or use drugs despite some kind of physical problem that it has caused, such as cirrhosis of the liver or hepatitis C?

105. _____

106. Do you drink or use drugs in situations that are potentially dangerous, such as while driving or working?

106. _____

107. Are you ashamed to tell your family or friends how much you really drink or use drugs?

107. _____

108. Review the questions you checked (✔) in this section. How severely does this group of symptoms distress you and affect your life? (Use the 0 to 4 scale.)

    These symptoms are commonly associated with drug and alcohol addiction problems. See page 72 for a detailed description.

108. _____

---

109. Do you often yell at people for doing things that irritate or offend you?

109. _____

110. Do you feel as though people do these things to you on purpose?

110. _____

111. Do you often get angry at people for breaking the rules, like when someone cuts you off in traffic?

111. _____

112. Does your anger escalate very quickly and easily?

112. _____

113. Does your anger last for a long time, even after the event has passed?

113. _____

114. When you get angry, do you take it out on someone or something, or do you hold in your anger and think of ways to take revenge?

114. _____

115. When you get excessively irritated, have you noticed that your face feels hot, your muscles tense up, and your heart starts pounding?

115. _____

116. After getting angry with someone, especially a friend or a family member, do you sometimes realize that you went too far?

116. _____

117. Review the questions you checked (✔) in this section. How severely does this group of symptoms distress you and affect your life? (Use the 0 to 4 scale.)

117. _____

These symptoms are commonly associated with anger control problems. See page 31 for a detailed description.

---

118. Are you afraid that your friends and family are going to abandon you or reject you in some way?

118. _____

119. Do you engage in dangerous activities, like cutting yourself, having unsafe sex, going on shopping sprees, or driving at high speeds?

119. _____

120. Do other people deeply disappoint you?

120. _____

121. Do you feel hollow or empty inside?

121. _____

122. Have you ever tried to kill yourself or made plans to kill yourself?

122. _____

123. Do you often get uncontrollably angry?

123. _____

124. Do you ever feel you have to get angry so that other people will understand you?

124. _____

125. Do you struggle to control your emotions? 125. _____

126. Do your emotions often explode and overwhelm you? 126. _____

127. Do you experience waves of depression or fear that you can't get rid of? 127. _____

128. Do you often worry that something bad is going to happen to you or someone else? 128. _____

129. Review the questions you checked (✔) in this section. How severely does this group of symptoms distress you and affect your life? (Use the 0 to 4 scale.) **129.** _____

These symptoms are commonly associated with emotion dysregulation. *See page 76 for a detailed description.*

---

130. Do you think about food or eating many times throughout the day? 130. _____

131. Are you afraid of gaining weight? 131. _____

132. Do you restrict your diet or engage in an excessive amount of exercise to burn off calories? 132. _____

133. Do you engage in any type of purging activity after eating, like forcing yourself to vomit or using laxatives? 133. _____

134. Before purging, do you eat an excessive amount of food, knowing that you'll soon be getting rid of it? 134. _____

135. Are you excessively concerned with how you look? 135. _____

136. Are you afraid that if you don't look a certain way, other people won't like you? 136. _____

137. Is your weight far below average, according to what is commonly accepted as a normal weight? 137. _____

138. Do other people think that you look too skinny, even if you don't agree with them? 138. _____

139. Have other people expressed their concern that you don't eat enough, even if you don't agree with them? 139. _____

140. If you're a woman, have you stopped having your period prematurely? 140. _____

141. Do you feel depressed or anxious? 141. _____

142. Do you have fine body hair growing unexpectedly on your stomach, back, chest, or pelvic region? 142. _____

143. Do you have a slow or irregular heartbeat? 143. _____

144. Do you often feel cold?   144. _____

145. Do you have frequent stomach pains or constipation?   145. _____

146. Do you have unexpected tooth erosion?   146. _____

147. Do you have small red spots on your arms or legs that later bruise?   147. _____

148. Review the questions you checked (✔) in this section. How severely does this group of symptoms distress you and affect your life? (Use the 0 to 4 scale.)   **148.** _____

These symptoms are commonly associated with anorexia. *See page 34 for a detailed description.*

---

149. Do you ever feel out of control and eat an excessive amount of food in a relatively short time?   149. _____

150. After eating so much, do you purge yourself of the food somehow, such as by vomiting, using laxatives, or taking enemas?   150. _____

151. Do you maintain your weight through some other type of activity, like excessive exercise or regular fasting?   151. _____

152. Do you sometimes feel ashamed about your behavior or are you afraid to tell people what you do? (Maybe you hide your eating and purging activities because you don't want people to know about them.)   152. _____

153. Are you very afraid of gaining weight?   153. _____

154. Are you excessively concerned with how you look?   154. _____

155. Are you afraid that if you don't look a certain way, other people won't like you?   155. _____

156. If you're a woman, have you stopped having your period prematurely?   156. _____

157. Have you experienced excessive tooth erosion, stomach problems, or heart trouble?   157. _____

158. Review the questions you checked (✔) in this section. How severely does this group of symptoms distress you and affect your life? (Use the 0 to 4 scale.)   **158.** _____

These symptoms are commonly associated with bulimia. *See page 52 for a detailed description.*

159. Do you worry excessively about a particular part of your body, or maybe many parts of your body?   159. _____

160. Do you think of yourself as flawed, ugly, or abnormal because of your body?   160. _____

161. Do you often feel upset, depressed, or angry?   161. _____

162. Do other people tell you that they don't notice your imperfections, or that you're imagining the defects to be bigger than they really are?   162. _____

163. Do you regularly look at yourself in mirrors, store windows, spoons, or other reflective surfaces to check the part(s) of your body that you're worried about?   163. _____

164. Do you cover all the mirrors in your home so that you can't see your reflection?   164. _____

165. Do you spend an excessive amount of time and effort trying to hide or cover the parts of your body that distress you with makeup, clothing, or styling?   165. _____

166. Are you considering cosmetic surgery or dermatology treatments to improve the parts of your body that distress you, or have you already had surgery or treatment to correct your flaws?   166. _____

167. Do you avoid social situations where others might notice your imperfections?   167. _____

168. Review the questions you checked (✔) in this section. How severely does this group of symptoms distress you and affect your life? (Use the 0 to 4 scale.)   **168. _____**

These symptoms are commonly associated with body dysmorphic disorder. *See page 49 for a detailed description.*

---

169. Is it very difficult or impossible for you to focus your attention on most tasks?   169. _____

170. Do you get easily distracted?   170. _____

171. Do you often daydream or does your mind easily wander?   171. _____

172. Do you have trouble listening to other people because of your inability to focus on what they're saying?   172. _____

173. Do you give up on many tasks because of your inability to complete them?   173. _____

174. Do you often think that no matter how much willpower or discipline you have, it's still not enough to accomplish most tasks?   174. _____

175. Do you often feel restless, fidgety, or find it hard to sit still for very long?   175. _____

176. Do you find it hard to control your behavior or hold back your impulses?   176. _____

177. Do you often do things that you later regret or do things for which you're later criticized?   177. _____

178. Do you often feel, or have you ever been described, as "hyperactive" or "out of control"?   178. _____

179. Have you experienced many of these problems since you were a child?   179. _____

180. Have these problems interfered with your relationships, schoolwork, or job performance?   180. _____

181. Review the questions you checked (✔) in this section. How severely does this group of symptoms distress you and affect your life? (Use the 0 to 4 scale.)   **181.** _____

These symptoms are commonly associated with attention-deficit/hyperactivity disorder. *See page 41 for a detailed description.*

---

182. Do you have continual physical pain that has not responded to medical treatments?   182. _____

183. Was your pain caused by an accident or an illness?   183. _____

184. Do you have chronic stomach problems, such as bloating, nausea, or a constant upset stomach?   184. _____

185. Do you have some kind of sexual or reproductive problem, such as a loss of interest in sex, painful sexual experiences, or an inability to perform sexual activities?   185. _____

186. Do you have problems with your vision, hearing, balance, movement, sense of touch, or any other physical difficulties?   186. _____

187. Have you experienced a loss of physical movement or a loss of one of your senses for which a medical professional has not been able to find a cause?   187. _____

188. Do you often feel ill, despite the fact that a medical professional has told you there is nothing wrong with you?   188. _____

189. Review the questions you checked (✔) in this section. How severely do any of these symptoms distress you and affect your life? (Use the 0 to 4 scale.)

    These symptoms are commonly associated with somatoform disorders. See page 119 for a detailed description.

189. _____

---

190. Do you see, hear, smell, taste, or feel things that other people can't? (This includes hearing voices or sounds, seeing hallucinations, or smelling scents that other people aren't able to perceive. This pertains only to your awake, daily experience, not to your dreams.)

190. _____

191. Are your thoughts often jumbled and confused?

191. _____

192. Is it hard for you to make decisions?

192. _____

193. When you speak, is it hard for other people to understand you?

193. _____

194. Do you sometimes think that someone is communicating with you in a secretive, special way, such as through codes transmitted over the radio or messages hidden inside books?

194. _____

195. Do you think that you're being singled out for punishment or spied on by God, the government, or someone else?

195. _____

196. Do you think that someone else is controlling your mind or body?

196. _____

197. Do you have other beliefs that no one else has or that you're too afraid to talk about?

197. _____

198. Do you sometimes behave in ways that are highly unusual and unpredictable? (This includes doing things in public that other people consider inappropriate.)

198. _____

199. Does your body ever become extremely rigid or impossible to move?

199. _____

200. Does your body ever become uncontrollably active?

200. _____

201. Are your emotional reactions or verbal responses much less expressive than those of other people?

201. _____

202. Do your emotional reactions often come at unusual or inappropriate moments, such as laughing when other people are being serious?

202. _____

203. Do you often find it hard to take care of yourself, such as eating regular meals and washing yourself?

203. _____

204. Do you often feel very sad or unhappy?

204. _____

205. Review the questions you checked (✔) in this section. How severely does this group of symptoms distress you and affect your life? (Use the 0 to 4 scale.)

These symptoms are commonly associated with schizophrenia. *See page 112 for a detailed description.*

205. _____

206. Do you think that other people are out to get you in some way?

206. _____

207. Do you think that other people are watching you all the time?

207. _____

208. Do people often say things that sound suspicious to you?

208. _____

209. Do you doubt the loyalty of your friends and family?

209. _____

210. Is it hard for you to make lasting friendships or to engage in family activities because of your suspicions?

210. _____

211. Review the questions you checked (✔) in this section. How severely does this group of symptoms distress you and affect your life? (Use the 0 to 4 scale.)

These symptoms are commonly associated with extreme suspicion of others. *See page 80 for a detailed description.*

211. _____

212. Do you have urges and impulses to do things that you can't stop or control?

212. _____

213. Do you steal things you don't need?

213. _____

214. Do you set fires for no apparent reason?

214. _____

215. Do you have fits of anger, aggression, or destructiveness that go beyond normal reactions to situations?

215. _____

216. Do you pull out your own hair, eyelashes, or eyebrows so much that it leads to hair loss?

216. _____

217. Do you gamble so excessively that it leads to problems with your family, relationships, work, the law, or your finances?

217. _____

218. Before doing something impulsively, do you feel pressure building up inside of you?

218. _____

219. Before doing something impulsively, do you notice physical sensations, such as your heart pounding, a tingling in your fingers, or headaches?

219. _____

220. After doing something impulsively, do you feel relieved, happy, excited, or satisfied?

220. _____

221. After doing something impulsively, do you regret your actions, because they cause you embarrassment, legal problems, or create problems for other people?

221. _____

222. Review the questions you checked (✔) in this section. How severely does this group of symptoms distress you and affect your life? (Use the 0 to 4 scale.)

222. _____

These symptoms are commonly associated with impulse control disorders. *See page 86 for a detailed description.*

---

223. Do you prefer to be alone, even if other people are around and ask you to participate in their activities?

223. _____

224. Is it very hard or embarrassing for you to form relationships?

224. _____

225. Have you stopped trying to form relationships?

225. _____

226. In general, do you not care what other people think about you?

226. _____

227. Have you been told that it's hard to tell how you're feeling or what you're thinking?

227. _____

228. Would you describe yourself as very shy or as a loner?

228. _____

229. Do you have a job that doesn't require much interaction with other people?

229. _____

230. Do you have few, if any, close friends?

230. _____

231. Review the questions you checked (✔) in this section. How severely does this group of symptoms distress you and affect your life? (Use the 0 to 4 scale.)

231. _____

These symptoms are commonly associated with schizoid personality disorder. *See page 109 for a detailed description.*

---

232. Is it impossible for you to make decisions without the constant assistance and approval of other people?

232. _____

233. Do you think that you aren't smart enough or competent enough to make your own decisions?

233. _____

234. Are you constantly afraid of upsetting other people?

234. _____

235. Do you make decisions to please other people?

235. _____

236. Do you tolerate unsatisfying friendships and romantic relationships because you're afraid of being alone?

236. _____

237. Do you often do things you don't want to do, just because you're afraid of hurting the other person's feelings?

237. _____

238. Is it very difficult for you to tell other people what you think because you're afraid that they'll criticize you?

238. _____

239. Review the questions you checked (✔) in this section. How severely does this group of symptoms distress you and affect your life? (Use the 0 to 4 scale.)

239. _____

These symptoms are commonly associated with dependent personality disorder. *See page 55 for a detailed description.*

---

240. Do you think that you possess many more exceptional characteristics than other people?

240. _____

241. Is it very important that other people acknowledge your talent, attractiveness, and intelligence?

241. _____

242. Are you often focused on your own success, intelligence, and beauty?

242. _____

243. Do you think you're more deserving than other people?

243. _____

244. Do you expect special treatment from other people?

244. _____

245. Do you manipulate other people to get what you want?

245. _____

246. Do you get angry with other people if they ignore you?

246. _____

247. Do you think of your romantic relationships as a game, where you control the other person to get what you want?

247. _____

248. Are you often jealous of other people?

248. _____

249. Review the questions you checked (✔) in this section. How severely does this group of symptoms distress you and affect your life? (Use the 0 to 4 scale.)

249. _____

These symptoms are commonly associated with self-focused personality disorder. *See page 116 for a detailed description.*

---

250. Do you manipulate, abuse, or lie to other people to get what you want?

250. _____

251. Do you often break the law?

251. _____

252. Do you have a history of violent behavior?

252. _____

253. Are your needs always more important than other people's needs?

253. _____

254. Would you describe yourself as an impatient person who gets frustrated easily?

254. _____

255. Do you think other people deserve to be taken advantage of because they aren't as smart as you are?   255. _____

256. Do you lose jobs because you stop showing up?   256. _____

257. Do you think you're charming enough to manipulate other people?   257. _____

258. Do you have few, if any, close friends or meaningful romantic relationships?   258. _____

259. Review the questions you checked (✔) in this section. How severely does this group of symptoms distress you and affect your life? (Use the 0 to 4 scale.)   **259.** _____

These symptoms are commonly associated with antisocial personality disorder *or* psychopathic personality traits. *See page 37 for a detailed description.*

---

260. Is it hard for you to remember a big part of your life, for no explainable reason? (Maybe there's a hole in your life's history.)   260. _____

261. Have you ever felt as if you had another life somewhere else, or discovered that you once lived somewhere else with a different name or family?   261. _____

262. Do you ever think that there might be more than one personality inside your body? (Maybe you've felt as if there's more than one "you" inside your body, perhaps even with different names and mannerisms. Here, too, there might be holes in your history that you can't explain.)   262. _____

263. Do you often feel as though you're living outside of your body, or like you're watching a movie about your own life instead of living it? (Sometimes during these detached moments, the world can feel very strange and unfamiliar.)   263. _____

264. Review the questions you checked (✔) in this section. How severely do any of these symptoms distress you and affect your life? (Use the 0 to 4 scale.)   **264.** _____

These symptoms are commonly associated with dissociative disorders. *See page 66 for a detailed description.*

Now read the directions at the beginning of chapter 2, Making Sense of Your Problem, to find the problems that are the most distressing in your life.

CHAPTER 2

MAKING SENSE OF YOUR PROBLEM

There is no normal life that is free of pain. It's the very wrestling with our problems that can be the impetus for our growth.

—Fred Rogers*

How to Use This Chapter

Now that you've completed the symptoms checklist, you're ready to get more information about the problems you're struggling with. Go back to the checklist and find the problems that you rated 3 "Very distressing" and 4 "Extremely distressing."

Write the names of those problems here to remind yourself:

_____

_____

_____

_____

_____

_____

*   From *The World According to Mr. Rogers: Important Things to Remember*. 2003. New York: Hyperion. p. 112.

These are the issues you'll want to read about first. Their descriptions in this chapter are arranged alphabetically. Find the problems you listed above and take your time reading their descriptions. Underline the sentences that stand out for you, so that you can share them with your mental health professional when you go to get help.

Again, the point of this chapter is to empower you with information and to help you find the best and most suitable treatment for yourself. Perhaps the disorder you read about will describe your problem exactly. That would be great. Then you would know what to seek treatment for. But maybe the description of the disorder describes only a part of what you've been struggling with. That's okay, too. You may need to read descriptions of several different disorders before discovering all of the symptoms that have been distressing you.

Sometimes people have only particular symptoms or traits of a disorder, or often people suffer from multiple disorders at the same time, especially when they've survived a traumatic event, or when alcohol and/or drugs are involved. Ultimately, you may need treatment for both problems, but don't get discouraged. The more information you have about your disorder, the better prepared you'll be to find the most effective treatment.

After you're done reading about your most distressing problem, go back to the checklist and find the problems that you rated 1 "Mildly distressing" and 2 "Moderately distressing" so that you can read those descriptions, too.

Write the names of those problems here to remind yourself:

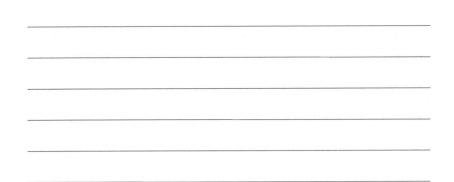

While you're reading about all of the problems you're struggling with, pay extra attention to the section called What Can You Do About It? This section will highlight some of the recommended treatments for each disorder. Write them down or circle them in the book. Then, when you're done reading about the disorders, you can read descriptions of their recommended treatments in chapter 3, Making Sense of the Treatments.

ADJUSTMENT DISORDER

WHAT IS IT?

An *adjustment disorder* is a reaction to a stressful situation that lasts longer than what is considered typical.[1] Events that can cause an adjustment disorder include having a serious illness, getting divorced, being fired from a job, leaving for school, relocating to a new home, or other life-changing situations like these. In response to these types of events, it would be normal for someone to feel upset or anxious. But if you're struggling with an adjustment disorder, the severity and length of your reaction has gone beyond what is considered usual.

For example, perhaps you lost your job, and as a result, you've spent the last three months sitting on your sofa watching television because you're so upset. Or, maybe your child recently left home to attend college and since then you've been so excessively worried about him or her that you haven't been able to function at work. Keep in mind that most people are distressed or saddened by these types of events. What makes an adjustment disorder a clinical problem is the amount of time you're affected or the severity of the distress in your life.

An adjustment disorder will begin within three months of experiencing a stressful situation and will usually disappear after six months.[1] However, if the stressful situation is ongoing, such as a chronic illness, a difficult divorce, or continuing financial problems, it isn't unusual for an adjustment disorder to last for as long as the situation remains unchanged.

There is no concise psychological definition of what an adjustment disorder will look like. In many ways an adjustment disorder may look similar to depression or anxiety. The difference is that an adjustment disorder can always be traced back to an activating circumstance or situation. By definition, if the symptoms of an adjustment disorder are caused by the death of someone you care about, your diagnosis would be defined more appropriately as "bereavement."

ARE THERE OTHER RELATED PROBLEMS?

In severe cases, an adjustment disorder might also lead to excessive alcohol or drug use, suicide attempts, or physical illness.[1]

WHO IS AFFECTED?

Some researchers have estimated that adjustment disorder is a widespread problem, affecting 12 percent of the people seeking mental health treatment in hospitals,[2] and as many as 10 to 30 percent of the people seeking treatment at other mental health centers.[1] Women are typically diagnosed with adjustment disorder twice as often as men.[1]

WHAT CAUSES IT?

An adjustment disorder is caused by the experience of a stressful situation. Unfortunately, despite the widespread prevalence of adjustment disorders, very little research has been done to determine what specifically happens to a person who experiences this problem or to investigate the problem any further.[3, 4]

WHAT CAN YOU DO ABOUT IT?

Fortunately, the prognosis for a person struggling with an adjustment disorder is good. Research has shown that people in treatment for adjustment disorders tend to need less treatment, return to work sooner, and are less likely to suffer from a relapse of the problem when compared to people with other mental health problems.[3, 5, 6] But, due to the lack of research, treatment recommendations are scarce. It does seem reasonable to assume, however, that many forms of psychotherapy will be effective if they help you examine your thoughts, emotions, and behaviors surrounding the stressful event. This will be especially true if you need help with bereavement issues.

Remember, too, that by definition, an adjustment disorder will not last longer than six months. Therefore, it's possible that the problems you're dealing with might disappear on their own. However, if your problems are exceptionally difficult or long lasting, you should seek immediate treatment.

Recommended treatments for adjustment disorder include:

· Any psychotherapy that provides you with support

ANGER CONTROL PROBLEMS

WHAT ARE THEY?

People with *anger control* problems often react in quick and aggressive ways when they feel insulted, wronged, or injured. If you have this problem, you get infuriated easily when you think that other people are treating you unfairly.[1] Maybe you've noticed that you often blow up or "explode" at others. People with this type of problem are also quick to blame other people for their problems, without looking at the role that they might actually be playing in the situation.[2]

Everyone gets angry sometimes. This is normal, and sometimes it's even necessary and helpful. If someone is hurting you, it's beneficial to your health and survival to get angry and tell that person: "Stop!" But in other less threatening situations, not everyone expresses their anger in the same way.[3] Some people try to communicate with the other person to work out a compromise, some people try to think of a non-threatening response, and some people try to distance themselves from the situation before reacting.

However, people with an anger control problem often react in a way that is more intense and aggressive than what the situation calls for. Some people physically hurt other people, or themselves. Some take their frustrations out on objects by punching walls or kicking garbage cans. Other people argue aggressively. They call others insulting names, give dirty looks, make threatening gestures, or even hold all their anger inside and stew in their own hostility, perhaps while plotting how to take revenge.[1]

If you're struggling with an anger control problem, either you or the other people in your life have noticed that you get angry very easily, frequently, and with great intensity. Probably your anger also lasts for a long time, sometimes, perhaps, as long as an entire day.[1,4] Maybe you frequently get angry with the other drivers on the road and yell at them for driving in ways that you think are stupid or insulting. Perhaps you even follow them down the road and try cutting them off in retaliation for what you perceive as bad driving.

You may also get into arguments with store clerks, and scream at them for not treating you the way you think you deserve to be treated. Or, maybe you frequently yell at your coworkers or employees for doing things you think are dumb. It's also possible that your anger leads to physical fights with your spouse or partner, your children, or maybe even strangers. In these situations, your anger control problem can be exceptionally violent and dangerous to yourself and others.

When you find yourself in these situations, you probably notice that your heart begins to race, your face gets hot and flushed, your muscles tense up, your breathing gets faster, your palms get sweaty, and you become edgy and nervous.[1] You might also feel a little sick, as if your stomach is bothering you or you're having heartburn. And when the situation is over, you might also notice that you've made other people feel very uneasy or upset, and maybe you even feel guilty about your excessive anger.

ARE THERE OTHER RELATED PROBLEMS?

An anger control problem is often very damaging for both you and the other people in your life. For the person with the problem, excessive anger has been linked to higher job stress, increased blood pressure,[5] an increased risk for heart disease,[6-10] and an increased potential for suffering. In a study of people with long-term lower back pain, higher levels of anger were associated with a less-frequent tendency to forgive others, greater psychological suffering, and, in some cases, greater physical pain.[11] Other researchers have found that people who report high levels of anger also experience greater sensations of physical pain, even if the anger is covered up and not expressed by the person.[12-14]

Having high levels of anger can also lead to problems sleeping at night, as well as increased daytime fatigue as a result of not sleeping.[15] It's also been widely reported that men who commit domestic violence against their spouses and partners consistently have higher levels of anger and hostility when compared with men who don't commit these acts of violence.[16]

Other studies have also suggested that excessive anger is often associated with other disorders, such as depression, bipolar disorder, antisocial personality problems, self-focused personality problems, and emotion dysregulation problems.[17-20]

WHO IS AFFECTED?

Unfortunately, there are no statistics on how many people are affected by anger control problems. However, one large study of 1,300 people who were seeking treatment at a mental health clinic found that anger control problems were just as prevalent as depression and anxiety for that group of people.[17] If this same comparison holds true for the general population, it would mean that millions of people around the world are affected by anger control problems.

WHAT CAUSES IT?

The exact cause of an anger control problem is unknown. However, it is known that it has both biological and social contributing factors. The emotion of anger activates the *behavioral activation system* within the larger human nervous system.[21-23] When a person is confronted with an anger-inducing situation, the behavioral activation system causes that person either to confront the situation and express the anger, or to escape the situation and suppress the anger. The choice someone makes in that situation is influenced by a combination of inheritable genetic tendencies to either express or suppress anger,[24] and other social factors.

Anger is a fundamental emotion that is expressed and recognized in every culture around the world.[25-27] However, the way in which a person expresses anger is largely determined by what is considered acceptable by that person's culture.[28-30] Some cultural groups are more likely to suppress their anger while other groups are more likely to express their anger.[31-33] Research has shown that children imitate aggressive behaviors that they observe in other people, especially when that type of behavior is rewarded.[34, 35] So, if a person grows up in a family, peer group, or culture where excessive anger is frequently displayed or accepted as normal, that person has a greater chance of developing an anger control problem.[36-40]

Other factors also influence anger. Someone who thinks that other people don't like him or her will more quickly blame others for their problems and is more likely to get angry with them.[41, 42] Many people get easily angered when they're already experiencing negative feelings caused by hunger, stress, nervousness, sadness, fatigue, illness, or boredom.[43, 44] A person is also more likely to become angry when the situation is perceived to be unfair, preventable, intentional, and someone else's fault.[1, 45]

WHAT CAN YOU DO ABOUT IT?

There are some very successful treatments to help people with anger control problems reduce but not eliminate their anger.[46] Remember, anger is a fundamental emotion that is often helpful, so it isn't realistic to try to completely get rid of your anger. Many of these treatments—often called anger management—help people to identify the triggers for their anger and then how to create distance between the trigger and the angered response.

Many people feel as though their anger washes over them very quickly and leaves them little choice but to get angry. Anger management treatment aims to create a gap of time between the moment you feel angry and the moment when you respond, in order to provide you with time to choose an alternative response. One of the treatments proven most effective is cognitive behavioral therapy.[47-50] This treatment often uses relaxation skills to help manage angry feelings, thought-processing to help reassess triggering situations, and skills training to learn new types of responses to angry situations.[1, 47]

Other forms of successful treatment include anger management group therapy,[51] forgiveness therapy,[52] and mindfulness therapy.[54] The antidepressant medications fluoxetine (Prozac) and nefazodone (Serzone) have also shown some effectiveness at treating the anger attacks that accompany depression.[55-57]

Recommended treatments for anger control problems include:

- Anger management/cognitive behavioral therapy, see page 136

- Mindfulness therapy, see page 165

- Antidepressant medications, see page 155

- Forgiveness therapy

ANOREXIA

WHAT IS IT?

Anorexia, also called anorexia nervosa, is an eating disorder characterized by an excessively low body weight. Officially, you would be diagnosed with anorexia if you weighed 85 percent or less of what is considered normal for someone your age, sex, and height.[1] People with anorexia refuse to gain any weight and try to maintain a low body weight (or lose more) by restricting what they eat or by purging themselves of food after they've eaten. Restriction is often accomplished with dieting and the use of diet pills, while purging is usually done through vomiting and/or the use of laxatives. Some people with anorexia indulge in eating binges right before they purge, meaning that they eat an excessive amount of food in less then a few hours and then immediately remove it before it can be digested. (See the section on bulimia, page 52, for more information about bingeing and purging practices.) Forty to 80 percent of people with anorexia also engage in excessive exercise practices in order to burn up the few calories they allow themselves to digest.[2]

If you're struggling with anorexia, most likely you're also battling an intense fear of gaining weight and becoming fat. You probably spend a lot of time analyzing the way you look in the mirror; and no matter how much weight you lose, you probably think it's never enough. People with anorexia never think that they look good enough, despite the excessive amount of time they spend focusing on the way they look and limiting the amount of food they digest. This inability to see the danger of their situation is part of the illness.

ARE THERE OTHER RELATED PROBLEMS?

The excessively low body weight of a person with anorexia is dangerous because it causes a wide variety of health problems. In actuality, anorexia is self-induced starvation, and the resulting health problems are the same ones that would be seen in a person suffering from starvation caused by poverty, war, or drought. Anorexia can lead to heart complications, such as an excessively slow heart rate,[3] mitral valve prolapse,[4, 5] and congestive heart failure.[6]

Other related problems include osteoporosis,[7] liver damage,[8] anemia, stomach pain, constipation, hypoglycemia, a sensitivity to cold, brittle nails, small bruises on the arms and legs, thinning hair on the head, and the development of fine downy hair on other parts of the body.[1, 9] The erosion of dental enamel is also common among people who purge after eating, due to the reflux of their stomach acids.[1] More than 95 percent of adult women with anorexia also stop having their periods.[9] However, many of these problems are reversible if anorexia is treated early in its course, and the person regains a healthy weight.[9] Unfortunately, despite these dangers, many cases of anorexia last as long as ten to fifteen years.[10, 11]

Many people with anorexia also struggle with other mental health problems, such as depression, anxiety, and substance abuse.[12] Because of these combined problems, it's an unfortunate fact that the rate of suicide among people with anorexia is higher than that of the general population.[13] Because of the serious health risks associated with anorexia, as well as its association with depression and suicide, anorexia is an illness that requires immediate and intensive treatment as soon as possible. In a twenty-one-year follow-up study on patients who had been hospitalized for anorexia, almost 16 percent of them had died from related complications, such as infection, dehydration, and suicide.[14]

Unfortunately, this mortality rate is more often the norm than the exception.[10] In fact, for women between the ages of fifteen and twenty-four, anorexia leads to more than twelve times as many deaths each year than do all other causes of death,[15] which also means, by some estimates, that it kills more Americans each year than any other mental health problem.[9, 12]

WHO IS AFFECTED?

Anorexia affects over 1 million Americans.[9] In most reported cases, it appears to affect women more than men. Over the course of their lives, less than 1 percent to almost 4 percent of women will develop the illness.[16] Overall, men report anorexia only one-tenth as often as women do,[1] and research seems to indicate that men who identify as gay or bisexual are often at a greater risk for developing anorexia than are heterosexual men.[17] However, it's believed that the general rate of anorexia for all men is higher than officially recognized, either because it goes undiagnosed by doctors[18] or because men are ashamed of reporting it.[19-21] In both men and women, anorexia usually develops between the ages of twelve and twenty-six, with the greatest frequency between the ages of fourteen and eighteen.[1, 22]

WHAT CAUSES IT?

The cause of anorexia is still not fully understood.[10] One theory is that the Western idealization of beauty and thinness has led many women to become depressed and anorexic,[23] and there is some research to suggest that the general messages we see on television and in magazines reinforce these ideas in women who already have anorexia.[24] However, anorexia is not confined to the Western world. Cases have also been recorded in places like sub-Saharan Africa,[25] where anorexic female students limited their food consumption for self-imposed religious reasons, not because they wanted to be thin. Some researchers think that anorexia is a form of restriction that certain people use to control their lives and their bodies,[26] while one study found that anorexic women thought of themselves as being less independent from their families than did their nonanorexic sisters.[27]

WHAT CAN YOU DO ABOUT IT?

Treatment of anorexia usually requires a team of medical and psychological professionals.[28] The immediate medical concern is to restore the lost weight of the anorexic person and to handle any related health problems. For some people, this may require hospitalization. In conjunction with this, intensive psychological treatment is also required. Successful treatments for adults have been achieved using cognitive behavioral therapy[29, 30] and some general forms of therapy that offer support.[29] Successes have also been reported using family therapy,[31] especially for children and adolescents.[32, 33] Overall, many of the psychotherapies outlined in this resource are thought to be helpful, especially if they include dietary advice.[28] Studies of medications also suggest that antidepressants can be helpful for people who also have symptoms of depression.[34, 35] However, when used as the sole means of treatment, antidepressants won't always work for everyone.

Recommended treatments for anorexia include:

- Medical care

- Cognitive behavioral therapy, see page 136

- Family therapy, see page 146

- Antidepressants for symptoms of depression, see page 155

- Any psychotherapy that provides you with support

- Professional dietary counseling

ANTISOCIAL PERSONALITY DISORDER

WHAT IS IT?

If you have an *antisocial personality* you manipulate and abuse other people for your own purposes.[1] Plus, you frequently lie to get what you want and show little or no consideration for the needs and safety of other people. A person with an antisocial personality can also be violent, destructive, impatient, egotistical, cunning, and easily agitated. If you have this type of personality, you most likely break the law when you want to and are often at risk for being arrested. Unfortunately, personality styles like this one create problems in your relationships, job, and other social situations. As a result, personality styles like this are officially referred to as "personality disorders."

At some point in most of our lives, most of us will hurt someone or take advantage of someone, either accidentally or on purpose. But unlike a person with an antisocial personality, most of us will feel guilty afterwards[2] and will try not to do it again. This is very different from a person with an antisocial personality, who usually feels no regret and will often hurt other people in physical, emotional, psychological, and financial ways.

If you have an antisocial personality, you definitely have a long history of taking advantage of other people, and you're probably very good at it. You might have learned how to be charming in order to make other people like you and forgive you, even after you've done something bad to them. Maybe you think that other people aren't as smart as you and deserve to be taken advantage of. Or, maybe you think that other people exist just to serve your needs. Whatever the case, you've probably been manipulating people since you were a child or a teenager.

Chances are good that you have a lengthy criminal record, or at least you should, but maybe you've been able to avoid being arrested. In comparison, your work history is probably very short, because you've been fired for not showing up on a regular basis. Perhaps you think that ordinary work is for people who aren't as smart as you are, and so you get by in life by taking what you need or engaging in illegal activities. Your history of relationships is also probably spotty. Most likely, you have few close friends and your romantic relationships feel more like sexual conquests, with you moving from one person to the next.

When referring to a person with an antisocial personality, the terms "sociopath" or "psychopath" are often used. However, there are some researchers who reserve the term "psychopathic" for a subgroup of people with antisocial personalities who are even more dangerous than most antisocial people.[3, 4] According to these researchers, psychopaths have certain personality features that make them particularly scheming and predatory. These types of people lie excessively, don't take responsibility for their own actions, are exceptionally charming, have overinflated ideas about their own value and abilities, show very little emotion, and have no pity for others.[5] In part, this clinical definition of a psychopath was created to more accurately predict which prisoners would engage in future violence once they were released.[6-8]

However, not all psychopaths are in prison. As the leading researcher in this area has noted, psychopaths find jobs not only as drug dealers, criminals, and terrorists, but also as dishonest politicians, corrupt lawyers, and powerful business leaders, among other careers.[3]

ARE THERE OTHER RELATED PROBLEMS?

Obviously, the most frequently related issue is breaking the law. In surveys of prisons, the rates of antisocial personality problems among men have ranged from approximately 33 to 62 percent of the population.[9-13] Similarly, the rates for women in prison have ranged from almost 12 to 60 percent of the population.[12-16] In comparison, people who have been identified as psychopaths, a smaller subgroup of antisocial personality, are estimated to make up 15 to 25 percent of prison populations.[3]

People with antisocial personalities are also at a higher risk of dying from unnatural causes. In one long-term study, people with this type of personality were almost four times as likely to die when compared with other people.[17] Among the many reasons for this likelihood are an increased risk for suicide,[18-21] an increased risk for accidents,[22] and an increased risk of experiencing a violent death.[23]

Many people with antisocial personalities also struggle with social phobia, specific phobia, post-traumatic stress disorder, panic disorder, generalized anxiety disorder, depression, bipolar disorder,[24-27] alcohol and drug problems,[28] and gambling addictions.[29]

WHO IS AFFECTED?

In a large study of American adults, it was estimated that almost 4 percent of that population, or almost 8 million people, have antisocial personalities, with men being affected more often than women.[30] In other studies, the estimates ranged from approximately 1 to 2 percent[31, 32] of the adult population. In comparison, it's estimated that 1 percent of the general population would be diagnosed as clinical psychopaths.[3] In general, almost 15 percent of all American adults, or almost 31 million people, struggle with personality disorders like antisocial personality,[30] and these types of long-term problems are often the cause of general unhappiness and disability in a person's life.[32]

WHAT CAUSES IT?

The exact cause of an antisocial personality is unknown. The problem always begins in childhood or adolescence in the form of early antisocial activities called conduct disorders.[1] Most likely, this type of personality is caused by both biological and social factors.[33, 34] In general, it appears that personality problems like this one have a strong chance of being passed on in families, due to influential genetic factors.[35] One study has even shown that certain elements of psychopathic behavior, like lack of empathy, also appear to be highly inheritable.[36] Another study has shown that antisocial personality problems tend to run through multiple generations of families,[37] suggesting that children can learn antisocial behaviors from their parents, inherit antisocial behaviors, or be mistreated by their parents and become antisocial themselves.

Interestingly, other studies have suggested that children who experience low levels of parental care and excessive levels of parental protection may also be at risk for developing antisocial personalities as adults.[38, 39] Some children, especially boys, are also born with aggressive personalities that seem to persist into adulthood, a factor that may put them more at risk for becoming antisocial.[40, 41] In a study of more than 1,000 three-year-olds who were reevaluated at the age of twenty-one, children who had been described as short-tempered and impulsive were almost three times more likely to be diagnosed with adult antisocial personalities, and were almost five times more likely to be convicted of an adult violent crime.[42]

Other numerous studies have suggested that antisocial personality problems might be linked to malfunctions in the part of the brain responsible for problem solving, memory, and the regulation of thoughts and behaviors.[43-46] This malfunctioning could be caused by accidents, traumas, or it may exist from birth.[47]

Many other childhood experiences are also thought to influence the development of later antisocial personalities. These early risk factors include the following: being born to a mother who experienced famine during pregnancy,[48] childhood hyperactivity,[49] being physically abused and neglected,[50] living with a mother who is depressed,[51] experiencing childhood depression oneself,[52] having low self-esteem,[53] having friends who also display antisocial behaviors,[54-56] and living in poverty.[30, 54]

WHAT CAN YOU DO ABOUT IT?

Unfortunately, there is little research to suggest which is the most effective treatment for an antisocial personality.[57, 58] People with antisocial personalities usually come to therapy because someone else has forced them, such as an employer, parent, or judge.[59] Needless to say, most people who are forced into psychotherapy don't want to be there and don't want to change. However, if a person with this type of personality does want to undergo psychotherapy, it might also be necessary to treat that person for drug and alcohol problems, due to the high association of substance abuse with antisocial personality.[60] One very small study suggested that cognitive behavioral therapy might be helpful for treating a person's antisocial habits.[61] Other reviews suggest that brief psychodynamic therapy, longer-term psychodynamic therapy, interpersonal therapy, and cognitive behavioral therapy may all provide at least some help to people with personality disorders like this one.[57, 62-64]

Ideally, all of these treatments should be able to help a person think beyond his or her own self-interests.[59] Disturbingly, it's been noted that psychotherapy for psychopaths can have a dangerous effect, because it can help these criminals learn how to manipulate people even better than they already do, while having little benefit on their own state of mind.[7]

Recommended treatments for antisocial personality disorder include:

· Cognitive behavioral therapy, see page 136

· Brief psychodynamic therapy, see page 135

· Psychodynamic therapy, see page 167

· Interpersonal therapy, see page 153

ATTENTION-DEFICIT/HYPERACTIVITY DISORDER

WHAT IS IT?

Attention-deficit/hyperactivity disorder (ADHD) is a problem characterized by an inability to focus your attention; an inability to control your impulses, behaviors, and emotions; and a recurring feeling of restlessness.[1-3] If you're struggling with ADHD, these problems get in your way all the time and prevent you from completing tasks at work in a quick and efficient way.[4]

Adults with ADHD typically have a low tolerance for frustration. You probably are easily distracted at home and at your job. Maybe you find it very hard to read or focus your attention on one thing, and so you frequently switch tasks. Perhaps others have described you as a "daydreamer" or as a person who is not "detail oriented." You probably also find it hard to control your impulses. Maybe you habitually speak without thinking and interrupt others' conversations. Perhaps you have a history of automobile crashes or other accidents, caused by impulsive behavior.[5] It's also probable that you find it hard to remain seated for a long time and find it difficult to work quietly.

The truth is that people struggling with ADHD are often restless and forgetful. This doesn't happen because they aren't trying hard enough or because they're lazy, it happens because they find it exceptionally difficult to concentrate on a single thought or topic for more than a few minutes. For adults with ADHD, no amount of will-power is ever enough to counteract the forces of the disorder.

Due to the inability to focus, many people with ADHD perform poorly at school and work, despite their qualifications and true abilities.[1] And, unfortunately, due to these same reasons, people with ADHD are more likely to lose their jobs, perform poorly in school, and have conflicts with their family and friends.[1]

Most adults with ADHD can remember having this problem since they were children. Frequently, they can remember being disciplined for not being able to sit still or finish their schoolwork. And while some people might outgrow these problems or have them become less severe over time, many adults remain burdened with these problems for most of their lives. Some research indicates that as adults with ADHD age, their hyperactive behaviors become less frequent; however, their disorganized behaviors often become more noticeable.[2, 6]

ARE THERE OTHER RELATED PROBLEMS?

Adults struggling with ADHD often come to a mental health professional for help with other related problems, rather than ADHD itself.[1, 6] These problems often include anxiety, depression, emotion dysregulation, sleep problems, and substance abuse.[7]

WHO IS AFFECTED?

ADHD is a disorder that affects both children and adults. For adults struggling with ADHD, the problem usually began when they were in preschool or in the early years of elementary school.[8] It's estimated that between 3 and 7 percent of school-aged children suffer with ADHD,[2] and boys are affected two to three times more often than girls.[9] Follow-up studies indicate that 30 to 80 percent of children who were diagnosed with ADHD continue to struggle with the disorder when they become adults.[10-15] As a result, it's estimated that 1 to 5 percent of all adults struggle with ADHD.[3, 16-20]

WHAT CAUSES IT?

ADHD research suggests that the cause of the disorder is largely due to biological factors, rather than environmental ones, such as where you grew up. Brain-imaging studies of people with ADHD have discovered differences in the part of the brain associated with the control of voluntary movements.[21, 22] Since biological factors like this tend to be inheritable, you have a greater risk of developing ADHD if one of your parents has the disorder.[23, 24] In fact, one study suggested that ADHD had a higher risk of being inherited than any other psychiatric disorder.[25]

However, just because you might have a genetic likelihood for developing ADHD, this doesn't mean that you will always be affected. Some genetic codes are expressed only under certain environmental conditions such as stress, injury, and toxic environments, which have also been associated with the development of ADHD.[23]

WHAT CAN YOU DO ABOUT IT?

Unfortunately, ADHD in adults isn't always recognized by mental health professionals.[5, 26] As a result, not everyone with the problem will receive proper care. If you suspect you have ADHD, it's important that you provide your mental health care provider with the details of the disorder. Even then, many mental health professionals will still want to verify that the disorder has existed since childhood, before making an official diagnosis.[2] For this reason, it might be necessary for other family members, especially older family members, to speak with your mental health care professional to verify the diagnosis.

If ADHD is properly identified, there are a number of effective treatments. In children and adolescents, the most common form of treatment is the medication methylphenidate (Ritalin).[27] Ritalin is a stimulant, but ironically, in children and some adults it has a calming effect that relieves many of the ADHD symptoms.[28, 29] However, not everyone responds well to Ritalin[30] and some people may find the side effects of the medication to be intolerable. Typical side effects of Ritalin include muscle tics, loss of appetite, and insomnia.[5] Antidepressant medications such as bupropion (Wellbutrin), imipramine (Tofranil), and the nonstimulant medication atomoxetine (Strattera) are also used to treat ADHD.[29, 31]

In conjunction with medication, many people with ADHD may find it helpful to also use psychotherapy, especially those people who find the medication ineffective or intolerable. Psychotherapeutic treatments for adults with ADHD typically focus on two goals: creating strategies to manage the symptoms of ADHD and learning how to cope with the emotional impact of the disorder.[32, 33] In general, treatments that provide little interaction between you and your psychotherapist will probably not be effective in treating your ADHD.[34] Typically, people with ADHD need interactive structured therapies to help them stay focused on their thoughts and tasks.

For example, cognitive behavioral therapy has been shown to be an effective ADHD treatment in a number of studies.[35-38] The people treated in these studies were able to improve their organization and time-management skills, as well as examine and partly change the way they think and feel. Similarly, a version of dialectical behavior therapy, modified specifically to treat ADHD, has also been shown to be an effective treatment.[1]

Recommended treatments for attention-deficit/hyperactivity disorder include:

· Medications, see page 155

· Cognitive behavioral therapy, see page 136

· A modified version of dialectical behavior therapy, see page 141

BIPOLAR DISORDER/MANIC DEPRESSION

WHAT IS IT?

Bipolar disorder, or *manic depression*, is a problem characterized by excessively energetic moods called mania or manic episodes, which are more intense and very different than normal excitement.[1] *Manic episodes* are uncontrollable periods of excessive energy that can begin at any time. During a manic episode, you can feel overly happy, restless, irritable, excessively self-confident, easily distracted, or some combination of these feelings.

If you experience mania, the excessive energy and mood swings will interfere with your life. During manic episodes, you often don't need to sleep because you have so much energy. However, you also can't control your thoughts because they are racing too fast, making it impossible to do any work. You probably feel confused during the mania, and can't remember things because you have so many thoughts. As a result, the speed with which you talk is so fast that it is hard for others to understand what you are saying.

You may have even noticed that some people look a little frightened or confused when they're with you, because they can't understand you or because you're moving at such a fast pace, they can't keep up. The overwhelming energy you experience might lead you to think that you're indestructible and cause you to become angry or irritable with others. Or, it might make you think you are irresistible to others, and lead you to aggressively seek out new relationships, or rekindle old relationships with people you haven't seen in years.

During the mania, you may also find yourself engaging in an excessive number of plans and activities. Some of these plans might get out of control because you don't consider all the possible pitfalls, while other impulsive activities, like shopping sprees and sexual encounters with strangers, may interfere with your long-term relationships.

Many times, someone with bipolar disorder also has episodes of depression or dysthymia in between periods of mania, resulting in very severe mood swings from very high to very low. In order to differentiate how severe a person's problem is, three different types of bipolar disorder have been identified: bipolar-I, bipolar-II, and cyclothymia.

A person with bipolar-I will have a manic episode that lasts for at least one week. On average, these episodes usually last from three to six months.[2, 3] Bipolar-I may also include episodes of depression or dysthymia in between the manic episodes. In severe cases of bipolar-I, you may even experience visual or auditory hallucinations or delusional thoughts, such as the belief that you possess great powers.[4] On average, a person with bipolar-I can expect a manic episode every two to four years,[4] and the odds of having a second manic episode after your first one are greater than 90 percent.[1]

Some people experience a less disabling degree of mania, called *hypomania*, which doesn't interfere with their lives as much. Typically, these hypomanic episodes last for at least a few days and include many of the same symptoms as in a manic episode.[1] In between these hypomanic periods, you might also experience depression or dysthymia, but hypomanic episodes never include hallucinations or delusions.[4] Someone who experiences hypomanic episodes and at least one depressive episode might be diagnosed with bipolar-II, while a person who experiences hypomanic episodes and less disabling depressive symptoms, such as dysthymia, might be diagnosed with *cyclothymia*.

If you experience hypomania, you might actually look forward to your hypomanic episodes, because you become excessively creative and/or productive during these periods. It's also possible that during hypomania your shyness disappears and you become more outgoing.[5] You might even be able to think a little more quickly and clearly than normal, and you might feel powerful and irresistible to others. However, these feelings can also lead you to make an excessive number of rash judgments, like going on impulsive shopping sprees.

Someone who experiences four or more manic or hypomanic episodes every year has *rapid cycling bipolar disorder*. An equally severe complication is called a *mixed episode*. This refers to a span of one week during which a person experiences both depression and mania almost every day. Officially, all of these bipolar disorders, along with depression and dysthymia, are collectively referred to as "mood disorders."

ARE THERE OTHER RELATED PROBLEMS?

The most dangerous problem related to bipolar disorder is suicide. Some studies have estimated that 25 to 50 percent of the people with bipolar disorder will attempt to kill themselves at least once during their lifetimes,[6-9] and 10 to 19 percent of those who have bipolar disorder will ultimately die from suicide.[7] Most of these suicides will occur during a depressive episode.[10] This rate of suicide is about fifteen times greater than the suicide rate for the general public.[11] These sobering statistics highlight the severity of bipolar disorder and the need to get professional treatment.

Another dangerous and related problem is alcohol and drug abuse.[12] In particular, the abuse of stimulants, such as methamphetamines, cocaine, and crack cocaine,[13] as well as the abuse of marijuana[14] appear to be especially common among people with bipolar disorder. In one very large study of more than 43,000 people in the United States, approximately 28 percent of those who experienced manic episodes also had a problem with drugs or alcohol, as did approximately 27 percent of those who had hypomanic episodes.[15] Sadly, the use of alcohol and drugs appears to increase the chances of suicide in people suffering from bipolar disorders.[16, 17]

Many people with bipolar disorders also have problems with anxiety disorders, such as panic disorder, social phobia, specific phobias, generalized anxiety disorder, post-traumatic stress disorder, and obsessive-compulsive disorder.[12, 14, 18-20] In addition, some studies have found relationships between bipolar disorders and anti-social personality problems and emotion dysregulation problems.[21, 22] Many people with bipolar disorder also have problems with eating disorders, such as bulimia and anorexia.[14, 23]

WHO IS AFFECTED?

A report published by the World Health Organization[24] stated that bipolar disorders were the sixth leading cause of disability in the world in 1990, trailing problems such as heart disease and depression. In the United States, bipolar disorders as a whole will affect approximately 4 percent of the adult population at some point in their lives.[25] In particular, bipolar-I affects under 1 percent to almost 2 percent of the adult population,[1, 2, 4, 10] or approximately 2 million Americans.[26] Men and women appear to be equally affected by bipolar-I,[2] with the first manic episode usually occurring when a person is in his or her early twenties.[1] However, children and adolescents can also be affected by bipolar disorders.[5]

Bipolar-II affects slightly fewer people at under 1 percent of the population,[2, 7] and it seems to affect men and women differently. Men tend to have an equal number of depressive episodes for every hypomanic episode they experience, while women have more depressive episodes.[1]

Cyclothymia affects from under 1 percent to 5 percent of the population.[1] Cyclothymia can begin as soon as adolescence or early adulthood, it's equally common in men and women, and the odds of it developing into either of the bipolar disorders are 15 to 50 percent.[1]

In general, women experience more rapid cycling[27] and are at a greater risk for experiencing a manic or a hypomanic episode during pregnancy or shortly after childbirth.[28]

WHAT CAUSES IT?

Most scientific researchers agree that there is no single cause of bipolar disorder.[5] However, the development of the disorder is strongly influenced by genetic risk factors.[29] If someone in your immediate family has bipolar disorder, your odds of developing the disorder are six to eight times greater than someone who is not related to a person with bipolar disorder.[4] However, first-degree relatives share more than just genetic makeup; they also share common experiences, socioeconomic status, and other life situations that might trigger bipolar disorder. Brain chemicals called *neurotransmitters* might also contribute to the development of bipolar disorder. In particular, the levels of the neurotransmitters serotonin, norepinephrine, and dopamine appear to influence the disorder.[30, 31]

Other theories suggest that the cause of the problem might lie in the way neurons in the brain transmit their signals, either transmitting too easily during mania or not transmitting enough during depression.[30] If you do have a genetic or a biological risk for developing bipolar disorder, certain environmental factors, such as stress, might trigger manic or hypomanic episodes.[32] These potential stressors include disrupting your daily routine, making changes in your sleep schedule, changing your work schedule, and participating in family conflicts.[33] Research has shown that changes in sleep patterns very often trigger manic episodes.[34]

WHAT CAN YOU DO ABOUT IT?

Regrettably, many people who need help for bipolar disorder don't get it.[35] In one large study of adults in the United States, within a year of the problem's onset, only 39 percent of those affected by the disorder sought help; and on average, people waited six years before seeking treatment for their manic symptoms.[36] This is unfortunate, considering that there are many treatments to control the disruptive course of the disorder.

Because of the strong biological factors associated with the disorder, the primary treatment for bipolar disorder is medication. Currently, the first-line of mood stabilizing medications for manic symptoms includes lithium (Eskalith), divalproex sodium (Depakote), carbamazepine (Tegretol), olanzapine (Zyprexa), risperidone (Risperdal), ziprasidone (Geodon), quetiapine (Seroquel), and aripiprazole (Abilify).[37] The second choice for medications includes the antipsychotic medications haloperidol (Haldol), chlorpromazine (Thorazine), and clozapine (Clozaril) as well as the anticonvulsant medications clonazepam (Klonopin) and lorazepam (Ativan).[37]

Although some evidence suggests that lithium might lower a person's risk of suicide,[38] the use of lithium also requires the person to undergo regular blood tests to prevent the buildup of toxins. Certain antidepressants are also used to control depressive symptoms related to bipolar disorder.[10] Some of the more commonly prescribed antidepressants used to treat bipolar disorder include fluoxetine (Prozac), bupropion (Wellbutrin), paroxetine (Paxil), venlafaxine (Effexor), sertraline (Zoloft), fluvoxamine (Luvox), and citalopram (Celexa) as well as the anticonvulsant medication lamotrigine (Lamictal).[37]

The type of medication, or the combination of medications, you receive will depend on the type of mania that is being experienced, the stage of the problem, and the activity of any hallucinatory or delusional symptoms.[37] Unfortunately, the use of any of these medications will result in some accompanying side effects that might make you want to quit using them.[10, 39] However, stopping your medication, no matter how good or bad you feel, almost always leads to the reoccurrence of manic symptoms. Don't stop taking your medications without first consulting your medical doctor to discuss alternative medications.

Due to the high numbers of people who stop taking their bipolar medications,[40, 41] psychotherapy is a necessary additional treatment for controlling the problem.[10] The primary goals of psychotherapy for bipolar disorder are to help you stick to your medication schedule, help you to recognize and avoid potential relapse factors, reduce life stressors, maintain your daily routines, improve family communication, and support you in your struggles with the disorder.[10, 32]

Among the many types of psychotherapy shown to be effective in controlling bipolar disorder, cognitive behavioral therapy has been the most widely researched.[42] Cognitive behavioral therapy aims to reduce the negative thoughts and behaviors that might add stress to your life in order to lessen the risk of manic episodes.[43] In clinical studies, people who both took medication and utilized cognitive behavioral therapy experienced improvements in their lives,[44, 45] some for as long as one year after treatment.[46] In one study, the participants who used medication and cognitive behavioral therapy stuck to their medication schedules better, had fewer bipolar episodes, experienced better social functioning, and developed better coping strategies for dealing with stress, when compared with the group that received general support and medication.[47] The use of group cognitive behavioral therapy has also been effective.[48, 49]

Another psychotherapeutic treatment that was shown to be effective was a form of family therapy.[32] This kind of treatment will help you identify and reduce family stressors that might bring on manic episodes, and also maintain a regular schedule of medication.[33] In clinical trials, family therapy has been shown to be effective at achieving these goals.[50, 51] Other therapies, such as interpersonal therapy,[52, 53] group therapy,[54, 55] and psychodynamic therapy,[56] as well as general psychoeducation,[57] have also demonstrated some successes in improving people's lives who are dealing with bipolar disorder.

Lastly, newer research has also given hope that omega-3 fatty acids can successfully control some types of depression and mania.[58-60] Omega-3s are commonly found in some fish oils, walnuts, flaxseeds, and soybeans, as well as nutritional supplements.

Recommended treatments for bipolar disorder include:

. Mood stabilizer and antidepressant medications, see page 155

. Cognitive behavioral therapy, see page 136

. Family therapy, see page 146

. Interpersonal therapy, see page 153

. Psychoanalytic/Psychodynamic therapy, see page 167

. Omega-3 fatty acids

BODY DYSMORPHIC DISORDER

WHAT IS IT?

Body dysmorphic disorder (BDD) is a problem characterized by an obsessive concern with a part of your body that you think is severely flawed or deformed.[1] The anxiety that this obsession causes is extremely troubling. People with BDD often think of themselves as ugly and abnormal. When these beliefs become strong enough, many people with BDD begin avoiding social events and other gatherings, like work, where other people might notice their "defects." In extreme cases, a person may become housebound or leave the house only at night.[1] If you have BDD, you probably spend a great amount of time checking your appearance in the mirror, store windows, spoons, or even the face of your watch.[2]

In one study,[2] people with BDD reported that they constantly checked their appearances because they hoped that when they did, they would either look better than they last remembered or finally feel comfortable with the way they looked. Some of the people reported spending as long as two hours and forty-five minutes in front of the mirror checking their appearances. Unfortunately, most of these people reported that they didn't feel better after spending any amount of time checking their appearances.

On the other hand, it's also possible that you are just the opposite. Maybe you avoid mirrors completely, or keep them covered, so that you don't have to look at yourself at all. Many people with BDD find faults with their skin, eyes, ears, nose, hair, thighs, hips, mouth, arms, feet, stomach, breasts, and genitals.[1, 3] You may even be extremely concerned with more than one part of your body. The imperfection can be very large or very small. Other people might say that they don't notice the imperfection or that you're imagining the problem to be bigger than it really is. But to you, the imperfection is glaring and embarrassing.

The obsessional concern may feel as though it's out of your control, and it might even occupy most of your thoughts throughout the day. You probably spend a lot of time and go to great efforts to change the imperfection or hide it from others. You might notice yourself picking the skin of the imperfection, constantly covering it with makeup, or seeking reassurances from other people that they can't see it.[4] Most likely, you also have either had plastic surgery or are currently considering it.[5]

ARE THERE OTHER RELATED PROBLEMS?

If people with BDD do seek help from a mental health professional, it's usually for some other problem.[4] Many people with BDD also struggle with depression, anxiety, social phobia, alcohol abuse, and substance abuse.[6, 7] Many others battle obsessive-compulsive disorder,[8] which shares similar characteristics with BDD.[9-11] Some evidence even points to a possible connection between BDD and the development of anorexia.[12, 13] In severe cases of BDD, suicidal thoughts and attempts are not uncommon.[3, 14]

WHO IS AFFECTED?

It's believed that BDD usually begins during adolescence, but it's also known to develop earlier in childhood.[1] The rate of BDD in the general population is unknown.[1] The best estimate is about 1 percent,[15-17] although one study of college students found the rate to be as high as 13 percent.[18] Unfortunately, a true estimate of the prevalence is not known because most people with BDD never seek treatment.[19]

WHAT CAUSES IT?

Most likely, BDD is caused by a mixture of risk factors and events.[20] Due to the similarities between BDD and obsessive-compulsive disorder, it's believed that BDD may also be partly triggered by biological factors.[20] However, it's still unclear if BDD runs in families, as does obsessive-compulsive disorder.[1] Some medical reports suggest that BDD can be triggered by the onset of an illness, such as Bell's palsy or colitis.[21] Other theories point to life events. One theory proposes that disruptive childhood experiences, such as being teased and having poor self-esteem, can make a person vulnerable to BDD.[3]

One of the most unfortunate influencing factors, however, is that many people, even those without BDD, are dissatisfied with the way they look.[22] Many women are concerned that they are not thin enough,[23] and many men are concerned that they are not muscular enough.[24] In one study,[25] 25 percent of the women and 19 percent of the men said that they had serious concerns about their appearances.

Unfortunately, many of these people probably have a distorted, unrealistic view of how they look. In clinical studies of female dieters[26] and males with eating disorders,[27] both men and women thought of themselves as being fatter than they really were. In further studies,[28] men and women with BDD reported very inflexible thinking styles that reinforced their distorted view of how they looked. They believed that their own view of themselves was accurate and that others saw them the same way. They were also unwilling to consider that their beliefs might be wrong. Not surprisingly, the people with more severe cases of BDD also had more inflexible styles of thinking.

Interestingly, one group of researchers proposed that the study of art or design might be an influencing factor in the development of BDD. In a study of 100 people with BDD,[29] 20 percent had an education or job in art or design. This finding led researchers to consider two possibilities. First, perhaps studying art during adolescence, when BDD develops most often, somehow contributes to the development of the illness. Or, the second possibility might be that people with BDD are more naturally drawn to the study of art and design.

WHAT CAN YOU DO ABOUT IT?

Unfortunately, many people try to treat BDD and their dissatisfaction with their body by having plastic surgery or dermatology treatments.[5, 30, 31] Sadly, most of these attempts fail. In a study of people with BDD who received plastic surgery or dermatology treatments, 72 percent reported no change in the severity of their BDD symptoms and 16 percent reported that their symptoms actually worsened.[5] This study highlights the fact that BDD is a problem in self-perception: that is, the problem isn't how you really look, but how you think you look. It's a very important difference, because successful psychological treatment for BDD can help only if you change the way you think about yourself and the world.

One of the most effective psychological treatments for BDD is very similar to the treatment for obsessive-compulsive disorder.[32, 33] Cognitive behavioral therapy for BDD typically involves two processes: (1) evaluating your beliefs about your body, and (2) safely and systematically exposing yourself to previously avoided situations while abstaining from body-checking behaviors.[34] In one test of this treatment, BDD was eliminated in 82 percent of the cases.[34] This therapy has also been shown to be effective in group therapy settings.[35]

Eye-movement desensitization and reprocessing therapy has also demonstrated positive results in treating BDD,[36] as has the use of antidepressants,[4] especially fluoxetine (Prozac) and fluvoxamine (Luvox).[37-41]

Recommended treatments for body dysmorphic disorder include:

· Cognitive behavioral therapy, see page 136

· Eye-movement desensitization and reprocessing therapy, see page 144

· Antidepressant medications, see page 155

BULIMIA

WHAT IS IT?

Bulimia (also called bulimia nervosa) is an eating disorder that involves binge eating followed by some type of behavior to prevent weight gain.[1] Usually, this means that you will purge yourself of food you've just eaten, in order to remove it before it can be digested. This type of behavior is also seen in some people with anorexia. However, unlike the dangerously low weight of someone with anorexia, most people with bulimia weigh approximately their normal expected weight.[1] *Binge eating* is an activity that takes place in the span of a few hours and usually involves a large consumption of high-calorie foods.

For example, this could mean that you eat multiple bags of candy and chips at home, or it could mean that you drive to a number of different fast-food restaurants in a short period of time eating multiple meals. Most often, this type of behavior is done in secret and alone.[1] Perhaps it even requires you to lie to the people who are closest to you. Many people binge because they feel stressed, depressed, or extremely hungry.[1] Once the bingeing starts, you may feel that you're out of control and can't stop eating, or maybe you even feel like you're outside of your body while your eating is going on.[1] Either way, you probably continue bingeing until you feel full.[1]

After eating such a large quantity of high-calorie foods, many people with bulimia feel guilty about what they've done and become fearful of gaining weight. So, immediately after eating, 80 to 90 percent of them will force themselves to vomit in order to prevent the food from being digested.[1] Purging can also be accomplished through the abuse of laxatives, diuretics, enemas, or syrup of ipecac. Other people with bulimia will offset their binge eating by engaging in excessive exercise habits or by fasting for a day or two.[1] A person who regularly binges without purging, exercising, or fasting might be diagnosed as suffering with *binge eating disorder*.[1]

If you're suffering from bulimia, most likely you're battling with an intense fear of gaining weight and becoming fat. You probably spend a lot of time analyzing the way you look in the mirror; but no matter how much weight you lose, you probably think it's never enough. People with bulimia never think they look good enough, despite the excessive amount of time they spend focusing on the way they look and limiting the amount of food they digest. This inability to see the danger of the situation is a part of the illness.

ARE THERE OTHER RELATED PROBLEMS?

Although the risk of dying from bulimia is much less severe than the risk of dying from anorexia,[2, 3] there are still many serious health problems that will persist for as long as the bingeing and purging continue. These problems include: sore throats, erosion of tooth enamel, swelling of the salivary glands, stomach acid reflux,[4] upset stomach,[5] severe constipation,[6] and severe fluid and electrolyte imbalances that can lead to heart arrhythmias.[7, 8] Additionally, the abuse of ipecac can lead to heart damage and general muscle weakness.[9] The good news is that most of these problems are reversible, especially if your bulimia is treated early in its course.[4]

In addition, many people battling bulimia also struggle with depression,[10, 11] obsessive-compulsive disorder,[12] alcohol and drug addiction (especially amphetamines, marijuana, and tranquilizers),[13] and emotion dysregulation problems.[14, 15]

WHO IS AFFECTED?

Bulimia usually begins during adolescence and has the greatest likelihood of starting around age eighteen.[16] It's estimated that approximately 3 percent of all women will develop bulimia at some point in their lives.[1, 17] However, for college-age women, the risk is slightly higher at 5 percent.[18] For men, the odds appear to be much less. Men are diagnosed with bulimia ten to twenty times less often than women.[19] However, it's believed that these numbers might be low, either due to the assumption that eating disorders affect only women and therefore go undiagnosed by doctors, or due to the fact that men are ashamed of reporting bulimia.[20-23] Some research does indicate, however, that men who identify as gay or bisexual are often at a greater risk for developing bulimia than are heterosexual men.[24]

WHAT CAUSES IT?

The exact cause of bulimia is still unknown.[4] Like many other mental health issues, it's probably caused by a mix of hereditary[25] and environmental issues.[26] In a study of developmental risk factors, women with bulimia were more likely to report past experiences of obesity, sexual and physical abuse, depression, substance abuse, low self-esteem, a sense of perfectionism, disturbed family relationships, and obese parents.[27] These findings seem to indicate that the development of bulimia is the result of being exposed to general risk factors for both mental health problems and extreme dieting.

However, the results of this one study are by no means definitive. Other theories suggest that the Western ideal of thinness[28] and the media's depiction of women[29] are at least partly responsible. Still another theory suggests that women of color may develop eating disorders when their cultural view of their own body image comes into conflict with that of the majority culture.[30]

WHAT CAN YOU DO ABOUT IT?

The most effective form of treatment for bulimia is cognitive behavioral therapy,[4] which, in some cases, is even more effective than the use of medications alone.[31] In various studies, cognitive behavioral therapy has resulted in 45 to 49 percent full-recovery rates,[31, 32] and a 70 to 94 percent[33] success rate in reducing bingeing and purging behaviors. Cognitive behavioral therapy for bulimia has been effective in both group and individual therapy settings,[34, 35] and the effects of the treatment appear to be long lasting.[36] Interpersonal therapy[32] and self-psychology[37] have also shown some success in treating bulimia.

Studies of antidepressants, especially fluoxetine (Prozac), have demonstrated some short-term success using the medication alone and in combination with cognitive behavioral therapy.[31] However, the long-term success of these drugs is still unknown.[38]

The advice of a certified dietician can also be beneficial. One study[39] added protein to the diets of women with bulimia and found that these women exhibited less binge eating, reported less hunger and greater fullness, and consumed less food in between meals over the two-week course of the study.

Recommended treatments for bulimia include:

- Cognitive behavioral therapy, see page 136

- Interpersonal therapy, see page 153

- Self-psychology, a form of psychoanalysis, see page 167

- Antidepressant medications, see page 155

- Professional dietary counseling

DEPENDENT PERSONALITY DISORDER

WHAT IS IT?

A person with a *dependent personality* is unable to make decisions without the constant assistance and approval of other people.[1] If you have this type of personality, you probably don't think you're good enough or smart enough to make decisions for yourself. Or, maybe you don't think you're worthy enough to make decisions that will benefit you. Instead, you try to make decisions that please other people, so you'll be liked and not abandoned. Unfortunately, personality styles like this one often create problems in your relationships, job, and other social situations. As a result, personality styles like this are officially referred to as "personality disorders."

We all want to be liked by other people. And there are certainly many appropriate times to ask others for help with a problem, especially when you really don't know what to do. However, if you have a dependent personality, you find it nearly impossible to make even small decisions without the help and approval of someone else, even when you do know what to do. The problem is that you are afraid of making a "wrong" decision—a decision that possibly might lead to criticism and abandonment.

If you have a dependent personality, it's likely you've given away a huge amount of the power to run your own life. You probably ask other people for advice to make small and large decisions every day. Your questions can range from "What kind of pants do you think I should wear?" to "What do you think I should do with the rest of my life?" Sometimes, it might seem as if it's impossible to make up your own mind. Every day, you probably find yourself checking in with other people about your plans and decisions, and as a result, it's hard to get anything accomplished.

It's also likely that it feels frightening to tell people what you really think and feel. Maybe you're afraid that if they saw "the real you" they wouldn't like you and they'd leave. As a result, you probably tolerate unsatisfying friendships and bad romantic relationships just to be sure you're never left alone. Maybe you even jump right into a new relationship as soon as the old one ends. One person with this problem summed it up when he said: "I'd rather be in a bad relationship than no relationship at all."

You probably even find yourself doing things that you don't want to do, maybe things that go against your values and better judgments, just so you don't hurt anyone's feelings or get left alone. Maybe your friends ask you to participate in activities you don't want to do. Or, maybe you volunteer to take on extra chores at your job, even though you don't have the free time, just to be sure you don't anger your boss and coworkers.

And yet, despite all your efforts to please other people, it's very likely that you still don't have many close, satisfying relationships—relationships in which your needs are met just as much as the other person's.[2]

ARE THERE OTHER RELATED PROBLEMS?

A person with this type of personality is also in danger of experiencing problems such as depression, dysthymia, bipolar disorder, panic disorder, generalized anxiety disorder, bulimia, and social phobia.[3-6] There's also an increased risk of suicide among people with dependent personalities.[7] Other studies have found relatively strong relationships between dependent personality and alcohol and drug problems, especially for men.[8, 9]

WHO IS AFFECTED?

It's estimated that less than 1 percent to almost 2 percent of the general adult population, or approximately 1 million American adults, have a dependent personality, with women developing the problem more often than men.[10-12] In general, almost 15 percent of all American adults, or almost 31 million people, struggle with personality problems like this one,[10] and these types of long-term problems are often the cause of general unhappiness and disability in a person's life.[12]

WHAT CAUSES IT?

A dependent personality is probably caused by a combination of biological and social factors. One study has shown that personality disorders in general have a strong chance of being passed on in families, due to influential genetic factors.[13] However, in this same study, the influence of environment might also have been a possible cause of dependent personality. Other studies have found that children who experience depression have greater odds of developing a dependent personality later in adulthood.[14, 15]

One social theory suggests that children learn to be excessively dependent by watching their excessively dependent parents, who get their needs met by constantly relying on other people. In contrast, studies of family influences have found that parents who are extremely protective and overly strict often cause their children to become excessively dependent adults.[16-19] This type of parenting style prevents a child from learning from his or her errors and it also prevents the child from developing any sense of independence.[20] If a child is consistently raised this way, believing that he or she is not capable of doing anything without others' help, while also believing that he or she will be punished when wrong, it is easy to foresee how that child might develop a dependent personality in adulthood.

WHAT CAN YOU DO ABOUT IT?

Unfortunately, there's little research to suggest which treatment is the most effective for helping someone with a dependent personality.[21] However, whichever treatment you choose, the ultimate goal should be to help you function more independently. In a study of many personality problems, including dependent personality, the use of brief psychodynamic therapy was helpful in improving people's lives, even a year and a half after the treatment ended.[22, 23]

In a similar study, cognitive behavioral therapy was also shown to be effective.[24, 25] One of the skills taught in cognitive behavioral therapy is assertiveness training, which helps you learn how to ask for what you need in life.[26] Longer-term psychodynamic therapy,[27, 28] couples therapy,[29] and family therapy[30] are also thought to be helpful treatments for this problem. In these last two therapies, other people in your life are included in the treatment to assess what roles they might be playing in your dependency issues.

Lastly, one group of researchers found some success using antidepressant medications such as fluoxetine (Prozac) to treat dependent personality issues.[31]

Recommended treatments for dependent personality disorder include:

- Brief psychodynamic therapy, see page 135

- Cognitive behavioral therapy, see page 136

- Psychodynamic therapy, see page 167

- Couples therapy, see page 139

- Family therapy, see page 146

- Antidepressant medications, see page 155

DEPRESSION

WHAT IS IT?

Depression, or unipolar depression, is a problem characterized by both an extremely sad mood that lasts for a long period of time and a lack of pleasure in doing things that usually make you happy.[1] Someone with depression also has problems sleeping, either sleeping too much or too little; trouble thinking and concentrating; low levels of energy; unexpected changes in weight; and feelings of nervousness or agitation. With severe depression, there can also be recurrent thoughts about dying or actual suicide attempts.

If you're experiencing these symptoms for at least two weeks, you might be diagnosed as having a major depressive episode. When left untreated, some major depressive episodes can last as long as nine months, on average.[2] After the depressive episode ends, you might return to feeling normal. However, after your first major depressive episode, the odds are 50 percent more likely that you'll experience another one, and with each new episode the odds only get worse that these episodes will keep coming.[3] This is why getting treatment for your depression is so important, even if your last depressive episode has already ended.

It's important to remember that depression is not a sign of weakness, or an inability to cope with normal problems. Most people with depression can't treat the problem effectively by themselves. People with depression usually have a very pessimistic view about themselves and life, and they think of themselves as incapable of handling problems.[4] This way of thinking is both a result of the disorder and, perhaps, part of the cause. Regardless, depression is a very serious problem that can affect anyone and is beyond the control of most people once it appears.

If you're suffering with depression, there are probably many days when you don't feel like getting out of bed. Either you feel too tired or maybe you think, "Why bother?" since your life feels hopeless or pointless. Throughout the day, you probably feel sluggish, unmotivated, and empty inside, like there's a part of you missing. You might even be experiencing headaches or body aches for which there are no apparent causes. You're also likely to be restless and agitated, which makes it even harder to concentrate. Most likely, you've given up your interest in activities that once excited you, possibly even sex. Instead, thoughts about death and dying occupy you more frequently than they once did. You might've thought about ways to kill yourself or you may have actually tried. Or, perhaps you take dangerous risks while driving, because you think that it wouldn't make a difference if you did die.

Depression can also cause many problems in your relationships, especially marriages and partnerships.[5] Often, people who are depressed have problematic beliefs about their relationships. Some people believe that they shouldn't disagree with their partners, which only puts added stress on both people.[6] Others who are depressed seek constant reassurance from their friends and partners.[7] People with depression will do this to determine if they're doing the "right" thing or to find out if they still are loved. Unfortunately, no amount of reassurance from the nondepressed partner or friend ever seems to be enough. And, eventually, in some cases, the constant reassurance-seeking can lead to the nondepressed partner or friend also becoming depressed.[8]

Another type of depression is called *dysthymia*.[1] This type of depression is a longer lasting depression that seems to stay with you for your entire life. In some ways, dysthymia might not be as severe or disabling as depression, because maybe you can still function in your everyday life, and you might not have as many problems with sleeping, thinking, or weight changes. But because dysthymia is so constant and long lasting, it becomes part of your personality style. If you have dysthymia, you might look generally unhappy or sad all the time, and your mood might never return to a balanced, healthy state. A person with dysthymia might also develop depression, a condition that is known as *double depression*. Officially, depression and dysthymia, along with the bipolar disorders, are collectively referred to as "mood disorders."

Lastly, it's important to note that depression is not the same as mourning. Many people will react in a way that resembles depression after someone they know dies. So, if you recently suffered the loss of someone in your life and are experiencing the problems described above, this would be considered normal. However, if the feelings persist for an extended length of time or become worse, you should consider consulting a mental health professional.

ARE THERE OTHER RELATED PROBLEMS?

Because untreated depression has the habit of repeating itself, and getting worse, one of the most serious consequences of the disorder is suicide. Twenty to 35 percent of all suicides are due to depression.[9] This doesn't mean that if you have depression you're going to kill yourself, but it does mean that depression is a serious problem that needs to be treated.

Many people with depression and dysthymia also struggle with other problems. In one large study, almost half of the people diagnosed with depression had some other problem.[10] Frequently, these problems include specific phobias, social phobia, generalized anxiety disorder, panic disorder, post-traumatic stress disorder, obsessive-compulsive disorder, dependent personality problems, and emotion dysregulation problems.[11-13] Many people with depression and dysthymia also battle drug and alcohol problems,[14, 15] which complicates the treatment of both the depression and the substance abuse. In one very large survey of more than 43,000 people in the United States, approximately 19 percent of those with depression also had a problem with drugs or alcohol, as did approximately 18 percent of the people with dysthymia.[16]

Many people with depression also have medical conditions, such as hypertension, arthritis, skin problems, cancer, speech disorders, heart disease, ulcers, and cardiovascular disease.[17-20] Often it's the development of one of these illnesses that leads to the onset of depression.[20] However, there's also evidence that the reverse can be true. If left untreated, depression can lead to problems like cardiovascular disease and heart disease, and if you already have had a heart attack, depression can increase your risk of having another one.[21-25]

WHO IS AFFECTED?

A 1996 report published by the World Health Organization[26] stated that the worldwide impact of depression has long been underestimated and it's only getting worse. The report stated that by the year 2020, depression will be the number one cause of disability for women around the world. Plus, when both sexes are considered, depression will be the world's second leading cause of disability, behind only heart disease. In the United States alone, it's been estimated that depression affects approximately 5 to 10 percent of the adult population every year, or approximately 10 to 19 million adults.[11, 27-29] However, over the course of a person's entire life the statistics get even higher.

During the course of a lifetime, 5 to 12 percent of all men and 10 to 25 percent of all women will probably experience an episode of depression.[1, 30] In general, women are usually diagnosed with the problem twice as often as men.[1] Some researchers think that women are more vulnerable to depression due to factors such as hormonal changes during puberty,[31] greater risk of experiencing anxiety,[32] greater number of life stressors,[33] and greater lack of social support.[34, 35] Depression usually begins between the ages of fifteen to thirty for both men and women, but depression and dysthymia can also affect younger children.[1, 36] In the United States, the average age of onset for depression is twenty-seven for men and twenty-eight for women, with similar ages in other Western countries.[37]

Dysthymia affects approximately 3 to 5 percent of the adult population at some point in their lives, or approximately 11 million Americans,[27, 28, 30] and, again, women are usually diagnosed with the problem twice as often as men.[38] Like depression, dysthymia can also begin at any point in a person's life, but it usually begins between childhood and early adulthood.[1]

WHAT CAUSES IT?

The exact causes of depression and dysthymia are still unknown. However, there are many biological, environmental, and social risk factors that are known to influence the development of the disorder.[39]

Heredity

Many people are born with a genetic risk for developing depression,[40] which can then be triggered by social or environmental factors such as stress.[41] Since the end of the twentieth century, scientists have been examining the genetic instructions that create the human body. One of the results has been the identification of similar genetic codes for depression in related family members. If you have an immediate family member who is depressed, such as a parent or a sibling, you are one and a half to three times more likely to develop depression than someone who is not related to your family.[1] Similarly, dysthymia is more common in people who have a parent or a sibling who is depressed or dysthymic.[1] However, keep in mind that heredity is only a risk factor and not a definite cause; it means only that you are more vulnerable to depression.

Biology

Brain chemicals called *neurotransmitters* also contribute to the development of depression. In particular, the neurotransmitters serotonin and norepinephrine appear to play key roles. Originally, it was thought that low levels of these chemicals in the brain caused depression, but more recent research suggests that it is more complicated than that.[42] It's now thought that these two chemicals might regulate other neurotransmitters, such as dopamine and acetylcholine, that might also contribute to depression.[43, 44]

Similarly, the hormone melatonin can play a role in depression. In winter, the decrease in sunlight causes the human body to produce more melatonin, which results in greater fatigue and the need to sleep more.[45] Some people are affected more strongly by this surge of melatonin, resulting in a form of depression called *seasonal affective disorder* (SAD).[46, 47]

Illnesses

Illnesses can also cause depression, especially life-threatening and chronic illnesses. Very few people who are battling cancer, for example, are going to do so and not feel depressed at some point. Facing disease, and possibly death, is enough to make even the strongest person feel depressed. Additionally, certain illnesses create real chemical changes in the body that cause depression or depression-like symptoms. Some of these illnesses include: multiple sclerosis, thyroid problems, cancer, the flu, hepatitis, tuberculosis, Parkinson's disease, tumors, stroke, dementia, Alzheimer's, and vitamin deficiencies.[48] Women who suffer from premenstrual syndrome (PMS) or who have recently had a baby may also experience symptoms of depression.[39] If you're experiencing one of these illnesses, or another illness that you suspect is leading to depression, you should consult a medical doctor in addition to a mental health professional.

Medications

Certain medications for other illnesses might also cause depression. These include the hepatitis medication interferon-alfa (Roferon) and the arthritis medication indomethacin (Indocin).[48-50] Additionally, some oral contraceptives can also cause depressive symptoms.[50] If you are taking any of these medications and are experiencing depression, contact your medical doctor. However, don't stop taking your medication without talking to your medical doctor first. Stopping your medication by yourself might lead to more complicated and severe problems.

Other Substances

Many other substances can also cause depression. Alcohol, by its nature, is a depressant. At first, it might make you feel good, but if consumed in large enough quantities, it will make you feel depressed. Many frequently used recreational drugs can also cause depression or depression-like symptoms. These drugs include marijuana, cocaine, heroin, Valium, Ecstasy, amphetamines, and others. An excessive use of caffeine, which causes increased heart rate, anxiety, and irritability, can worsen your depression. Many environmental toxins are also suspected of being linked to depression. These chemicals include: pesticides, copper, aluminum, mercury, lead, formaldehyde, and others.[39] If you believe that you are being exposed to one of these chemicals, or to another toxic chemical, consult a medical doctor for a checkup.

Trauma

Depression can also be caused by traumas in your life. A *trauma* is any event that causes severe emotional or physical injury and leaves long-lasting damage. Some of the more common causes of trauma include war, crime, rape, accidents, abuse, natural disasters, and relationship problems. However, other causes are definitely possible and it's not necessary for the trauma to have occurred recently for it to affect your mental health. It's also possible that older traumas are causing your depression.

For example, children who experience any form of abuse are more likely to develop depression as adults, possibly due to the effects of stress on the nervous system caused at the time of the abuse.[51] Another study has shown that people who experience the childhood loss of a parent, to either death or divorce, are much more likely to develop depression as adults.[52] Interestingly, in this study, it was the early loss of a parent due to divorce, rather than death, that was a stronger predictor of depression. Both of these types of experiences have very long-lasting impacts on a person. They may cause you to look at life and relationships in a very negative way, which eventually might lead to depression.

Other research has shown that, in general, traumatic events have long-lasting impacts on the brain, especially on the parts of the brain associated with memory and emotions.[53] These results occur no matter when the trauma took place in your life. But because the brain is very fragile and still developing as a child, any trauma that occurred during that time is bound to leave some impact on your life, no matter how inconsequential you think that trauma is to you now.

Self-Defeating Thoughts

Depression can also be caused by repetitive self-defeating thoughts.[54-56] The messages we replay in our heads are some of the most powerful obstacles we must overcome in our lives. Sadly, many of these self-defeating thoughts don't even originate with us. Instead, they were told to us by our parents, friends, or society. Some of these thoughts might include "I'm not good enough," "I'm unlovable," or "I should take care of others instead of myself."[57] Anyone who hears messages like these often enough will usually begin to believe them. In other contexts, this process is called propaganda, brainwashing, and advertising, and we are all capable of being affected by it.

Interpersonal Conflicts

Depression is also caused by feelings of not being connected with others or being in conflict with others.[39] The feelings of being alone or unwanted are, perhaps, two of the most powerful emotions we can experience. So, it's not strange that feeling them can lead to depression. These are very difficult feelings to deal with, especially if you're by yourself or in an unsatisfying relationship. Trying to cope with the problem of loneliness while you're alone hardly ever leads to a solution. In fact, social isolation and lack of social support are two predictors of suicide in people with severe depression. People who think they have no one else to live for often don't want to live for themselves.

Loss of Meaning

Lastly, depression can also be caused by the loss of meaning in your life.[39] The meanings we give life can be religious, spiritual, community-based, or personal. Sometimes, these beliefs are challenged. Most of the time, the belief will remain strong or adjust to accommodate new information. However, sometimes meanings and beliefs fail, and we lose faith in our religion, country, society, or job. When this happens, it's understandable that depression follows. If you spend years investing time, energy, and commitment into something, that something becomes very powerful in your life. Then, if that something is suddenly shown to be wrong, or if you begin to have doubts about what you were investing in for all those years, that realization may have a major negative impact on your life. It might even cause you to doubt yourself: "What was I thinking for all those years?"

WHAT CAN YOU DO ABOUT IT?

Regrettably, more than half the people who need treatment for depression don't seek help.[27, 58] In one large study of adults in the United States, only 37 percent sought help for their depression within a year of the problem's onset; and, on average, people waited eight years before seeking treatment.[59] This is unfortunate, considering that there are very effective treatments for depression that could help people avoid the long-term disability associated with the disorder.[60] In general, more than 80 percent of the people who do seek help for depression experience an improvement in their lives.[61]

The majority of people who seek help for depression initially choose to take antidepressant medications.[62-64] For some causes of depression, such as heredity, biology, illnesses, medications, and other substances, antidepressant medications might be the best initial treatment. Or, a combination of psychotherapy and antidepressants might be necessary, especially to treat chronic depression.[65]

Among the more commonly prescribed antidepressants are a group of medications called selective serotonin reuptake inhibitors (SSRIs), which includes fluoxetine

(Prozac), sertraline (Zoloft), fluvoxamine (Luvox), paroxetine (Paxil), and citalopram (Celexa). Other newer types of antidepressants include venlafaxine (Effexor), nefazodone (Serzone), mirtazepine (Remeron), and bupropion (Wellbutrin).

In general, both these and other types of antidepressants need to be taken regularly for six to eight weeks before the therapeutic effects begin to take effect, and all of the medications induce additional side effects.[66]

Due to these complications, many people seek psychotherapy as an alternative or additional treatment. In many studies, certain types of psychotherapy have been shown to be just as effective as antidepressant medications,[65] for both moderate and severe depression,[67] and in some cases, psychotherapy succeeds where antidepressants fail.[68] In clinical studies, some treatments have been shown to be more effective than others at treating depression. These successful treatments include behavioral therapy, cognitive behavioral therapy, interpersonal therapy, and brief psychodynamic therapy.[65, 69, 70]

Both behavioral therapy and cognitive behavioral therapy focus on the ways your actions can contribute to your problems,[71] while cognitive behavioral therapy also focuses on your habitual negative thought patterns.[54] For these reasons, these two types of therapy are often successful in treating depression caused by illnesses, other substances, trauma, self-defeating thoughts, interpersonal conflicts, and loss of meaning. Cognitive behavioral therapy has probably received the most research of all the treatments. In one study, cognitive behavioral therapy for depression was shown to leave lasting improvements in the brain, similar to the effects of taking antidepressant medication.[72] Also, in one comparative study with medication, cognitive behavioral therapy was shown to be twice as effective in preventing relapses of depression one year after treatment ended.[73]

Interpersonal therapy for depression focuses on relationships and how they might be contributing to your depression.[74, 75] For this reason, interpersonal therapy is often effective in treating depression caused by relationship conflicts and the mourning of a lost loved one.

Brief psychodynamic therapy focuses on resolving internal struggles and relationship problems caused by personal interactions and historical conflicts.[76, 77] For these reasons, brief psychodynamic therapy is often effective in treating depression caused by trauma, interpersonal conflicts, and loss of meaning in your life.

Couples therapy and family therapy have also been shown to be effective in treating depression caused by interpersonal conflicts, although they have not received as much clinical support as the other therapies.[78-80]

Many people have also found relief using many of the other psychotherapies highlighted in this book, such as long-term psychodynamic therapy and humanistic therapy. These and other types of psychotherapies can often be helpful in treating depression caused by interpersonal conflicts and loss of meaning in your life.

Other people have found relief using alternative treatments for depression. For depression caused by seasonal affective disorder, light therapy—exposure to sunlight or special sun lamps—is often effective.[47] Exercise can also be effective. One study of 156 adults over the age of fifty compared the use of antidepressants versus participation in an exercise regimen.[81] Interestingly, the volunteers in both treatments improved and were no longer depressed at the end of the study. However, ten months after the study ended, volunteers in the exercise group had less of a chance of relapsing into depression, especially if they had continued to exercise on their own.

Additionally, some people have sought treatment for depression by using over-the-counter remedies such as Saint-John's-wort. While there is some evidence that this can be effective in treating mild to moderate forms of depression,[82, 83] one large scale study sponsored by the National Institute of Mental Health found that the herb was no more effective than a placebo pill.[84] In addition, Saint-John's-wort has been known to interfere with the effectiveness of other medications, such as antidepressants and some oral birth control pills.[66]

Lastly, perhaps the most drastic form of treatment for depression is electroconvulsive therapy (ECT),[85] which is known more commonly as "electroshock therapy." Usually, this is used as a last alternative for treating depression when the disorder hasn't responded to other forms of treatment. ECT is a hospital procedure in which you are given a muscle relaxant and anesthesia before having an electric current sent through your body for half a second. This treatment is usually conducted six to twelve times and spread out over the course of two to four weeks.[86] Many patients find relief for their depression using this treatment when other methods have failed,[87, 88] especially when a person's depression also includes delusions.[89]

Recommended treatments for depression include:

- Antidepressant medications, see page 155

- Behavior therapy, see page 133

- Cognitive behavioral therapy, see page 136

- Interpersonal therapy, see page 153

- Brief psychodynamic therapy, see page 135

- Couples therapy, see page 139

- Family therapy, see page 146

- Exercise

- Light therapy

- Electroconvulsive therapy

- Saint-John's-wort

DISSOCIATIVE DISORDERS

WHAT ARE THEY?

Dissociative disorders are a group of disorders characterized by a strange feeling of being detached from reality. By definition, the word "dissociate" refers to a state of cutting yourself off from something, such as your memories, your surroundings, or even from yourself. Typically, this group of problems includes dissociative amnesia, dissociative fugue, dissociative identity disorder, and depersonalization disorder.[1] In each of these disorders, some form of dissociation takes place.

Everyone experiences some form of mild dissociation on a regular basis,[2, 3] like daydreaming. However, what makes this common experience different from a dissociative disorder is the severity and length of the dissociation. If you experience some form of dissociative disorder, the experience is very disturbing and beyond your control. Maybe you can't remember a significant part of your life, which goes beyond normal forgetfulness or old age. This problem might be related to *dissociative amnesia* or a *dissociative fugue*. (A fugue is a long period of dissociation during which you forget all or most of your personal identity.)

If you also experience pieces of missing time for which you can't account, and sometimes feel as though there are a number of distinct personalities living inside your body, this might be a *dissociative identity disorder*, formerly known as "multiple personality disorder." Or, maybe you often feel detached from your body, as if you're watching yourself in a movie. This might be a *depersonalization disorder*.

ARE THERE OTHER RELATED PROBLEMS?

Many people suffering with a dissociative disorder also have other mental health problems, like emotion dysregulation problems,[4, 5] depression, or drug or alcohol abuse.[5]

WHO IS AFFECTED?

The prevalence of dissociative disorders is unknown. The best estimates vary widely from 5 to 58 percent of hospital patients[4-6] and 2 to 6 percent of the general population.[7, 8]

WHAT CAUSES THEM?

Sadly, many people who struggle with a dissociative disorder have also suffered from extreme traumas in their lives, such as physical and sexual abuse as a child,[4, 9-11] rape,[12] war,[13] natural disasters,[14] witnessing a murder,[15] and other such frightening experiences.[16] In these cases, some researchers believe that dissociation acts as a protective psychological defense, which prevents the victim from being overwhelmed by the experience or memories of the experience.[17] However, other research has indicated that less traumatic events might also trigger dissociative disorders.

In one study of adult men and women,[18] patients who were diagnosed with a dissociative disorder had all recently experienced difficulties getting their basic needs met for living, needs such as health, safety, love, self-esteem, and self-determination. [19, 20] The patients had all experienced difficulties in their relationships, marriages, or employment, and later, as their difficulties improved, their dissociative problems also lessened. Here, too, the dissociation might have been a protective mechanism from the overwhelming pain of the frustrating experience.

WHAT CAN YOU DO ABOUT THEM?

Unfortunately, the research on treating dissociative disorders is not as extensive as the treatment literature for other problems. This might be because some mental health care professionals don't think that dissociative disorders are a true, verifiable problem.[21, 22] So, if you suspect you have a dissociative disorder and are seeking treatment, be sure to shop around for a mental health professional who has experience treating your problem.

Fortunately, there have been several effective treatments reported. Some people may be treated on an outpatient basis, while others with more severe cases may require a hospital stay.[23] The common goal of most of these successful treatments is to help you recover lost memories, integrate disconnected elements of your personality, and ground you in the present moment when you start to dissociate. Some successes have been achieved using psychodynamic treatments,[24] hypnotherapy,[25, 26] eye-movement desensitization and reprocessing,[27] cognitive behavioral therapy,[28, 29] antidepressants, anti-anxiety medications,[30] and diazepam (Valium).[31]

Recommended treatments for dissociative disorders in general include:

- Psychodynamic therapy, see page 167

- Hypnotherapy, see page 152

- Eye-movement desensitization and reprocessing, see page 144

- Cognitive behavioral therapy, see page 136

- Medications, see page 155

- Family therapy, see page 146

The following pages contain specific information on each of the dissociative disorders. Please find the one(s) that most pertain(s) to you, and then continue reading.

DISSOCIATIVE AMNESIA AND DISSOCIATIVE FUGUE

What are they? Dissociative amnesia and dissociative fugue are two similar disorders characterized by the inability to remember significant episodes of your life.[1] These memory losses aren't caused by brain damage; old age; normal forgetting; or the use of drugs, medication, or alcohol. Instead, they usually follow the experience of a traumatic situation.

Dissociative amnesia is the mysterious loss of your memories. In its most severe form, this loss is very disturbing because it can involve many memories of various aspects of your life. As described earlier, most people who experience this loss of memory do so after being involved in a severe trauma, such as an accident, a crime, or combat.[15, 16] This loss of information can appear either quickly and unexpectedly, such as when following a trauma, or one day you may simply notice that there's an inexplicable gap in your memory of your life.

In the case of traumas, the time span that's often forgotten is the period during which the trauma took place. In all cases, it's possible that your memory is either completely blank or only partially impaired. It's also possible that the time span you forgot is extensive, stretching back years, or it may be selective, relating only to specific categories of information, such as your family. The length of time that is forgotten can range from minutes to years.[1] In one case study,[25] a fifty-one-year-old woman couldn't remember the twelve-year time span between the ages of thirty-seven and forty-nine, a memory loss caused by a car accident.

Similarly, *dissociative fugue* involves a different form of incomprehensible memory loss. If you're experiencing a dissociative fugue, you will forget all, or most, of your personal information, such as your name, family, and job. In addition, you will often inexplicably travel to a new place far from where you once lived. During this period of forgetfulness, you will act and appear normal. However, quite suddenly, you may become very confused and distressed by the sudden disconnection from your original personal identity and memories. It's at this point that the problem usually becomes identifiable.[1]

In most cases of reported dissociative fugues, the person doesn't take on a new name and identity.[1] However, it has been known to happen. Following recovery from a dissociative fugue, you may have no memory of what happened to you when you were in your fugue state.

Who is affected? It is unknown how many people experience dissociative amnesia in the general population. However, in one very small study of psychiatric hospital patients,[5] 42 percent of them met the criteria for dissociative amnesia, but only one of the patients had experienced a dissociative fugue. Similarly, in the general population, less than 1 percent is estimated to experience a dissociative fugue.[1] Both disorders may occur at any age, but most cases of fugue are reported in adults.[1]

What causes them? Both dissociative amnesia and fugue are often associated with the experience of a severe trauma, such as combat, accidents, abuse, and crimes.[1]

Stressful life events, such as relationships and job difficulties, also have been known to trigger these disorders.[18]

What can you do about it? As previously stated, dissociative amnesia and dissociative fugue have been successfully treated using many psychotherapeutic techniques found in this book. Often, these techniques can help recover lost memories and resolve conflicts that might have led to the memories' original departure.

DISSOCIATIVE IDENTITY DISORDER

What is it? *Dissociative identity disorder* is a problem characterized by severe splits in a person's sense of self.[1] Formerly, dissociative identity disorder was called "multiple personality disorder." If you suffer from dissociative identity disorder, you experience two or more distinct alternative personalities in your body that emerge at certain times. In reported cases, the number of personalities has ranged from two to over a hundred, but most people report ten or fewer.[1]

Often, the appearance of these alternative personalities is triggered by stressful situations.[1] These alternative personalities are far different than the normal shifts in behavior a person makes to adapt to new situations in life. Usually, these alternative personalities have their own unique names, behaviors, memories, and traits. In addition, the individual alternative personalities are often unaware of each other[32] and they're also unaware of information learned by other personalities.[33, 34]

It is often the case that the alternative personalities display behaviors that are far different than the original personality. For instance, perhaps one of the alternative personalities likes to go to parties and dance, while the original personality is more of a shy homebody. Even more puzzling, the alternative personalities sometimes insist that they are a different age, gender, race, or sexual orientation than the original personality.[35]

If you're suffering from dissociative identity disorder, perhaps some of your friends have commented on your strange behavior. Maybe they've told you that you weren't acting "like yourself," or perhaps they told you stories about yourself that you think are impossible; stories you can't remember, but which your friends can prove. Also, you probably experience episodes of lost time, that is, times when you find yourself in a strange situation and have no idea how you got there.[33] It might also be true that there are lengthy periods of your childhood that you can't remember.[36] These types of amnesia are key characteristics of dissociative identity disorder.[1] And again, as with the other dissociative disorders, these memory losses are not caused by brain damage, old age, normal forgetting, or the use of drugs, medication, or alcohol.

Are there other related problems? Often, many people suffering from dissociative identity disorder also suffer from other problems, such as depression and suicidal thoughts,[37] anxiety, substance abuse, somatization disorders[38] (which affect the body), emotion dysregulation problems,[39] post-traumatic stress disorder,[1] and auditory hallucinations.[40]

Who is affected? The rate of dissociative identity disorder in the general population is unknown. However, in studies of psychiatric patients in hospitals, estimates have ranged from less than 1 percent to 12 percent,[6, 41] and in one very small study of psychiatric patients, the rate was 25 percent.[5] In case studies, women are frequently diagnosed with dissociative identity disorder more often than men.[1, 30]

What causes it? Dissociative identity disorder has been called the most severe type of dissociative disorder.[42] Sadly, it's often associated with cases of severe childhood trauma, such as physical abuse, sexual abuse, a dysfunctional home environment, and parental rejection.[3, 42-45] As a result, some researchers believe that the process of dissociating and creating multiple personalities is an unintentionally defensive act to protect yourself from both the trauma and the memories of the trauma.[43] However, the exact cause of the disorder is unknown.

What can you do about it? Dissociative identity disorder has been successfully treated using many of the psychotherapeutic techniques found in this book, such as cognitive behavioral therapy, psychodynamic therapy, hypnotherapy, eye-movement desensitization and reprocessing, and the use of medication. However, the research literature doesn't support one treatment as being better than another. In general, the goal of all of these treatments is to help bring relief from symptoms associated with the disorder and to help you incorporate the many personalities into one integrated whole.[28]

DEPERSONALIZATION DISORDER

What is it? *Depersonalization disorder* is a problem characterized by a feeling of being disconnected from your body and/or your thoughts.[1] Some people who struggle with depersonalization disorder feel as though they're watching themselves from outside their bodies or that they're watching themselves perform on television. Yet, despite these feelings, people suffering from depersonalization disorder aren't hallucinating. They're able to distinguish reality from their dissociation and they find the experience very disturbing.[46] The disorder can come on quite suddenly within hours, or it can slowly worsen over the course of weeks or months.[47]

In a large study of people with depersonalization disorder,[47-49] many of them reported feeling as if their surroundings were not real. In addition, they also felt like they were looking at the world through a fog, as if their bodies didn't belong to them, and that once-familiar places suddenly felt foreign. Some of them even reported that sometimes they felt as if they were outside of their bodies looking at themselves or that they didn't recognize themselves when looking in a mirror.

If you're suffering from depersonalization disorder, most likely you can relate to some of these symptoms. In addition, perhaps you often feel emotionally and physically numb, isolated, without motivation, unable to concentrate, unable to remember things, weightless, and dizzy.[50] Maybe you also experience a distortion of your senses, like the loss of sound, color, or taste. Or maybe, sometimes, you feel as though the world is two-dimensional or not solid.[50]

Are there other related problems? In addition, people with depersonalization disorder often suffer with other problems, such as depression, panic disorder, phobias, generalized anxiety disorder, and drug or alcohol abuse.[47]

Who is affected? Many people experience this type of depersonalization phenomena at least one time in their lives. In studies of the general population, 34 to 70 percent of the people interviewed had experienced some type of depersonalization, usually caused by stress, exhaustion, exposure to a life-threatening situation, or drug use.[1, 51-54] However, in depersonalization disorder, the episodes of dissociation are more severe; they are continual, upsetting, and they interfere with your life. Unfortunately, the number of people suffering from depersonalization disorder is unknown.[1]

In a study of 117 people with depersonalization disorder,[47] men and women were affected equally, the average age of onset for the illness was sixteen years old, and the people interviewed had been suffering with the illness for as little as three months to as long as fifty-eight years.

What causes it? One study of depersonalization disorder found that there were some common triggers that brought on the feeling of being disconnected from one's body and/or thoughts.[47] These triggers included: stress, fear, depression, marijuana use, and the use of hallucinogenic drugs. However, as with the other dissociative disorders, depersonalization disorder is also strongly associated with the experience of severe traumas, such as combat, accidents, childhood emotional abuse, and crimes.[1, 55] Factors like stress, depression, fatigue, and alcohol and drug use are also reported to make the feelings of disconnection worse.[47]

What can you do about it? Depersonalization disorder, its cause, and its treatment are still not fully understood.[47] Unfortunately, not much research has been done to investigate effective treatments. However, among the little research that does exist, one study found cognitive behavioral therapy to be somewhat effective.[56, 57] Cognitive behavioral treatment for depersonalization disorder attempts to analyze the catastrophic thoughts that accompany episodes of depersonalization and correct any behaviors that might contribute to the illness, such as behaviors formed to ward off the episodes of depersonalization.[50] In a study of this treatment,[56] patients reported significant improvements in the severity of their symptoms.

In addition, other smaller studies have had success using psychodynamic therapy,[58] family therapy,[59] hypnotherapy, and the use of antidepressant and antianxiety medications.[47]

DRUG AND ALCOHOL ADDICTION PROBLEMS

WHAT ARE THEY?

The repeated use of drugs or alcohol can cause you many problems, such as physical and psychological addiction, family difficulties, legal complications, health problems, problems with your job, and relationship troubles.

One of the first signs that you have an alcohol or drug problem is the development of a pattern of usage called *substance abuse*.[1] Substance abuse might first be noticeable when your life or work begins to suffer because of your alcohol or drug use. Maybe you've been skipping work and staying at home to get high, or maybe your grades in school have dropped because you show up drunk.

Another indication of substance abuse is that your alcohol or drug use has begun to cause problems with your relationships, like arguments with your wife when you're high, physical fights with friends when you're drunk, or arguments with people about your substance use.

A third indication is the occurrence of legal problems caused by your use, like being arrested for driving under the influence (DUI) or possession of drugs.

A fourth indication that you have a substance abuse problem is that you use drugs or alcohol in potentially dangerous situations, like driving while intoxicated, or caring for your children when you're high.

Beyond the level of substance abuse is an even more dangerous level of alcohol and drug use called *substance dependence*.[1] One of the first warning signs of substance dependence is *tolerance*. This means there is the need to use an increased amount of drugs or alcohol in order to achieve the same "high" or feeling you once did with smaller amounts.

A second indication is that you spend a lot of time getting and using drugs or alcohol.

A third sign of substance dependence is that you miss important family and social events because you're too busy drinking or using drugs.

A fourth indication is that you realize you're unable to cut down on your drinking or drug use.

A fifth warning sign is that you realize you've been using or drinking in larger amounts and for a longer period of time than you originally thought you would be.

A sixth indication of substance dependence is that you continue to use drugs or drink alcohol despite the fact that you have problems caused by your use, like ulcers or alcohol-induced depression.

And, finally, a seventh indication of substance dependence is withdrawal, which occurs when you reduce the amount you use or stop using completely. *Withdrawal* is typically experienced as physical discomfort, emotional distress, or mental anxiety that makes you want to restart your habit. Some substance withdrawals, like those experienced from addiction to alcohol, can be potentially life-threatening and include uncontrollable body tremors and hallucinations. The long-term dependence on certain medications like phenobarbital, diazepam (Valium), and lorazepam (Ativan) can also lead to dangerous withdrawal symptoms and should be supervised by a medical professional.

ARE THERE OTHER RELATED PROBLEMS?

Although some of the problems of long-term alcohol and drug use might seem obvious, other potential health dangers aren't often thought about. Here is a partial list of health risks associated with frequent and/or extended use of alcohol and drugs.[2]

Alcohol can cause depression, anxiety, sleep problems, liver and throat cancer, dementia, heart failure, cognitive processing problems, digestive problems, anemia, fetal alcohol syndrome, and accidents.

Stimulants, such as cocaine ("crack"), amphetamines, methamphetamines ("crystal meth," "crank"), and Ritalin can cause depression, psychosis, irreversible brain damage, seizures, heart failure, stroke, skin damage inside your nose, and nutritional problems.

Opioid drugs, such as heroin, codeine, opium, and morphine, often include other habits, such as needle use, that can lead to problems like hepatitis, tuberculosis, tetanus, HIV, and abscesses.

Inhalants, solvents, and anesthetics, such as amyl/butyl nitrate ("poppers") and ketamine ("special K"), can cause severe memory problems, severe confusion, extreme fearfulness, and violence.

Cannabinoids, such as marijuana and hashish, can cause lung problems, lack of motivation, a lack of pleasure, and fatigue.

Psychedelics, such as MDMA ("Ecstasy"), LSD ("acid"), and PCP ("angel dust"), can cause memory problems, intense fear, and psychological dependence.

Depressants, such as the barbiturates secobarbital and phenobarbital, can cause depression, weight loss, irritability, and nutritional problems.

Anti-anxiety medications, such as diazepam (Valium), triazolam (Halcion), and lorazepam (Ativan), can cause confusion, a decrease in physical functioning, and difficulties with learning.

Many people with drug and alcohol problems also suffer with other related mental health problems, such as depression, dysthymia, bipolar disorder, panic disorder, social phobia, specific phobias, generalized anxiety disorder, and post-traumatic stress disorder.[3-5] Many others also suffer with personality disorders such as emotion dysregulation, antisocial, obsessive-compulsive, schizoid, dependent, and self-focused personalities.[6, 7] Plus, many people use both drugs and alcohol, and suffer from the effects of both substances.[8]

WHO IS AFFECTED?

A 1996 global study of disease found that alcohol use was the fifth leading cause of disability in the developed world among both physical and mental health problems.[9] It's estimated that approximately 9 to 13 percent of the adult population in the United States will struggle with an alcohol abuse problem at some point in their lives, and approximately 5 to 14 percent of the adult population will struggle with alcohol dependence during their lifetimes.[10, 11] In general, it appears that men are twice as likely as women to develop either problem.[10]

It's estimated that almost 4 to 8 percent of the adult population in the United States will struggle with a drug abuse problem at some point in their lives, and approximately 3 to 8 percent of the adult population will struggle with drug dependence during their lifetimes.[10, 11] And again, it appears that men are more likely to develop either problem.[10]

WHAT CAUSES IT?

Research has discovered a number of probable causes for addiction. Your genetic characteristics can make you more vulnerable to drug addiction[12] and alcohol consumption.[13] Plus, if you come from a family with alcoholism problems, your own chances of developing a problem with alcohol[14] and drugs increase,[15] especially if both of your parents have drinking problems.[16]

The use of alcohol and drugs also causes a chemical chain reaction in your brain, which leads to pleasurable feelings similar to the ones experienced with food and sex.[17, 18] This chemical reward system has been shown to be an important key to understanding the power of addiction, because the longer the addiction continues, the harder it becomes to feel good without the use of drugs or alcohol.[19] Many people continue their addiction for this reason.

Other people continue using to avoid the harsh feelings of withdrawal or the unpleasant side effects of their habit, such as the depression caused by alcohol and cocaine. In short, many people originally use drugs or alcohol to feel good and continue their habits in order to not feel bad.[20-22]

Many people have serious problems with alcohol, drugs, and mental health problems. In these cases, it's very difficult to determine what the original problem was. Some people report that they first began to use drugs or alcohol because they were feeling depressed or anxious and they wanted to ease their pain.[23] However, alcohol and drugs tend to make depression and anxiety worse. Plus, if you don't already have a problem with depression or anxiety, the long-term use of alcohol or drugs can create one.[1] This often makes it difficult to determine what came first, the substance problem or the mental health problem.

WHAT CAN YOU DO ABOUT IT?

Usually fewer than 50 percent of those who need help for drug and alcohol problems seek treatment,[24] and those who do seek treatment often wait as long as five to nine years before doing so.[25] This is unfortunate considering that there are many programs and treatments available to help people with both problems. Initially, many people find help for alcohol and drug problems in 12-step programs such as Alcoholics Anonymous and Narcotics Anonymous. These programs view addiction as a disease and focus on complete abstinence from drugs and alcohol. Many of these 12-step programs are centered on a belief in a "higher power" or God, but non-spiritual 12-step programs also exist.

An alternative to 12-step programs is the harm-reduction model of treatment.[2] Harm-reduction treatment doesn't demand abstinence from the very beginning of treatment. Instead, it will help you cut down your drinking or drug use while simultaneously investigating the issues that are maintaining your addiction. Other treatment facilities such as detoxification centers and residential treatment centers also can provide structured support for the early stages of sobriety and medical assistance to ease the symptoms of withdrawal.

In conjunction with these treatments, all of the psychotherapies found in this book will provide additional support for your recovery. In research studies, cognitive behavioral therapy, motivation-enhancement treatment, interpersonal therapy, and couples therapy have all been shown to be especially effective in treating substance abuse problems.[26, 27]

A number of medications have also demonstrated some effectiveness at treating substance abuse problems. Certain antidepressant medications can help reduce alcohol consumption[28] and cocaine consumption,[29, 30] while medications such as methadone (Dolophine), levo-alpha-acetylmethadol (LAAM), buprenorphine (Buprenex, Suboxone), and naltrexone (ReVia) can effectively reduce heroin addiction.[31, 32]

Recommended treatments for drug and alcohol addiction problems include:

· Twelve-step programs, such as Alcoholics Anonymous and Narcotics Anonymous

· Harm-reduction treatment programs

· Detoxification and residential treatment centers

· Cognitive behavioral therapy, see page 136

· Interpersonal therapy, see page 153

· Couples therapy, see page 139

· Motivation-enhancement treatment

· Any psychotherapy that provides you with support

· Antidepressant medications, see page 155

· Addiction-reducing medications

EMOTION DYSREGULATION/BORDERLINE PERSONALITY DISORDER

WHAT IS IT?

Emotion dysregulation is a disorder characterized by quick, frequent, and painful mood swings that are beyond the control of the person with the problem.[1, 2] If you're suffering with emotion dysregulation, you also have great difficulty forming and maintaining relationships, problems controlling your own spontaneous and reckless behavior, and a fluctuating idea about who you are.[1, 3] The overall theme for this illness is rapid and unpredictable change, in your thoughts, moods, behaviors, relationships, and beliefs about yourself.[4, 5]

Very often, these rapid changes are caused by recurring fears of being criticized or deserted by other people, or by the actions of other people that feel like criticism, such as small disagreements or changes in plans.[1] In response to these types of situations, a person with emotion dysregulation can suddenly become very sad, nervous, angry, or short-tempered.[3] You might also engage in self-harming behaviors, like cutting yourself or suicidal acts. Unfortunately, personality styles like this often create problems in your relationships, job, and other social situations. As a result, personality styles like this one are officially referred to as "personality disorders," and in many other references, this particular problem is referred to as "borderline personality disorder."

If you're suffering with emotion dysregulation, you most likely have a history of intense relationships that begin and end very quickly. When you form a relationship, you probably think very highly of the other person and want to spend as much time with that person as possible. But, at the first sign of a potential problem, such as the other person not making time for you, you start to think that the person is going to desert you. Maybe you even think that the other person doesn't like you as much as you like him or her. You suddenly feel intensely afraid, hurt, anxious, angry, sad, or ashamed. And, possibly, you feel this way for a few hours or maybe even as long as a few days. Then, just as suddenly, you end the relationship and begin to think of that person in a very negative way. Or, maybe you do something very extreme to try to keep that person from leaving you, such as calling him or her all the time, or threatening to kill yourself if he or she doesn't stay with you.[3]

It's also likely that when frustrating situations like this happen, you become overwhelmed with anger and either lash out at others or keep the anger bottled up inside yourself. Maybe you do something to punish yourself during times like these, such as cutting yourself on the arms and legs, using drugs and alcohol excessively, engaging in unsafe sexual encounters, going on shopping sprees you can't afford, gambling excessively, or engaging in an unhealthy eating habit like bingeing and purging.[4] Similarly, in other more hopeless situations, you might have tried to kill yourself or thought about suicide in a detailed way.

These quick fluctuations in emotional states and relationships are very common for people with emotion dysregulation. Most people with this problem are constantly examining their relationships for problems and are constantly expecting to be deserted by other people.[6] People with emotion dysregulation also tend to categorize themselves, others, and things into classes of either "all good" or "all bad," with no middle ground in between.[3] This is why small problems can often lead to the end of a relationship. Yet, despite how quickly these relationships can be terminated, many people with emotion dysregulation are actually afraid of being alone, because they think that they're not capable of coping with problems by themselves.[6]

Battling emotion dysregulation can be very tiring and confusing. People with this problem are in severe physical,[7] emotional,[2] and psychological pain[8] almost all the time. They also lack a stable sense of who they are.[1] One minute you may think of yourself as a good person and the next minute you think of yourself as evil and flawed. Thoughts about other people fluctuate rapidly, as well. You may want to trust others, but at the same time, you don't think other people are trustworthy.[6]

All of this confusion can very easily leave you feeling empty, sad, and hollow inside. Adding to the bewilderment of the disorder, you may sometimes feel as though you leave your body during times of stress and can't recall what happened. These severe periods of dissociation only add to your unstable sense of self. Similarly, and equally disturbing, are periods of hallucinations that occur during times of stress or depression.[1, 9]

ARE THERE OTHER RELATED PROBLEMS?

Of all the problems related to emotion dysregulation, the most severe is suicide. It's estimated that as many as 75 percent of the people with emotion dysregulation will attempt to kill themselves at some point,[10] and as many as 10 percent eventually will take their own lives.[11-14] Not surprisingly, it seems that the level of emotional instability is the most accurate predictor of suicide, rather than the person's level of depression.[15] However, many people with emotion dysregulation also suffer with depression, dysthymia, post-traumatic stress disorder, eating disorders, social phobia, specific phobia, panic disorder, and drug and alcohol problems.[16-19]

Males suffering from emotion dysregulation seem to be more likely to develop drug or alcohol problems than female sufferers. But female sufferers appear to be more likely to develop bulimia, anorexia, and other eating disorders.[19, 20] People with emotion dysregulation also frequently suffer with other personality disorders, such as a dependent personality and an extreme suspicion of others.[21] In addition, they often endure chronic medical conditions such as fibromyalgia, chronic fatigue syndrome, obesity, diabetes, hypertension, arthritis, and back pain.[7]

WHO IS AFFECTED?

Studies have estimated that approximately 1 to 5 percent of the general population is affected by emotion dysregulation,[22-25] while as many as 15 percent of psychiatric hospital patients are thought to be affected.[26] The disorder sometimes begins as early as childhood or adolescence,[27] but many people first seek treatment around the age of eighteen.[28] Many studies report that almost 75 percent of the people diagnosed with emotion dysregulation are women.[25, 26] However, this striking outcome isn't always found,[20, 22] and a few researchers have uncovered evidence that some mental health professionals diagnose women with emotion dysregulation more frequently than men, even when both sexes have the same symptoms.[29, 30]

WHAT CAUSES IT?

The exact cause of emotion dysregulation is unknown, but most likely it has both biological and social causes.[31] In general, personality problems like this one have a strong chance of being passed on in families, due to influential genetic factors that can be inherited.[32] Certain personality traits like emotional instability also appear to be highly inheritable.[33] Using brain-imaging technology, researchers have determined that certain behaviors related to emotion dysregulation, such as impulsivity, are related to low levels of the brain chemical serotonin.[34] Using similar techniques, researchers also found that people with emotion dysregulation interpret other people's facial expressions in an overreactive way when compared to people without the disorder.[35] This makes it hard for some people to interpret neutral facial expressions, and sometimes it leads them to misinterpret neutral faces as having threatening expressions.

In addition, some brain-imaging studies have found that people diagnosed with emotion dysregulation also exhibit smaller sizes in certain brain areas involved with emotional functioning.[36, 37] The most alarming research findings have linked emotion dysregulation with a history of being abused, especially sexual, physical, emotional, and verbal abuse.[38] In one study, 91 percent of those with emotion dysregulation had been the victim of some type of abuse and 92 percent had experienced severe neglect as a child.[39]

In another study, 40 percent had been sexually abused,[40] with both men and women affected.[41, 42] In many cases, the victims reported being sexually and physically abused as children by more than one person.[43, 44] In another report, 50 percent of the people with emotion dysregulation reported being sexually abused as children on a weekly basis for at least one year by a parent or a friend of the family.[45] In this same study, it was discovered that the severity of the sexual abuse and overall neglect was related to the severity of the emotion dysregulation. Similarly, in another study, the severity of the sexual abuse experienced was proportional to the victim's history of suicidal behavior.[46]

Yet, despite how devastating these abusive events can be to an individual, not everyone who experiences them will develop emotion dysregulation.[47] Another theory suggests that a person who develops emotion dysregulation is naturally defenseless against emotional reactions, and is unable to react in a healthy and helpful way to emotional experiences.[3] This vulnerability is then made worse when the person is placed in an abusive situation, like the ones just described. Similarly, if you grew up with an abusive parent who always criticized you and invalidated your emotions, it's not hard to imagine that you would grow up very confused and doubtful about your own emotional reactions.

WHAT CAN YOU DO ABOUT IT?

The treatment of emotion dysregulation most often involves a long-term commitment. On average, most people with emotion dysregulation go to at least six mental health professionals seeking the right person to help them.[48, 49] Many seek individual psychotherapy, group therapy, or family therapy, but in severe cases, hospitalization or inpatient care may be necessary.[4] Many types of treatments have been used to help people with this problem. Among them, psychodynamic therapy has been shown to be effective for some cases.[50, 51]

However, the treatment that has received the most validation for its effectiveness is dialectical behavior therapy,[3, 52-54] which was developed specifically to treat emotion dysregulation. This treatment has been shown to relieve symptoms of emotion dysregulation, decrease the tendency to commit suicide,[55, 56] and decrease the tendency to misuse drugs.[57, 58] This last factor is especially important, because in one study, the absence of an alcohol or drug problem was the best predictor of symptom reduction.[18] Dialectical behavior therapy balances the need for change with an acceptance and understanding of your current behavior.[3] The treatment aims to broaden your ability to be mindful of the present, while also decreasing your self-harming behaviors. Also it will teach you new skills to regulate your emotions, behaviors, and thoughts.

Many people with emotion dysregulation are also prescribed multiple medications.[59] For example, small studies of some antidepressants have demonstrated some benefits. Fluvoxamine (Luvox) can decrease quick mood changes,[60] while fluoxetine (Prozac) can decrease impulsive anger[61] and impulsive hostility.[62] Studies of antipsychotic medications, such as clozapine (Clozaril), risperidone (Risperdal), and olanzapine (Zyprexa), have also shown some benefits, including reduced hallucinations,[63] reduced self-harming behaviors,[64] reduced hostility and depression,[65] and an overall feeling of improvement,[66] especially when used in conjunction with dialectical behavior therapy.[67]

Similar small studies of the mood stabilizer valproic acid (Depakote),[68] the anticonvulsant topiramate (Topamax),[69] the anticonvulsant lamotrigine (Lamictal),[70] and omega-3 fatty acids[71] have also showed some evidence for reducing hostile behavior in people with emotion dysregulation.

Recommended treatments for emotion dysregulation include:

· Dialectical behavior therapy, see page 141

· Medications, see page 155

· Psychodynamic therapy, see page 167

EXTREME SUSPICION OF OTHERS/PARANOID PERSONALITY DISORDER

WHAT IS IT?

Someone with an *extreme suspicion of others* is very mistrustful of other people and their motives, even when there is little or no evidence to support the suspicion.[1] A person with this problem is also constantly on the lookout for being attacked, hurt, or tricked by other people.[2] Unfortunately, personality styles like this often create problems in a person's relationships, job, and other social interactions. As a result, personality styles like this are referred to as "personality disorders," and in many other references, this problem is referred to as "paranoid personality disorder." Most of us have had the experience of meeting someone we just don't trust. Maybe the person has done something to us in the past or maybe he or she acts in a "shifty" way. In these specific instances, our distrust is a normal defensive reaction to protect us from being hurt. However, someone with an extreme suspicion of others is highly mistrustful of most people almost all the time.

If you have an extreme suspicion of others, it's probably very hard for you to trust anyone, including your friends, family, and coworkers. It's also probably difficult for you to share details about your life with other people, due to the fear that they'll use that information to hurt you in some way. Maybe you suspect that your friends and family are talking about you behind your back or somehow making plans to humiliate you. People with this problem are always questioning the loyalty of others, and any deviation from 100 percent loyalty is interpreted as a betrayal. As a result, you've probably found yourself with few close friends, damaged family relationships, and few social interactions—additional problems that tend to make you feel worse.

People with this problem often hold grudges, are extremely jealous, are quickly angered if they think they've been insulted, and often try to control other people's lives.[1] If this way of viewing the world is maintained over a period of many years, and studies have shown that it often is,[3] it can become a major problem in your social and professional life.

ARE THERE OTHER RELATED PROBLEMS?

Many people with an extreme suspicion of others also suffer with other problems, such as drug and alcohol addictions,[4] depression, dysthymia, bipolar disorder, panic disorder, social phobia, specific phobia, and generalized anxiety disorder.[5-7]

WHO IS AFFECTED?

It's estimated that almost 2 to 6 percent of the general adult population, or approximately 9 million American adults, have an extreme suspicion of others,[8, 9] with women reporting the problem more frequently than men.[10] In general, almost

15 percent of all American adults, or almost 31 million people, struggle with personality disorders like this,[10] and these types of long-term problems are often the cause of general unhappiness and disability in a person's life.[9]

WHAT CAUSES IT?

Extreme suspicion of others is probably due to a combination of biological and social factors. One study has shown that, in general, personality disorders have a strong chance of being passed on in families, due to influential genetic factors that can be inherited.[11] However, an extreme suspicion of others appears to be less inheritable than other personality disorders. Some research points to a possible link between schizophrenia and an extreme suspicion of others. In one study, people who had an immediate family member with schizophrenia had a much greater risk of developing an extreme suspicion of others, possibly caused by inheritable genetic factors.[12] Other studies have shown that there is also some connection between childhood anxiety problems and the development of an extreme suspicion of others in adults.[13]

Studies of social factors also have found many potential causes for this problem. In one study, children who experienced severe verbal abuse from their parents were three times as likely to develop an extreme suspicion of others than were children who were not verbally abused.[14] Other traumatic childhood events have also been linked to the problem.[15] Sadly, an extreme suspicion of others has been highly linked to childhood histories of sexual, physical, and emotional abuse.[16] From these examples, it's easy to understand how you might have become very distrustful of other people if you were severely abused as a child.

Other studies show that many of those affected by personality disorders like this one are also single, young adults, minorities, unemployed, poor, lack family and social support, live in cities, and experience more everyday problems than the general population.[8-10] Needless to say, some of these characteristics suggest that poor, inner-city minorities are at a greater risk for developing personality disorders than are white Americans living in the suburbs. In some studies, African-Americans and Native Americans have reported more extreme suspicion of others than white Americans have.[10, 17, 18] But considering that many inner-city minorities also have been the targets of racial discrimination and hostility, it might be expected that some of the people in this group would naturally behave in a way that is more suspicious of others.[19]

WHAT CAN YOU DO ABOUT IT?

Unfortunately, many people with this problem don't want to seek treatment.[20] However, some of them do seek help for other problems, such as depression.[21] As a result, there's little research to refer to in order to find out which treatment is most effective for an extreme suspicion of others.[22] Some researchers have suggested that the best treatment would be a long-term therapy that helps an individual learn how to accurately interpret the potential threat from other people.[22, 23] Other researchers have found some success using antidepressant medications, such as fluoxetine (Prozac).[6]

Despite the lack of research, many of the psychotherapies found in this reference have been shown to be effective treatments for other personality disorders, and possibly would be effective for this problem, too. Some of these treatments include psychodynamic therapy, interpersonal therapy, dialectical behavior therapy, and cognitive behavioral therapies.[24-28] These treatments will help you gain insight into the nature of the problem, develop coping skills for handling stress, and develop relationship skills to build healthier connections with other people.

Recommended treatments for extreme suspicion of others include:

. Psychodynamic therapy, see page 167

. Interpersonal therapy, see page 153

. Dialectical behavior therapy, see page 141

. Cognitive behavioral therapy, see page 136

. Antidepressant medications, see page 155

GENERALIZED ANXIETY DISORDER

WHAT IS IT?

Generalized anxiety disorder (GAD) is a disorder characterized by an excessive number of unmanageable worries that don't go away by themselves and last for a minimum of six months.[1] The concerns that cause the anxiety are usually very numerous and broad in scope, which is why the problem is referred to as "generalized."

The thoughts that cause the worrying aren't usually life-threatening. If you were in immediate danger, your emotional and physical reactions would more accurately be described as fear. Fear and anxiety are related emotions, but anxiety more precisely describes a situation where the cause of concern isn't imminent. Everyone experiences normal, temporary periods of anxiety in life, such as worrying about an upcoming test. However, a person with GAD worries excessively almost every day and, typically, the worrisome thoughts jump from one cause of concern to the next, making them uncontrollable, time-consuming, and very distracting.[1] Overall, GAD is a an intolerable and painful disorder.[2]

If you're struggling with GAD, you have numerous troubling thoughts that you can't control throughout the day. The causes of concern might not even be related to one another. Maybe you worry that someone you know is in danger, about your future career, or about some task that you're trying to complete at work. In these cases, you're probably afraid that you won't be able to cope with some future event if the worst outcome should occur.[3] But as these worries accumulate, you also begin to think of the world as a very unsafe and unpredictable place.[4, 5] For most people with GAD, this inability to predict what will happen in life is very disturbing.[6, 7]

In some instances, you might recognize that your worries are excessive and go beyond what might realistically happen. For example, perhaps you worry that someone you know is going to be hurt in a boating accident, but that person doesn't even own a boat. On the other hand, maybe you think that none of your thoughts is beyond the scope of what might realistically happen, but you do recognize that you can't stop these thoughts, and they're constantly bothering you. These are both forms of GAD. Most likely, you also find it very hard to focus on tasks, especially tasks that require a lot of concentration. Moreover, you probably suffer from frequent muscle aches, tension, and difficulties sleeping, as well as a general feeling of being uneasy most of the time.[8]

ARE THERE OTHER RELATED PROBLEMS?

GAD is often associated with many other problems.[9] Some surveys have shown that GAD is equally as burdensome as depression[10] and, unfortunately, many people suffer with both GAD and depression.[2] Many people with GAD also struggle from drug and alcohol problems,[11, 12] specific phobias, social phobias, post-traumatic stress disorder, dysthymia, bipolar disorder, attention-deficit/hyperactivity disorder, and dependent personality problems.[13-15] Physical illnesses related to stress are also common, such as chest pain,[16] irritable bowel syndrome, frequent headaches,[17, 18] diabetes, and cardiovascular disease.[19, 20]

WHO IS AFFECTED?

A survey of over 9,000 adults in the United States estimated that 6 percent of them would develop GAD at some point in their lives.[21] Other estimates suggest that in any given year, 3 percent of all adults in the United States are suffering with GAD,[13, 22] with women reporting the illness twice as frequently as men.[22] By far, GAD and the other anxiety disorders (including phobias, panic disorder, obsessive-compulsive disorder, and post-traumatic stress disorder) are the most common mental health problems in the United States.[13, 21] Other studies have suggested that over the course of a person's lifetime, the odds of developing GAD are approximately 1 in 20.[9] Many people with GAD report that they've been suffering with the illness since they were children,[23] but other estimates suggest that GAD often begins during adulthood,[21] especially when stressful events are experienced.[24]

WHAT CAUSES IT?

Although the exact cause of GAD is unknown, it's believed that the development of the disorder is influenced by biological, psychological, and social factors. Studies of family members indicate that the odds of inheriting GAD from a parent with the illness are almost one in three.[25, 26] Other research suggests that some people with GAD are born with a natural vulnerability to the illness that makes them more easily irritated and prone to muscle tension, restlessness, sleep problems,[27] and bodily discomfort.[28]

Some researchers believe that the act of excessive worrying may actually help you avoid feeling sad emotions, as well as help you avoid thinking about images of future negative events.[29, 30] Nonetheless, despite these temporary benefits, this excessive worrying can become overwhelming and lead you to become afraid of your own emotions, which can then lead to avoiding certain negative experiences.[31] Complicating the situation even more, some evidence suggests that people with GAD pay more attention to the negative emotional stimuli in their lives, such as threatening words and angry faces, than they pay to positive stimuli, even when they aren't aware that they're doing it.[32]

Studies of environmental and psychological factors suggest that childhood experiences can also make a person vulnerable to developing GAD. These early, influential experiences include trauma, abuse, or unstable and insecure relationships with parents.[30, 33] And of course, these same types of stressful events can cause GAD later in adulthood.

The development of GAD is also often associated with poverty and minority status. For example, in 1991, it was estimated that the rates of GAD were twice as high among people whose yearly income was below $10,000, when compared to people with incomes above that amount.[34] Furthermore, when women under thirty years old were compared, African-American women were almost twice as likely as white Americans to develop GAD, as were Hispanic-American women between the ages of forty-five and sixty-four when compared with white American women of the same age.[35]

WHAT CAN YOU DO ABOUT IT?

Unfortunately, many people with GAD don't seek treatment when they're first affected by the disorder, and often wait as long as nine years before doing so.[36] This is regrettable, especially when considering that there are many effective treatments for GAD.

Cognitive behavioral therapy for GAD has received much research support. In some treatment studies, cognitive behavioral therapy was helpful to approximately 50 percent of the participants.[37, 38] This treatment for GAD will help you to relax, assess the potential risks of your fears, and then safely help you confront those fears.[39, 40] Sometimes, even the relaxation techniques alone can lead to a significant reduction of GAD symptoms.[41]

Personal reports of patients also suggest that treatments such as psychodynamic therapy, control mastery therapy, interpersonal therapy, humanistic therapy, and many of the other forms of therapy outlined in this resource can be very effective. However, there has been little research done on these treatments for GAD.

Anti-anxiety medications such as alprazolam (Xanax), diazepam (Valium), lorazepam (Ativan), and buspirone (BuSpar) have all been shown to be effective, short-term treatments for GAD.[42] However, some of these medications can lead to dependence, as well as withdrawal symptoms if they're abruptly discontinued after long-term use. So, if you are prescribed any of these medications, it's very important that you follow the dosage recommendations of your medical professional. Some antidepressant medications, such as escitalopram (Lexapro), paroxetine (Paxil), sertraline (Zoloft), and venlafaxine (Effexor), have also been shown to be effective treatments, especially to relieve accompanying depressive symptoms.[43]

Recommended treatments for generalized anxiety disorder include:

· Cognitive behavioral therapy, see page 136

· Anti-anxiety and antidepressant medications, see page 155

GENERALIZED
ANXIETY DISORDER

IMPULSE CONTROL DISORDERS

WHAT ARE THEY?

If you have an *impulse control disorder*, you can't avoid doing something that might bring harm to yourself or others.[1] Typically, a person with this problem feels some type of increasing anxiety before committing the action, like pressure building up. Then, after the action, the person feels relief or even happiness, despite the possibly dangerous consequences. Among the officially recognized impulse control disorders are pathological gambling, kleptomania, pyromania, trichotillomania, and intermittent explosive disorder.[1] However, more recently, some researchers have suggested that other problems such as Internet addiction[2] and computer game addiction[3] share similar traits to the other impulse control disorders. In general, all of these problems have an extremely negative influence on your life,[4-7] as well as on the lives of the people around you.

Pathological gambling is repeated betting behavior that interferes with your finances, job, family life, or other relationships. If you're a pathological gambler, your betting activities greatly disrupt your life and the lives of the people around you. Your family relationships are frequently interrupted and maybe even ended.[8] You might also have lost your job because you missed too many days at work, or, perhaps you had to sell your car or house to pay off your gambling debts. Many pathological gamblers are constantly looking for a "system" to make back the money they've lost, and often, this leads to losing even more money.

As with some of the other impulse control disorders, many pathological gamblers will often hide their actions from their friends and family; however, in desperate financial times, these pathological gamblers often will go to those same people to borrow money to continue their gambling.[1]

If you have *kleptomania*, you steal things that are of no financial or personal value. Many thefts by kleptomaniacs are unplanned,[9] and the items stolen are sometimes put away without ever being used, while other items are given away, thrown away, or even returned.[10] If you have kleptomania, it's very likely that your thefts have become rituals you perform when you get anxious.[10] However, it's also possible that you have strong random urges to steal that only seem to go away after you perform the act.[11] Immediately following your theft, you might feel better or even pleasantly excited. But later on, it's very possible that you start to feel guilty about what you've done, or you see your actions as senseless and harmful to yourself and others.[10]

Pyromania is the repeated act of deliberately setting fires, usually at random locations,[5] after which you feel relieved or excited. The motive for setting these fires doesn't have to be to harm someone, but that harm is often the result of your actions.[12] By definition, the motive for setting a fire when suffering from pyromania is not for personal gain, such as collecting insurance money. If you have pyromania, you're probably very interested in all aspects of fire. Maybe you're interested in how fires start, what fires do, and how fires are stopped.[1] Perhaps you're even interested in the fire department. Some people with pyromania even scan the fire department's radio for calls, so they can go to the scene and watch the fire get extinguished.

A person with *trichotillomania* experiences a release of tension or satisfaction by pulling out his or her hair. Many people with trichotillomania pull out the hair from their heads, eyelashes, eyebrows, legs, arms, faces, and pubic region.[13] If you have trichotillomania, you've probably pulled out enough strands of hair to notice an area of hair loss on your head or on another part of your body. This noticeable balding probably causes you much discomfort, especially when you're in social situations where it can be noticed. As a result, you probably go to great lengths to hide your loss of hair, either by wearing hats and wigs, long-sleeve shirts, or covering the bald area with makeup.[14]

You may not even be aware that you're pulling out your hair. Many people with trichotillomania say that they feel bored or nervous before pulling out their hair, but after pulling it out, they feel guilty, sad, or angry.[13] Some of the same people also report that they pull out their hair when they're watching television, reading, talking on the telephone, and driving.[13]

Lastly, a person with *intermittent explosive disorder* will suddenly and unexpectedly lash out at other people in a very hostile way. By definition, the result of these aggressive behaviors is injury to other people or damage to their property.[1] The actions of people with intermittent explosive disorder are much bigger and more aggressive than what the situation requires. If you have intermittent explosive disorder, you probably feel very angry, energized, and nervous when you lash out, and then feel depleted of strength, relieved, embarrassed, and maybe even depressed when the event is over.[1, 15]

ARE THERE OTHER RELATED PROBLEMS?

People with impulse control disorders often suffer from many other problems. Among the issues reported with pathological gambling are suicide and suicide attempts,[16, 17] alcohol and drug problems, nicotine addiction, depression, bipolar disorder, obsessive-compulsive disorder, phobias, antisocial personality problems, and an extreme suspicion of others.[18, 19] People with kleptomania, intermittent explosive disorder, or trichotillomania often experience many of the same problems, plus additional problems. People with kleptomania commonly experience panic disorder, bulimia,[11, 20, 21] and being arrested.[22] Likewise, people with intermittent explosive disorder also commonly experience post-traumatic stress disorder, social phobia, and bulimia.[15, 23] Trichotillomania and obsessive-compulsive disorder are often experienced together.[24] In fact, trichotillomania is sometimes thought to be a form of obsessive-compulsive disorder.[25] Unfortunately, the research on pyromania is completely lacking.

WHO IS AFFECTED?

Most of the impulse control disorders are believed to be uncommon problems.[1] Pathological gambling is thought to affect 1 to 3 percent of the general population.[26, 27] Kleptomania is estimated to affect less than 1 percent of the general population.[28, 29] Trichotillomania is estimated to affect 1 to 4 percent of the general population.[30, 31] Estimates of intermittent explosive disorder have ranged from approximately 4 to 5 percent of the general population.[32, 33] And again, the research on pyromania is scarce and gives little estimate of the problem's prevalence.

WHAT CAUSES IT?

Although the exact cause of impulse control disorders is unknown, it's believed that the development of these problems is influenced by both biological and social risk factors.[14, 20, 34, 35] For people with pathological gambling and intermittent explosive disorder, defects have been found in the way the brain processes chemicals called *neurotransmitters*.[36, 37] Other research suggests that some problems might be at least partly explained by genetic factors that can be inherited.[38-40] Disruptive and violent childhood experiences have also been linked to the development of some of these problems.[41-45] Plus, some researchers believe that problems such as trichotillomania can be learned.[31] They assert that a person continues to pull out hair because this action temporarily relieves his or her tension, and so, naturally, the action is repeated.

WHAT CAN YOU DO ABOUT IT?

The research on treatments for impulse control disorders has largely focused on the use of cognitive behavioral therapy and medications. Cognitive behavioral therapy can help you relax, cope with stress, combat negative thoughts, and prevent damaging behaviors. In small studies, this type of treatment has been shown to be effective for kleptomania,[46, 47] pathological gambling,[48] and trichotillomania.[49, 50] Although no studies have yet investigated psychotherapeutic treatments for intermittent explosive disorder, cognitive behavioral therapy is often an effective treatment for general anger issues.[51] There's little research to suggest which treatment is best for pyromania, although one study helped children stop setting fires by getting them to chart the relationship between their feelings, stress levels, and actions.[52] Twelve-step programs such as Gamblers Anonymous can also be effective for providing support to someone who is trying to control gambling behaviors.[53]

Antidepressants, such as fluoxetine (Prozac), fluvoxamine (Luvox), sertraline (Zoloft), and venlafaxine (Effexor), have often been used to treat trichotillomania,[54] kleptomania,[22, 55, 56] intermittent explosive disorder,[57] and pathological gambling.[58] The antipsychotic medication olanzapine (Zyprexa) has also shown some effectiveness at treating trichotillomania.[59, 60]

Recommended treatments for impulse control disorders in general include:

. Cognitive behavioral therapy, see page 136

. Medications, see page 155

. Support groups, such as Gamblers Anonymous

OBSESSIVE-COMPULSIVE DISORDER

WHAT IS IT?

Obsessive-compulsive disorder (OCD) is characterized by uncontrollable, disturbing thoughts and urges called *obsessions*, which make you feel extremely anxious.[1] Then, in response to these obsessions, repetitious behaviors called *compulsions* are performed, which temporarily relieve your anxiety. However, the obsessions soon return and the compulsions are repeated. As the disorder intensifies, this repetitious cycle becomes very disturbing,[2] time-consuming, and it often leads to job interference, relationship difficulties, and the avoidance of feared situations.

There are a number of common obsessions. Among the most frequently reported is the fear of contamination by germs, dirt, chemicals, or diseases.[3] If you have this obsession, you're probably overwhelmed with thoughts about harming yourself or others, through contact with some type of surface, dirt, or bacteria. In response to this, you probably perform many compulsions, such as frequently washing your hands, changing your clothes, and avoiding dirty objects like doorknobs, shoes, and newspapers.

Repetitious uncertainty is another common obsession. This can include doubts about whether or not you turned off your stove, made a mistake in your work, or hit someone while you were driving. This type of obsession is extremely time-consuming because the compulsions that follow include checking and rechecking your actions. Typically, these compulsions include returning home to make sure you turned off your oven, or turning your car around to make sure you really didn't hit someone.

Obsessions of perfection are thoughts that require you to arrange objects perfectly or to perform tasks in a rigid systematic fashion. Often, people with this compulsion can't complete a task if they can't perform every step of that task in sequential order.

Obsessions about causing harm to others lead you to think about hurting other people, including strangers. This type of obsession may cause you to perform *reassurance behaviors*, in order to make sure that other people are safe.

Sexual obsessions often involve intrusive pornographic thoughts. This type of disturbing imagery may cause you to play mental games to distract yourself, like counting or drawing pictures in your imagination. Or, perhaps these thoughts lead you to pray in order to relieve yourself of guilty feelings.

Religious obsessions tend to focus on the fear that you're not doing what is morally right and the thought that you're going to be punished by God. Religious obsessions can also include uncontrollable, blasphemous thoughts in which you curse God. In these cases, you also might perform a praying ritual, or maybe you draw some type of religious imagery in a notebook.

Other obsessions include urges to do things that might seem aggressive or very much out of the ordinary, like screaming at your boss. Afterwards, you probably feel compelled to do something to relieve yourself of guilty feelings.

These are just a few examples of different types of obsessions. In all of these cases, the worries are highly unusual. They are not obsessional worries about common, daily occurrences, like paying the bills or getting to work on time. For each one of these obsessions, there are numerous types of compulsions, not just the ones listed here. In fact, your obsessions and compulsions may not even be related to each other in any realistic way. You may do anything after the intrusive thought to relieve yourself of anxiety. For example, a woman with a fear of contamination might obtain just as much relief from singing a song each time she feels dirty as she does from washing her hands. The point is that the obsession and the action that follows become habitual, time-consuming, and disturbing to you.

ARE THERE OTHER RELATED PROBLEMS?

Many people with OCD also suffer with other related problems, such as depression,[4] body dysmorphic disorder,[5, 6] bipolar disorder,[7, 8] phobias, panic disorder,[9] alcohol problems, post-traumatic stress disorder,[10] emotion dysregulation,[11, 12] anorexia,[13] depersonalization disorder,[14] and trichotillomania.[15, 16]

Another problem that is related to OCD is called *obsessive-compulsive personality disorder*.[1] Officially, this is considered a separate diagnosis but, in reality, it's a very similar problem. A person with an obsessive-compulsive personality disorder also has rigid, internal demands for organization and precision, but these demands are usually much more widely spread throughout the person's entire life. Someone with this problem may not appear as outwardly anxious as a person with OCD, but the person with the personality disorder still can't complete a task, unless following an internal set of rules.

People with this personality disorder are often described as collectors who never throw anything away or as misers who live in poverty while they hide their money away for emergencies.

WHO IS AFFECTED?

A 1996 global study of disease found that OCD was the tenth leading cause of disability in the world among both physical and mental illnesses; plus, it's the fourth most disabling mental health problem in the developed world.[17] It's estimated that almost 2 to 3 percent[4, 18] of adults in the United States suffer from OCD at some point in their lives. By some estimates, that's approximately 3 million adults in the United States alone.[19] In adults, OCD is equally common in men and women.[1] However, research has shown that OCD begins earlier in males than in females. Typically, males develop OCD between the ages of six and fifteen, while females develop it later, between the ages of twenty and twenty-nine.[1]

WHAT CAUSES IT?

It's estimated that 85 to 90 percent of all ordinary people experience intrusive thoughts and desires similar to the ones experienced by people with OCD.[20] So, what allows one person to ignore the obsessive thoughts while another person develops ritualized compulsions in response to them? Although the exact cause of OCD is unknown, the disorder is believed to have both biological and social risk factors. Research has shown that the chances of developing OCD are greater if someone in your family has it.[1] The development of OCD can also be triggered by medical conditions, such as head injuries[21] and epilepsy,[22] as well as by the birth of a child, which can make both the mother and the father vulnerable to the disorder.[23] Researchers have also observed physical differences in the brains of people with OCD. The areas affected are associated with emotional memories,[24] voluntary movement,[25] motivation,[26] and learning.[27, 28]

A group of OCD treatment experts concluded that people with OCD possess six unique qualities that might contribute to the development of the disorder.[29] These traits include: (1) the tendency to overestimate the danger of a situation, (2) the inability to tolerate uncertainty, (3) the belief that thoughts are controllable, (4) the belief that every thought is important, (5) the belief that perfection is both attainable and necessary, and (6) the belief that the person has the power to create or prevent dangerous outcomes.

In combination with these characteristics, one developmental theory points to the fact that OCD behaviors are largely learned over time. This behavioral model highlights the understanding that compulsions remove the person's anxiety quickly, but only for a short amount of time.[30] This temporary solution prevents you from learning to tolerate the discomfort of your anxiety, and it conditions you to use the compulsion each time you feel discomfort. Interestingly, other related research has shed light on one of the reasons why it's so hard to control unwanted thoughts. This research has demonstrated that the harder you try not to think about something, the more you actually think about whatever it is that you're trying to forget.[31]

WHAT CAN YOU DO ABOUT IT?

Almost 1.5 million people seek treatment for OCD in the United States alone.[32] However, some people wait as long as seven years before doing so.[9] This is very unfortunate, considering that there's a very effective treatment for OCD. The "gold standard"[33] of treatment for OCD is a form of cognitive behavioral therapy called *exposure and response prevention* or *exposure and ritual prevention*. This treatment safely and systematically exposes you to the feared circumstances and then helps you refrain from performing your compulsions, resulting in an anxiety level that decreases naturally over time.

Researchers have found that this form of therapy can result in an 80 percent success rate in the treatment of OCD,[34, 35] a treatment that's often more successful than the use of medications.[35] Amazingly, the research also suggests that exposure and response prevention causes the same beneficial changes in brain chemistry that have been observed when patients used pharmaceutical treatments.[36-38] Often, it's beneficial to include your family members in the exposure and response prevention treatment sessions, so that they can help you to overcome the disorder.[39]

Antidepressants are often the first medications chosen to treat OCD and they can be used successfully in conjunction with cognitive behavioral therapy.[40-42] Frequently used medications for OCD include clomipramine (Anafranil), fluvoxamine (Luvox), fluoxetine (Prozac), paroxetine (Paxil), sertraline (Zoloft), and citalopram (Celexa).[43] In severe cases, when a person fails to respond to either cognitive behavioral therapy or medication, brain surgery is sometimes a successful option.[44, 45] A procedure called a *cingulotomy* makes a microscopic cut in the part of the brain that's suspected of being involved with OCD. One study, which assessed the success of cingulotomy procedures, found that 32 to 45 percent of the patients showed long-term improvements.[46]

Recommended treatments for obsessive-compulsive disorder include:

· Cognitive behavioral therapy, see page 136

· Antidepressant medications, see page 155

· Surgery

PANIC DISORDER

WHAT IS IT?

Panic disorder is a problem characterized by extremely powerful feelings of fear that quickly overwhelm you.[1] Most often, a panic attack will intensify over a ten- to fifteen-minute period and will usually end within thirty minutes.[2] These very frightening experiences are called *panic attacks* and many people will have one in their life, due to fear or stress. Other people with anxiety problems, such as generalized anxiety disorder and social phobia, will also experience panic attacks when they're forced to do something that they're afraid of, like speaking in public, driving in traffic, or shopping in a crowded store.

However, if you have panic disorder, you experience multiple, unexpected panic attacks that seem to come out of nowhere. You also worry about the possibility of the attacks reoccurring and will often change your behavior to try to prevent the attacks.[1] In severe cases of panic disorder, you might not leave your home due to a fear of being stranded somewhere while having a panic attack. This additional problem is called *agoraphobia.*

Severe physical symptoms accompany panic attacks, such as intense heart-pounding, an inability to move, a feeling of being separated from reality, dizziness, stomach sickness, numbing of the senses, tightening in the throat, an inability to breathe, hot and cold sensations, excessive perspiration, and shaking.[1] Many people who experience panic attacks think that they're having a heart attack, going insane, or dying.[1] In fact, many people who experience panic attacks first seek treatment at hospital emergency rooms[3] or from their general medical provider.[4]

Although it's often the case that many people who have panic attacks mistake their problems for medical conditions,[5, 6] it's always necessary to have a medical examination to identify any real physiological problems. Some medical conditions can cause symptoms that are very similar to panic attacks. One of these conditions is thyroid disease; another is *mitral valve prolapse*, which is a common heart condition that can cause chest pains and palpitations similar to those experienced during panic attacks.[7, 8]

If you're suffering with panic disorder, you may experience panic attacks quite frequently or they may occur irregularly. Perhaps your last one was many months ago. Either way, you're probably very frightened of having another one, and this fear limits your ability to live the way you want to live. Maybe you no longer travel for vacations or shop at your favorite store because you're afraid of having a panic attack in front of other people. Your fear can also cause you to miss time at work or interfere with your relationships. If your panic disorder is severe, perhaps you've confined yourself to your home. Most people with agoraphobia are afraid of having a panic attack in a social situation that they can't escape or in an unfamiliar place where they can't find help.[9]

ARE THERE OTHER RELATED PROBLEMS?

Many people with panic disorder also suffer with other related problems, such as drug and alcohol problems,[10] specific and social phobias, generalized anxiety disorder, post-traumatic stress disorder, depression, dysthymia, bipolar disorder, attention-deficit/hyperactivity disorder, and intermittent explosive disorder.[11] Panic disorder is also common for people suffering with many of the personality disorders mentioned in this book, including an extreme suspicion of others, dependent personality, obsessive-compulsive personality, antisocial personality, and schizoid personality.[12]

WHO IS AFFECTED?

A 1996 global study of disease found that panic disorder was the fifth most disabling mental health problem in the developed world.[13] It's estimated that almost 1 to 2 percent of the general population will suffer with panic disorder in any given year,[10, 14] and as many as approximately 5 percent of the population will experience panic disorder at some point in their lives.[14, 15] By some estimates, approximately 2 million adults in the United States suffer with panic disorder each year.[16] Most often, panic disorder develops in the teenage or early adult years.[1] One-third to one-half of the people with panic disorder will also develop agoraphobia, usually within the first year of experiencing recurrent, untreated panic attacks.[1]

However, not everyone who has panic attacks will develop panic disorder. It's been estimated that 3 to 5 percent of the general population have panic attacks every year without worrying about the recurrence of the attacks and without changing their behaviors.[17]

WHAT CAUSES IT?

The exact cause of a panic attack is unknown. However, it's believed to have both biological and social risk factors. Your body's reaction during a panic attack is the same reaction it's designed to have during an encounter with any sign of danger. This reaction is called the *fight-or-flight response*. In the face of immediate threat, the human body is designed to automatically prepare itself to fight the danger or to run away from it. During the fight-or-flight response, the body becomes physically prepared to react to danger. The adrenal glands release increased amounts of adrenaline, which increases your heart rate, blood pressure, and energy level. This is the same thing that happens to the body during a panic attack. Normally, this adrenaline surge will last only two to three minutes.[18] However, during a panic attack, further worry and anxiety can cause your adrenal glands to initiate another surge of adrenaline, creating a longer-lasting sense of fear and panic.

The research on panic disorder suggests that most people remember experiencing some type of stress during their first panic attack.[19] In response to this initial attack, you might begin to closely monitor your body for signs of a second panic attack. This constant monitoring develops into a heightened awareness and sensitivity to even minor body sensations, especially changes in heartbeat.[20, 21] When this occurs, a slight fluctuation in heartbeat can be enough to trigger another panic attack.[22] Then, if you also have a real problem with your heart, such as mitral valve prolapse, or you consume even modest amounts of caffeine (which can cause symptoms of anxiety), a second panic attack is even more likely.

Excluding genuine medical problems, like mitral valve prolapse, the usual cause of recurring panic attacks is the fear of having another panic attack, along with the mistaken assumption that you're going to die during that attack.[22] Add to this problem the fact that most panic attacks take place outside the home, and it's easy to see why many people with panic disorder eventually develop agoraphobia and stay indoors.[23]

WHAT CAN YOU DO ABOUT IT?

Over 1 million people are treated for panic disorder each year in the United States.[24] Sadly, many people wait as long as ten years before seeking treatment for this illness.[25] This is unfortunate, considering that cognitive behavioral therapy is a very effective treatment for panic disorder with or without agoraphobia. In one study, cognitive behavioral treatment for panic disorder helped 85 percent of the patients become panic-free,[26, 27] and two years later 81 percent of them were still panic-free,[28] all without using medication.

The cognitive behavioral treatment for panic disorder focuses on four main areas: breathing skills to resist hyperventilation, thinking skills to develop coping statements, safe and systematic exposure to panic-inducing symptoms, and exposure to feared events.[29]

However, despite the successes of cognitive behavioral therapy, most patients are initially prescribed medications for their panic attacks[22] because they first seek treatment from their medical doctors.[4] Antidepressant medications such as fluoxetine (Prozac), fluvoxamine (Luvox), and sertraline (Zoloft) are usually the initial medications prescribed;[30] however, faster acting anti-anxiety medications such as diazepam (Valium) and alprazolam (Xanax) are also used.

These medications can all be effective for the short-term treatment of panic attacks. However, in long-term treatment studies, the use of cognitive behavioral therapy was superior to the use of medications and provided more benefits,[31, 32] including lower relapse rates.[22] In fact, unless it is immediately necessary, anti-anxiety and antidepressant medications are not recommended for the treatment of panic attacks. A patient on medications will rely on them for relief instead of relying on the skills developed in cognitive behavioral therapy.

Recommended treatments for panic disorder include:

· Cognitive behavioral therapy, see page 136

· Antidepressant and anti-anxiety medications if necessary, see page 155

PHOBIA

WHAT IS IT?

There are two different kinds of phobias, specific phobia and social phobia (also known as social anxiety disorder).[1] A *specific phobia* is an intense fear of something identifiable, like an object, animal, situation, or place. This fear is much different and more intense than normal worrying, and if you have a specific phobia, you will usually recognize that your fear is excessive.[1] For example, many people are afraid of animals, such as snakes or dogs, and they do their best to avoid them in everyday life. However, a person with a specific phobia of snakes becomes extremely anxious when other people even talk about snakes or when looking at pictures of snakes. This quick feeling of terror can overwhelm you and leave you feeling paralyzed. It's also likely that you experience a panic attack when this type of fear occurs.[1]

Your specific phobia also causes you to avoid the feared situation or object, no matter how extreme that avoidance might be. For example, a person with an elevator phobia will walk up twelve flights of stairs instead of using an elevator. In cases where an object or event can't be avoided, someone with a specific phobia will endure the situation with extreme agitation or anxiety. For example, one patient was known to have a phobia of bridges, but he could not avoid crossing a river every day to get to work. In order to cope with the situation, he would climb into the trunk of a coworker's car twice a day, five days a week, before crossing the bridge to and from his job.

Among the more commonly feared objects and situations are animals and insects, water, heights, blood, injections, elevators, driving, flying, bridges, telephones, and illness.[1]

If you're struggling with a specific phobia, you probably go to great extremes to avoid encountering your feared situation. Maybe you drive miles out of your way to avoid going through a tunnel or perhaps you don't take vacations with your family to avoid flying.

However, it's not possible to avoid your feared situation all the time. So, if you know ahead of time that you'll be encountering a feared situation, you probably worry about it for days before the event takes place. Then, when you do encounter the situation, you're quickly overwhelmed with a feeling of fear, and maybe you experience a panic attack, during which you feel as if you are also going to die. These feelings come on very quickly and they are overpowering. Most likely, you recognize that other people don't react to the situation the way you do, and maybe you can admit that your reaction is too extreme. Yet, you still feel completely helpless and very afraid when confronted with the situation.

The second type of phobia is *social phobia*, or social anxiety disorder. Social phobia is an extreme fear of being in social situations. These situations can include specific situations, like speaking or performing in front of people, or they can be more generalized, like interacting with people and meeting new ones. This debilitating fear can prevent you from forming and maintaining friendships and romantic relationships; furthermore, it can interfere with your career. One problem related to social phobia is *avoidant personality disorder*.[1] Officially, avoidant personality disorder is considered a separate problem. However, in reality, it's the same fear of social interactions defined in a different way.

If you're suffering with social phobia, you might be extremely nervous for days or weeks in anticipation of a feared occasion. This fear of social interaction is much more severe than just normal nervousness; it's excessive. In order to prevent this excessive fear, maybe you try to avoid all social situations, or, if that's impossible, maybe you endure the situations with great anxiety. Most people with social phobia are afraid that they'll be publicly humiliated or embarrassed in the social situation. Perhaps you're afraid that others will see you're nervous or sweating, or that they'll judge you as stupid or crazy. Or, maybe you're afraid of fainting or losing control of your bodily functions.[2]

ARE THERE OTHER RELATED PROBLEMS?

Many people with specific and social phobias also suffer with other problems such as generalized anxiety disorder, post-traumatic stress disorder, depression, dysthymia, bipolar disorder, obsessive-compulsive disorder, attention-deficit/hyperactivity disorder, intermittent explosive disorder, and drug and/or alcohol problems.[3, 4] Sometimes, people with social phobias will use alcohol to ease their anxieties and "loosen up" around other people. However, this often leads to the development of an alcohol problem on top of the social phobia.[5] Also, people with both types of phobias sometimes suffer from one of the personality disorders discussed in this book, such as an extreme suspicion of others, dependent personality, obsessive-compulsive personality, schizoid personality, or antisocial personality.[6]

WHO IS AFFECTED?

Specific and social phobias are two of the most common mental health problems in the United States.[4, 7] Every year, approximately 7 to 9 percent of the adult general population suffer with a specific phobia,[3, 4, 8, 9] and over the course of their lifetimes, approximately 11 to 13 percent will be affected by one.[9, 10] Similarly, every year, approximately 3 to 8 percent of the adult general population will suffer with social phobia,[3, 4, 9] and over the course of their lifetimes, approximately 12 to 13 percent will be affected.[9, 10] Women are almost twice as likely to struggle with a specific phobia, but the sexes are equally afflicted by social phobia.[9] Typically, both disorders begin in childhood, although specific phobias can also start in a person's midtwenties.[2]

WHAT CAUSES IT?

There are many possible causes of specific phobia.[11] One theory links specific phobias to traumas in a person's life. For example, people with driving phobias often have a history of bad car accidents, and some people with dog phobias have been attacked. However, it's also possible that someone can develop a specific phobia after witnessing something tragic happening to someone else. Another theory holds that parents with phobias unknowingly teach their fearful reactions to their children—who then imitate their parent's actions.

Social phobia can also be caused by many of the same mechanisms just described. It's also thought to develop from childhood shyness and social discomfort that persists into adulthood and becomes worse with aging.[12]

WHAT CAN YOU DO ABOUT IT?

Without treatment, phobias rarely go away by themselves.[2] Most people who aren't in treatment simply do their best to avoid their feared circumstance or object. In one study, people waited, on average, as long as twenty years before seeking treatment for their specific phobia and sixteen years before seeking treatment for social phobia.[13] This is very unfortunate, considering that cognitive behavioral therapy is a very successful treatment for both types of phobia.[14]

In studies of cognitive behavioral therapy for specific phobia, the effectiveness has been as high as 80 percent.[15] Cognitive behavioral therapy for specific phobia begins by teaching breathing and relaxation exercises to help you manage your anxiety level, and then proceeds progressively to expose you to the feared situation in a safe and systematic way.[11] Rarely does this treatment require the use of medication. For social phobia, there are two effective cognitive behavioral treatment models.[14] The first treatment helps you build social skills, such as conversational abilities and body language, through role-playing. The second form of treatment takes place in a group therapy environment, where participants help each other and provide feedback on their social interactions.[16]

Generally, people with both types of phobia initially seek treatment from their primary care physician.[17] In many of these cases, it can be expected that they'll be prescribed medication. Currently, there are no known medications that effectively treat specific phobias, but among the medications that have demonstrated effectiveness for treating social phobia are the antidepressant medications phenelzine (Nardil), fluvoxamine (Luvox), sertraline (Zoloft), and paroxetine (Paxil) as well as the anti-anxiety medication clonazepam (Klonopin).[18] Some people will find relief from taking these medications for their social phobia. However, the negative aspect is that the person's relief then becomes dependent on the continual usage of the medication.

Recommended treatments for specific and social phobia include:

- Cognitive behavioral therapy, see page 136

- Antidepressant and anti-anxiety medications for social phobia, see page 155

POST-TRAUMATIC STRESS DISORDER

WHAT IS IT?

Post-traumatic stress disorder (PTSD) is a problem that occurs after you experience a life-threatening event that makes you feel extremely frightened and vulnerable.[1] Such events can include war, crime, rape, abuse, accidents, natural disasters like floods and earthquakes, and other potentially deadly and dangerous circumstances. But, the traumatic event doesn't have to happen to you directly for you to develop PTSD. You might develop the disorder after witnessing someone else have their life threatened, or even after hearing about someone else's tragedy. Usually, symptoms of PTSD begin within three months of experiencing the trauma. However, it isn't unusual to experience a delay of several months or even years before the symptoms begin.[1]

The major symptoms of PTSD can be divided into three categories.[1] First, the traumatic event is re-experienced in some way, even after it has ended. This could mean that you have vivid and frightening dreams about the event, weeks or months after the event has taken place. Or, maybe throughout the day you experience intrusive thoughts and memories about the event that you can't get rid of or control. In severe cases, you might even feel as though you're once again reliving the event. Such experiences are called *flashbacks*. During a flashback, you might suddenly feel strange and unreal, like you're somewhere else.

It's also possible that you might become extremely frightened or agitated when you're in a situation similar to the traumatic event, or when you see or hear something that reminds you of the trauma. For example, if you experienced an event that involved gunshots, you might become frightened whenever you hear the sound of a car backfiring.

The second category of symptoms involves different kinds of avoidance behaviors caused by the trauma. Maybe you stay away from the site where the event took place and avoid conversations or thoughts about the event. Or perhaps your brain has blocked out all memories of the event. You might also find yourself avoiding things, events, or people that made you happy before the traumatic event. Or, you might even experience a generalized numbing of your emotions.

The third category of symptoms includes various kinds of heightened anxiety. This could mean that you experience trouble falling asleep, difficulty thinking and concentrating, a heightened sense of being on the alert for potential danger, or increased anger, agitation, and frustration.

In addition, it's also common for people with PTSD to think about death frequently, either their own or other people's deaths. For example, one client with PTSD remarked that she felt like she was living in "the land of the dead" more often than she felt alive.

ARE THERE OTHER RELATED PROBLEMS?

Many people with PTSD also suffer with other problems, such as obsessive-compulsive disorder, depression, dysthymia, bipolar disorder, attention-deficit/hyperactivity disorder, and intermittent explosive disorder.[2] In addition, the estimates of alcohol abuse among people with PTSD range from 16 to 68 percent,[3-5] which is much higher than the estimated alcohol abuse rate in the general population, which is approximately 7 to 18 percent.[6] Furthermore, men with PTSD are five times more likely than the general population to develop a drug abuse problem, and women with PTSD are almost two times more likely.[7]

Many people with PTSD frequently experience strong guilt feelings, especially if they've survived a trauma in which someone else has died.[1] Other people with PTSD sometimes experience chronic pain and poor physical health.[8, 9]

WHO IS AFFECTED?

A 1996 global study of disease found that PTSD was the sixth most disabling mental health problem in the world,[10] affecting approximately 5 million American adults every year.[11] It's estimated that 70 percent of American adults will experience a severe traumatic event at some point in their lives,[12] and an estimated 14 to 25 percent of those will develop PTSD.[13] For the overall general population, this translates into approximately 4 percent of all adults developing PTSD every year,[2] and approximately 7 percent of all adults developing PTSD at some point in their lives.[1, 14] In general, women appear to develop the disorder twice as often as men.[12]

However, women are also more likely to be the victims of certain violent crimes. Women are ten times more likely than men to be the victims of rape and sexual assault, and women are six times more likely to have violence committed against them by a spouse or romantic partner.[15] Refugees are also particularly at risk for developing PTSD. It's estimated that between 5 to 35 percent of the world's refugees have been tortured,[16] and some studies have found the rate of PTSD in torture survivors to be as high as almost 74 percent.[17]

WHAT CAUSES IT?

PTSD arises after experiencing a life-threatening situation, either directly or indirectly. People who experienced earlier traumas in their lives are also at a greater risk for developing PTSD if they experience newer traumas.[18] In fact, the children of parents who have PTSD are even at a greater risk for developing the disorder themselves, perhaps due to the level of stress hormones in both the parents and the children.[19, 20]

Research of the disorder strongly suggests that trauma causes physical changes in the brain. These changes include shrinkage in the part of the brain associated with certain kinds of memories, an increased activation in the part of the brain responsible for emotional processing, and decreased activation in the area of the brain responsible for language processing.[21]

The research also suggests that PTSD might be the unfortunate result of a natural survival process. When you experience a traumatic event, your brain releases chemicals that reinforce the memory of that event to help you avoid similar traumas in the future.[22] In the case of PTSD, this process seems to be frequently activated, which might explain the intrusive memories and dreams associated with the disorder. Similarly, another theory suggests that your fear response system is broadly expanded after suffering a trauma to help you avoid being traumatized again, thus causing general avoidance of anything slightly resembling the event.[23] Yet another theory suggests that the intrusive memories, flashbacks, and dreams associated with PTSD result from an inability to integrate the traumatic experience into your belief system about the world.[24] Many people wonder how such a bad thing could have happened to them or to someone they love.

WHAT CAN YOU DO ABOUT IT?

Despite the devastating effects that PTSD can have on a person's life, many people with the disorder wait as long as twelve years before seeking treatment.[25] This is unfortunate, considering that there are three very effective cognitive behavioral treatments for PTSD.[26, 27] On average, 67 percent of the people who complete one of the following treatments recover from the disorder.[28] *Stress inoculation training* is an effective treatment designed to teach a variety of coping skills to help manage the fears associated with the trauma.[29, 30] *Exposure therapy* also helps build coping skills, but in addition, it incorporates imaginative and real-life exposures to feared situations in a safe, step-by-step process.[31-33] *Cognitive processing therapy* utilizes writing exercises to neutralize thoughts, feelings, and memories about the traumatic event. Many of the other treatments found in this book are also believed to help relieve at least some of the symptoms associated with PTSD. In particular, eye-movement desensitization and reprocessing,[30, 36] brief psychodynamic therapy,[37, 38] hypnotherapy,[38] and acceptance and commitment therapy[39, 40] have all demonstrated some effectiveness in small studies.

Because many people suffering with PTSD first seek treatment from their primary care physicians,[41] medication is often prescribed as the initial treatment. Among the medications that are recommended for the treatment of PTSD are the antidepressants sertraline (Zoloft), paroxetine (Paxil), fluoxetine (Prozac), fluvoxamine (Luvox), citalopram (Celexa), nefazodone (Serzone), and venlafaxine (Effexor).[27] The short-term use of certain anti-anxiety medications such as clonazepam (Klonopin) might also be prescribed for certain symptoms related to PTSD,[27] as might certain antipsychotic medications such as risperidone (Risperdal) and olanzapine (Zyprexa).[42]

Recommended treatments for post-traumatic stress disorder include:

. Cognitive behavioral therapy, see page 136

. Medications, see page 155

. Eye-movement desensitization and reprocessing, see page 144

. Brief psychodynamic therapy, see page 135

. Hypnotherapy, see page 152

. Acceptance and commitment therapy, see page 129

SCHEMA-FOCUSED RELATIONSHIP PROBLEMS

WHAT ARE THEY?

A *schema* is a strongly held belief you have about yourself that is either positive or negative in nature.[1] In both cases, the schema is accepted as being true, even if a negative schema causes harm or difficulties in your life. A *schema-focused relationship problem* is a pattern of difficulties you have with other people that is caused by the negative beliefs you have about yourself.[2] The theme of these problems often remains the same over time, and repeats itself in different types of relationships, such as romantic involvements, business relationships, and friendships.

Most often, negative schemas develop at an early age. Children who are abused, mistreated, or criticized often think they've done something sufficiently bad to deserve their mistreatment. None of these unkind comments or actions is ever deserved. Nevertheless, children often will think poorly of themselves as a result of such actions. Later, as adults, these same people continue to think poorly of themselves, and their negative schemas continue to grow stronger. Sadly, if left untreated, negative schemas don't change very much throughout life [3, 4] and become harmful, both to self-esteem and relationships.

One leading researcher has defined eighteen common negative schemas that develop early in life.[5]

1. **Abandonment or instability.** If you have this schema, you're constantly afraid of relationships ending. Either you believe that you'll easily lose a relationship—caused by fights, breakups, divorces, affairs, or death—or you believe that anyone who would want you must be physically, mentally, or emotionally unhealthy, and will therefore be unable to take care of you.

2. **Mistrust or abuse.** If you have this schema, you're constantly afraid of being physically or emotionally hurt by other people, through direct force, deceptions, or lies. You might even believe that other people do this to harm you on purpose.

3. **Emotional deprivation.** If you have this schema, you believe that you will never get the care and support that you need.

4. **Defectiveness or shame.** If you have this schema, you believe that you're physically, emotionally, or psychologically defective, and therefore unworthy of being loved or cared for by anyone.

5. **Social isolation or alienation.** If you have this schema, you believe that you're so different from everyone else in the world that you'll never be able to fit in or be accepted.

6. **Dependence or incompetence.** If you have this schema, you believe that you're incapable or not smart enough to do anything without great assistance from other people.

7. **Vulnerability to harm or illness.** If you have this schema, you believe that you are exceptionally at risk for getting hurt or contracting some type of disease or illness.

8. **Enmeshment or undeveloped self.** If you have this schema, you believe that you can't live or enjoy life without the constant emotional support of someone else, usually someone of great importance in your life like a parent or spouse. In some instances, you don't even feel whole without that other person close by.

9. **Failure.** If you have this schema, you believe that you've never succeeded, nor can you ever succeed, no matter what the task.

10. **Entitlement or grandiosity.** If you have this schema, you believe that you're more important than other people and are therefore more deserving of privileges and rewards not given to others. Often, you seek fame, power, or control at the expense of other people's safety and needs.

11. **Insufficient self-control or self-discipline.** If you have this schema, you're unable to tolerate any type of discomfort or setback when trying to achieve something, and so you simply give up. In other instances, you're unable to control your emotional outbursts and impulses.

12. **Subjugation.** If you have this schema, you're constantly forced to give up your own needs by someone else who threatens to do something or withhold something if you don't.

13. **Self-sacrifice.** If you have this schema, you willingly give up your own needs in order to meet someone else's needs. Often, you feel guilty and are afraid that if you don't meet the needs of the other person, that person will suffer in some way.

14. **Approval-seeking or recognition-seeking.** If you have this schema, you're constantly trying to gain the appreciation and support of others. As a result, you fail to develop a sense of valid self-worth, because all of your value is dependent on what other people think of you.

15. **Negativity or pessimism.** If you have this schema, you pay attention only to the sad and difficult parts of life, such as troubles, grief, pain, destruction, and the loss of life. You also fail to see, or purposely ignore, anything good that might be taking place; plus, you usually expect that the worst will always happen.

16. **Emotional inhibition.** If you have this schema, you stop yourself from saying, doing, or feeling certain things that you're afraid might bother or offend someone else. In essence, you "stuff" all of your true feelings and opinions to satisfy other people.

17. **Unrelenting standards or excessive criticism.** If you have this schema, you set excessively high goals for yourself that are often impossible to meet or very damaging to the rest of your life. You also strive to do everything perfectly, and anything short of that, even 99 percent perfection, is considered a failure.

18. **Punitiveness.** If you have this schema, you believe that anyone who makes an error, large or small, should be criticized or disciplined. You are also quick to get angry with others, as well as with yourself, and you fail to think about reasonable circumstances that could explain why the error was made.

Most people recognize that they've dealt with at least one of these negative schemas at some point in their lives. If you recognize that you're still struggling with one or more of these schemas, it's easy to understand why you're having difficulties in your relationships. These negative schemas are like distorted fun-house mirrors that you've been using to view yourself since you were a child. At first, it might have been hard to believe that you really looked that way, but after seeing it often enough, you believed it. These schemas are so strong that even when good-natured people tell you that these negative things about you are untrue, you don't believe them. That's because each time you go home and look in the mirror, you still see that familiar distorted view of yourself.

Negative schemas can affect you and your relationships in three different ways.[1] In each situation, the schema causes you to do something that you're not even aware of. The first action is called *schema maintenance*. This refers to the actions you take to preserve the power of your negative schema, even when those actions make you feel worse about your relationships and yourself. For example, if you have a self-sacrifice schema you're constantly giving up your needs for the needs of other people. You probably pick romantic partners who are very demanding of you, as well as overcontrolling and bossy. As a result, you never get any satisfaction in your relationships and probably spend all of your free time helping other people.

The second way in which schemas affect relationships is called *pain avoidance*. Simply put, all negative schemas have unspoken rules, and when a rule is broken it causes frustration and pain in your life. To avoid this, you'll do anything to not break the rules; and again, most of this happens on a unconscious level. For example, the rule of a self-sacrificing schema says, "If you do anything for yourself, you're selfish and hurting somebody else." As a result, you never do anything for yourself and never break the rule.

However, while avoiding hurting someone else you never get any of your own needs met. In the worst-case scenario, you might even stay in a dysfunctional or dangerous relationship because you don't want to upset the other person by leaving. Unfortunately, surrendering your decision-making power like this to avoid immediate pain and discomfort actually increases the strength of your negative schema and makes it harder to change the schema in the future.

Finally, the third way in which schemas disrupt relationships is called *schema compensation*. In this process, you do the exact opposite of what the schema demands of you. For example, again, if you have a self-sacrificing schema you might suddenly get angry at other people and refuse to help anyone ever again. Naturally, this extreme opposite reaction will shock the people in your life who are accustomed to you doing everything they want you to do, and so it will certainly disrupt your relationships.

ARE THERE OTHER RELATED PROBLEMS?

There are no official estimates of other related disorders for people with schema-focused relationship problems. However, psychological research and theory have demonstrated that dysfunctional schemas account for many illnesses, such as depression,[6-8] drug and alcohol problems,[9-11] anxiety problems,[12, 13] eating disorders,[14, 15] and personality disorders.[16-18]

WHO IS AFFECTED?

There are no official estimates of how many people have been affected by schema-focused relationship problems. However, it seems obvious that we all have our own unique collection of both helpful and dysfunctional schemas that govern our lives and our relationships.[16]

WHAT CAUSES THEM?

The preceding information about schema-focused relationship problems is based on the theory of psychology found in cognitive behavioral therapy[16, 19] and schema-focused therapy.[1] Other clinicians from different schools of psychotherapy will have different ideas about what causes conflicts in a relationship. Using the schema model, however, it's clear that the dysfunctional schemas are themselves the problem.[20] They repeatedly make you think and feel the same way about yourself, others, and the world, whether or not those judgments and conclusions are correct or helpful. Moreover, most of us tend to develop at least one dysfunctional schema when we are young. As a result, relationships can be very complex. Each person enters a relationship with his or her own negative schemas, and this results in two active groups of schemas in each relationship, not just one.[21]

WHAT CAN YOU DO ABOUT THEM?

Both cognitive behavioral therapy and schema-focused therapy can improve these types of relationship problems. Cognitive behavioral therapy can help you test the rules of the schema by helping you to break those rules safely and systematically to see what the effect is on your relationship.[22] It will also help you challenge the truth of the schema by looking for evidence that contradicts it as well as help you replace pain-avoidance behaviors with new skills to handle confrontation.[16] Schema-focused therapy also uses some of the same methods. Plus, it uses imagery techniques to uncover suppressed emotions and interpersonal techniques to highlight just how your schema affects your relationships.[1] In some cases, treatment can be effective even if just one person from the relationship seeks help. In other cases, a couple may need joint [23] or family [4] cognitive behavioral therapy.

Many people in troubled relationships have also found help using other treatments found in this book, especially couples therapy and family therapy.

Recommended treatments for schema-focused relationship problems include:

- Schema-focused therapy, see page 172

- Cognitive behavioral therapy, see page 136

- Couples therapy, see page 139

- Family therapy, see page 146

SCHIZOID PERSONALITY DISORDER

WHAT IS IT?

If you have a *schizoid personality type*, you aren't interested in seeking social contacts or relationships and you often prefer to be alone.[1] You also aren't concerned about approval or criticism from others, and you show little emotional reaction to other people and events.[2] As a result, some people might describe you as very shy, reclusive, or even unfriendly; despite how you really feel. The word "schizoid" comes from the Greek prefix *schizo*, meaning "split," and "schizo" here applies to the way a person disconnects from other people. Unfortunately, personality styles like this one often create problems in your relationships, job, and other social situations. As a result, personality styles like this are officially referred to as "personality disorders."

In truth, everyone likes to spend some time alone. This is a normal and healthy desire. However, if you have a schizoid personality, you prefer to be alone almost all the time. This doesn't mean that you hate other people. It might just mean that you don't know how to interact with them,[3] or perhaps you feel extremely uncomfortable when you do try to interact.[4] Either way, most likely you avoid unnecessary interactions with people.

You might even have a job that requires little contact with other people, and chances are good that the other employees know very little about you.[5] It's also likely that you live by yourself, and if you do have relationships, they're probably not very intimate. Maybe the closest people in your life are your parents and siblings. If you do have a few other people in your life, such as a friend or a spouse, most likely your relationships with them are often difficult.[6] They probably ask you how you're feeling or what you're thinking because you don't offer the information voluntarily. Or, maybe they're constantly asking you why you don't want to participate in more family events or social gatherings.

Almost certainly, you're not interested in the same types of activities as other people. You probably prefer to do things by yourself, and don't seek activities where you might be noticed, praised, or criticized. Often, you probably just feel like hiding and being ignored.

ARE THERE OTHER RELATED PROBLEMS?

Many people with this type of personality also have bipolar disorder, depression, dysthymia, panic disorder, generalized anxiety disorder, and social phobia.[1, 7, 8] There's also an association between schizoid personality and drug and alcohol problems, especially for women.[9-11] One study found that some people with schizoid personalities later developed schizophrenia,[1, 12] and these two problems are considered to be related in some ways.[13] For example, people with schizoid personalities may develop short-term hallucinations and delusions when under stress.[1] There also appears to be a strong link between schizoid personality and homelessness.[14] In one study of homeless people, an association was found between the number of schizoid personality traits that a person had and the length of time that the person was homeless.

WHO IS AFFECTED?

In a large study of American adults, it was estimated that 3 percent of that population, or almost 7 million people, had schizoid personalities, with men and women being affected equally.[15] In other studies, the estimates have ranged from almost 1 to 2 percent of the general population.[16-18] Overall, almost 15 percent of all American adults, or about 31 million people, struggle with personality problems like this one,[15] and these types of long-term problems are often the cause of general unhappiness and disability in a person's life.[16]

WHAT CAUSES IT?

The exact cause of schizoid personality is unknown. The problem usually begins as early as childhood or adolescence[1] and it's possible that it has both biological and social causes. In general, it appears that personality problems like this one have a strong chance of being passed on in families, due to influential genetic factors that can be inherited.[19] Some researchers have suggested that schizoid personality might be related to another biological illness, *Asperger's syndrome*, which is a type of autism.[20, 21]

Like children with autism, children with schizoid personalities often take longer to develop language and motor skills, which makes interacting with other people more challenging.[22] Other researchers think that schizoid personality disorder might be related to early experiences of depression. In two studies, children who experienced depression had six to ten times the risk of developing schizoid personalities later in adulthood when compared with children who had not experienced depression.[23, 24]

Other researchers have uncovered possible links between schizoid personality and nutritional deficits. One group found that male children and teenagers with schizoid personalities were significantly underweight,[25] and another group of researchers found that male teenagers who had survived a period of famine as children had a greater risk for developing schizoid personalities.[26]

Some studies have looked at possible causes in a person's family history. One study discovered that children who experienced high levels of verbal abuse from their parents had a greater risk of developing schizoid personalities.[27] Another study found a possible connection with early emotional neglect by the person's parents.[28]

WHAT CAN YOU DO ABOUT IT?

Unfortunately, there is little research to suggest which treatment is the most effective for helping a person with a schizoid personality.[29] Many people with this problem usually come to treatment only when they're experiencing some other type of problem.[30] However, many mental health professionals believe that many types of long-term psychotherapy can help a person with a schizoid personality lead a healthier, more fulfilling life.[31] Reviews of different types of psychotherapies for the treatment of personality problems like this one suggest that brief psychodynamic therapy, longer-term psychodynamic therapy, interpersonal therapy, and cognitive behavioral therapy may all provide at least some help to people with schizoid personalities.[29, 32-34] Ideally, any one of these treatments should help you establish satisfying relationships and decrease your feelings of loneliness.[4]

Recommended treatments for schizoid personality disorder include:

· Brief psychodynamic therapy, see page 135

· Long-term psychodynamic therapy, see page 167

· Interpersonal therapy, see page 153

· Cognitive behavioral therapy, see page 136

SCHIZOID
PERSONALITY
DISORDER

SCHIZOPHRENIA

WHAT IS IT?

Schizophrenia is a disorder characterized by severely disorganized thoughts, emotions, and behaviors.[1, 2] The word "schizophrenia" means "split mind" and originally the disorder was given this name to call attention to the divided thought processes of the people affected by it.[3] Unfortunately, over the years, many people have confused schizophrenia with dissociative identity disorder and think that people with schizophrenia have multiple personalities. This isn't true. A person with schizophrenia suffers from a collection of different kinds of problems that make it very difficult to function at home, work, and in other social situations. And yet, despite these various problems with their thought processes, many people with schizophrenia have an average or above average intelligence.[4]

If you're suffering with schizophrenia, you probably experience some kind of hallucination. *Hallucinations* are visual, auditory, or other sensory events that only you can perceive. Your hallucinations might include seeing people or things that aren't really there, hearing voices speaking to you that only you can hear, or smelling scents that don't really exist. These hallucinations might happen frequently and are often very disturbing.

Another common experience in schizophrenia is delusional thinking. A *delusion* is a strongly held, but mistaken, belief. Perhaps you sometimes think that the television newscaster is talking directly to you, or that someone is sending you secret messages in the newspaper. Or, maybe you think you're being punished by a secret government organization, or that someone other than yourself is controlling your thoughts. These are all types of delusions.

Most likely, you also suffer from other serious problems with your thought processes. Typically, problems probably occur when you try to think of words you want to use, when you try to remember information, and when you try to maintain your focus on something.[5] These types of thought problems can often lead to problems in speaking, which are noticed by other people. Perhaps you, or others, have noticed that you have difficulty talking about one topic at a time. Maybe your mental focus and speech pattern switch from one subject to another very quickly and frequently. Or, maybe others have told you that sometimes they can't follow you or understand what you're talking about.

Most people with schizophrenia also suffer from some kind of severe behavior difficulty. This could mean that you have problems doing regular daily activities, like eating and bathing. Or, perhaps you can't control your impulses, and so you behave in unpredictable and inappropriate ways, like screaming at people in public. In more extreme cases of schizophrenia, a person might be unable to move and appear to be rigid, like a statue; or conversely, the person might engage in some type of strange, but constant, motion.

Other common problems associated with schizophrenia include difficulties interacting with others. Some people with schizophrenia appear to have an expressionless face and often seem unable to display their emotions, while others display emotions that are very different from what would be appropriate, like laughing during a serious conversation. Other problems can include an inability to participate in social or work activities, or to enjoy activities that provided entertainment before the person became ill with the disorder.

In a study that tried to identify the early warning signs of schizophrenia,[6] certain problems were frequently reported by people who later developed the disorder. These early problems included: hallucinations, becoming exceptionally suspicious of others, experiencing changes in sleep patterns, feeling very anxious, experiencing problems with thinking, becoming excessively angry, developing delusions, and experiencing depression. In additional studies,[7-9] the sudden development of very strange behaviors also preceded occurrences of schizophrenia. However, this development by itself isn't enough to predict the beginnings of the disorder.

ARE THERE OTHER RELATED PROBLEMS?

In addition to the severe problems associated with schizophrenia itself, as many as 50 percent of the people with the disorder have additional health problems.[10] Among the most common problems is cigarette smoking. It's estimated that up to 90 percent of people with schizophrenia smoke heavily,[1] making themselves vulnerable to many related health problems. People with schizophrenia also have a greater risk for developing diabetes,[11] and many of them also suffer with depression, obsessive-compulsive disorder, drug and alcohol addictions, anxiety, social phobia, and panic attacks.[12-14]

The greatest health risk associated with schizophrenia, however, is suicide. Suicide is the number one cause of premature death for people with schizophrenia.[15] Nearly 50 percent of people with schizophrenia will attempt to end their lives.[16] For these reasons, it's extremely important to seek help from a professional mental health care worker if you or someone you know has symptoms of schizophrenia.

Besides affecting individuals and families, schizophrenia also has a wide-ranging social impact. Many people with schizophrenia who lack family or social support become homeless and live on the streets[17] or end up in jail due to vagrancy.[18] In fact, it is believed that one-third of the estimated 350,000 to 1 million homeless people in the United States suffer from a severe mental disorder, and often it is schizophrenia.[18, 19]

WHO IS AFFECTED?

Schizophrenia is one of humankind's most serious health problems. In 1990, it was estimated that schizophrenia was the ninth leading cause of disability in the entire world,[20] trailing problems such as depression, accidents, alcohol use, and heart disease. On the whole, schizophrenia affects approximately 1 percent of the world's population,[21-23] a statistic that translates into almost 3 million people in the United

States alone.[24] Men have a slightly greater risk of developing schizophrenia than women.[25] Typically, people develop schizophrenia between their late teenage years and their early thirties, with men developing the disorder a little earlier in life than women.[1]

WHAT CAUSES IT?

Although the exact cause is unknown, it's generally agreed that schizophrenia is a brain disorder caused by biological factors, rather than by environmental or social risk factors.[2] However, environmental factors such as stress can trigger the disorder's onset or make it worse.[26] Schizophrenia appears to be inheritable. Your chances of developing the disorder increase from 1 in 100 to 13 in 100 if one of your parents has schizophrenia,[27] and the risk is higher if it's your mother who has the disorder, rather than your father.[1] This suggests that genetic factors can create a vulnerability to developing the disorder, and these factors can be passed on from generation to generation.[21]

The leading theory about schizophrenia is that it's caused by high levels of dopamine, a chemical neurotransmitter produced in the brain.[28] Some researchers believe that an inheritable genetic code produces an ineffective nerve receptor in the brain that disrupts the transmission of dopamine.[29] Other possible causes of schizophrenia have been identified using brain-imaging techniques, such as magnetic resonance imaging (MRI).

Also, researchers have observed that certain areas of the brain are sometimes smaller than expected in people with schizophrenia.[30-32] However, the differences are sometimes as small as 2 percent,[33] the results aren't always the same for men and women,[34] and sometimes such results are found only in 25 to 30 percent of the people observed.[5]

WHAT CAN YOU DO ABOUT IT?

The most important first treatment for schizophrenia is medication.[2] Some commonly used medications include risperidone (Risperdal), olanzapine (Zyprexa), quetiapine (Seroquel), ziprasidone (Geodon), clozapine (Clozaril), and aripiprazole (Abilify).[2, 35] If you're prescribed one of these medications, you'll need to take it for the rest of your life in order to control the symptoms of the disorder. This may seem unfair and burdensome, but the truth is that people who don't take medication for schizophrenia lead very unhealthy, unfulfilling lives.

Making this situation even more complicated is the fact that all of these medications have side effects. Some of them, like clozapine, have severe side effects that require monitoring with weekly blood tests.[35] Nevertheless, despite these complications, medication is still the best treatment for controlling the symptoms of schizophrenia. If you've already been prescribed medication for schizophrenia, it's critically important that you continue taking it. Stopping your medication without the advice and supervision of your medical doctor is never a safe decision, despite how good you might feel when you make that decision. If you do stop taking your medication, your chances of having a severe schizophrenic episode in the near future are much higher than they would be if you continued taking your medication.[26]

Psychotherapy is also necessary to control the symptoms of schizophrenia.[2, 36] Unfortunately, the truth is that many people with schizophrenia do stop taking their medications.[37] One of the goals for your treatment, therefore, is to help you adhere to your medication regimen. Specific types of psychotherapies, such as family therapy,[38] can educate your family members about the disorder and thus help to create a more positive environment in which you can live. In studies of family therapy, it has been shown to help prevent relapse, to lessen readmissions to hospitals, and to help you continue the use of medications.[39]

Cognitive behavioral therapy, in both individual and group settings, has also proven to be an effective treatment.[24, 40, 41] Cognitive behavioral therapy for schizophrenia is designed to help you relieve stress, understand the nature of your disorder, evaluate your hallucinations and delusions, adhere to your medication schedule, and prevent relapses.[42] In studies comparing the use of cognitive behavioral therapy with and without medication, people who used cognitive behavioral therapy with medication experienced fewer symptoms of schizophrenia and fewer relapses.[43-47]

In two small studies, acceptance and commitment therapy has also been shown to be an effective treatment when used in conjunction with medication.[48, 49] In both studies, the patients receiving this treatment were rehospitalized less frequently for their symptoms, reported greater overall improvements, and were able to cope with their hallucinations in less distressing ways.

Other kinds of treatments have also been successful at providing specific skills training to people with schizophrenia, such as social skills training[50] and supportive work training.[51] For people with more severe forms of schizophrenia, a residential living facility or a community-based care program may be an alternative to hospitalization. Assertive community treatment is one such program that offers the support of a team of health care workers twenty-four hours a day, and has been shown to reduce hospitalizations and improve the use of services.[52, 53]

Recommended treatments for schizophrenia include:

· Medications, see page 155

· Family therapy, see page 146

· Cognitive behavioral therapy, see page 136

· Acceptance and commitment therapy, see page 129

· Social skills training

· Supportive work training

· Assertive community treatment

SELF-FOCUSED PERSONALITY DISORDER

WHAT IS IT?

If you have a *self-focused personality*, you think you have many more exceptional characteristics than other people have, and you expect to be treated in a special way.[1] You also have an extreme overconfidence in your abilities[2] and you are often preoccupied with your own success, intelligence, and attractiveness. You criticize other people for their faults; and you will often demand that other people recognize your achievements.[1] Unfortunately, personality styles like this often create problems in your relationships, job, and other social situations. As a result, personality styles like this are officially referred to as "personality disorders," and in many references this particular problem is referred to as "narcissistic personality disorder."

As a rule, we all need to spend some time focusing on our own needs. This is important and most of us wouldn't survive if we didn't. The degree to which you believe that you deserve care and attention, from yourself and others, is called *self-esteem*,[3] and self-esteem is an essential element of a healthy life.[4] While developing your own self-esteem, it's usually natural to help other people get their needs met, too. However, people with self-focused personalities often get their own needs met at the expense of others.

If you have a self-focused personality, it's very important that other people see you as influential, talented, attractive, intelligent, persuasive, and an excellent employee or boss.[5, 6] Many people with self-focused personalities also consider themselves to be risk-takers[2] and are highly motivated to succeed in situations that will bring them praise from other people.[7] But although praise from others is desirable, criticism and mistakes are impossible to tolerate. Most likely, it's not easy for you to forgive someone who has criticized or harmed you,[8] and you might even seek revenge.[9]

In general, there appear to be two different types of people with self-focused personalities: those who are outgoing in social situations and those who are not.[10] If you're one of those who is outgoing, you probably like to show off and be the focus of attention. You also probably put a lot of time into the way you look, and expect other people to pay you compliments, but when they don't, you become offended or angry.[11] Others with this type of personality aren't outgoing, and like to keep to themselves. If you're more like this, chances are good that you become greatly upset when you are criticized, and you put a lot of energy into protecting yourself from disapproval.

Due to the characteristics of this type of problem, it's often very hard for someone with a self-focused personality to maintain romantic relationships.[12] Maybe your romantic partners disappoint you because they don't compliment you enough, or, maybe you're on the constant lookout for a better, more attractive partner. People with self-focused personalities are also known to turn romantic relationships into power "games,"[13] and many partners often grow tired of these games and leave.

ARE THERE OTHER RELATED PROBLEMS?

Many people with self-focused personality problems also suffer with bipolar disorder,[14, 15] depression,[1] and anxiety problems.[16] There is also a danger of developing problems with substance abuse,[17, 18] gambling addiction,[19] and eating disorders.[20, 21]

However, the greatest threat for people with self-focused personalities is the possibility of suicide.[22] Although there are no statistics on how many people with this problem try to take their own lives, it's been observed that suicide attempts can arise very quickly and without warning in people with self-focused personalities.[22] The risk of suicide is even possible when the person looks happy,[23, 24] meaning that it's not necessary for the person to be depressed.[25] It may be that a sudden injury to the person's self-esteem is a sufficient cause to attempt suicide.[26]

WHO IS AFFECTED?

It's been estimated that approximately 1 to 3 percent of the general population have self-focused personalities,[1, 27-29] with men being diagnosed with the problem 50 to 75 percent more often than women.[1, 30] In general, almost 15 percent of all American adults, or almost 31 million people, struggle with personality problems like this,[31] and these types of long-term problems are often the cause of general unhappiness and disability in a person's life.[29]

WHAT CAUSES IT?

The exact cause of a self-focused personality is unknown. The problem usually begins as early as childhood or adolescence[1] and it's possible that it has both biological and social causes. In general, personality problems like this have a strong chance of being passed on in families, due to influential genetic factors that can be inherited. And in one study, a self-focused personality appeared to have the highest chance of being inherited among all the other similar personality problems.[32] Other studies have observed that children who experience depression have greater odds of developing a self-focused personality later in adulthood.[33, 34]

In a study of social causes, one team of researchers found that self-focused personality traits in young adults were associated with having parents who were either too strict or too indulgent.[35] Other researchers think it's possible that some people develop self-focused personalities to protect themselves from feeling ashamed about who they are.[36] Despite all of the overconfidence and pride that is worn on the outside, many people with this type of personality style are not really as confident as they appear to be. People with self-focused personalities depend on their own continual success and praise from others to maintain their self-esteem, and when they don't get this, their self-esteem declines.[37, 38] It also declines when people with self-focused personalities recognize that their own popularity and social skills are less than their peers.[39]

WHAT CAN YOU DO ABOUT IT?

Self-focused personality problems are often very difficult to treat,[24, 40] partly because personality problems like this one are so long-standing. Due to the characteristics of this problem, a person with this type of personality will usually seek treatment for some other difficulty, such as depression.[41]

Unfortunately, there is little research to suggest which treatment is the most effective for helping a person with a self-focused personality.[42] However, in reviews of treatments for personality problems like this, brief psychodynamic therapy, psychodynamic therapy, and cognitive behavioral therapy all showed some effectiveness at improving people's lives.[43, 44] And in one very small study, interpersonal therapy also helped a person with self-focused personality traits.[45]

In general, if you do seek help for problems related to a self-focused personality, one of the treatment goals should be to help you develop a sense of self-worth that doesn't depend on praise received from others nor on criticism applied to other people.[46]

Lastly, one group of researchers found some success using antidepressant medications such as fluoxetine (Prozac) to treat self-focused personality problems.[47]

Recommended treatments for self-focused personality disorder include:

- Brief psychodynamic therapy, see page 135

- Long-term psychodynamic therapy, see page 167

- Cognitive behavioral therapy, see page 136

- Interpersonal therapy, see page 153

- Antidepressant medications, see page 155

SOMATOFORM DISORDERS

WHAT ARE THEY?

The root "soma" refers to the physical body. *Somatoform disorders*, therefore, are a group of illnesses characterized by physical problems, such as pain, immobility, or discomfort. Typically, this group of disorders includes: somatization disorder, conversion disorder, pain disorder, and hypochondriasis.[1] (Body dysmorphic disorder is also a somatoform disorder, but it's described elsewhere in this book; see page 49.) In all of these illnesses, the problems are serious enough to interfere with your daily life, your work, and your relationships. The problem is also usually bad enough to cause you to seek medical treatment.

However, for many of these problems there are no medical explanations or successful medical treatments. As a result, many people with somatoform disorders are referred to mental health professionals for additional assessment, explanations, and treatments. But just because you might be referred to a nonmedical professional doesn't mean that your pain isn't real. People with somatoform disorders aren't pretending to be sick; their pain is very real despite the fact that there is no known cause.

People with somatoform disorders are often referred to mental health professionals for treatment, instead of to medical professionals, for a number of reasons: (1) these problems are often made worse by psychological stress, (2) these problems can be made worse by a person's behaviors, (3) these problems often lead to emotional issues such as depression, and (4) in some cases, the cause of the problem is psychologically related.

WHO IS AFFECTED?

The prevalence of somatoform disorders appears to be high. As a group, somatoform disorders have been called the most common psychiatric problems seen by general practice medical professionals.[2] In a study of over 1,000 patients examined by their general practitioners, 16 percent met the criteria for severe somatoform disorders, and when mild impairment was included, the rate jumped to 22 percent.[2] Many of these people also suffered with depression and anxiety. In a study of hospital patients,[3] approximately 36 percent of the people who met the criteria for any somatoform disorder also had other mental health problems, such as depression and anxiety.

WHAT CAUSES THEM?

The cause of a pain disorder is usually a clearly identifiable event, such as an accident or the onset of a disease. However, the causes of somatization disorder, conversion disorder, and hypochondriasis are still largely unknown. Some evidence suggests that relatives of people with these problems are sometimes at a greater risk for developing them.[1] However, it's not clear if this is due to inheritable factors or to the fact that these people often live in the same environments. Clearly, there are other factors involved. For example, in some cultures it's more acceptable (or more common) to express psychological pain, such as sadness or suffering, either as physical pain or unexplained fatigue.[4]

WHAT CAN YOU DO ABOUT THEM?

Cognitive behavioral therapy has been shown to be an effective treatment for somatoform disorders.[5] This type of treatment might be used by itself to relieve some of the physical pain and discomfort, or it might be used in conjunction with conventional medical treatments, such as medication. Most likely, if you seek cognitive behavioral therapy, your psychotherapist will help you examine the possible ways your thoughts can ease your pain, explore the ways your behaviors are limiting your life because of your pain, and experiment with changes to increase your activities and social connections.[5]

Not only is this form of therapy effective for treating the pain associated with somatoform disorders, it's also been shown to be cost-effective when compared with the long-term costs of requiring constant medical care for these illnesses.[6] In a two-year study, some patients saved 64 percent more on their medical expenses than those in the group who didn't receive cognitive behavioral therapy.

The following pages contain specific information on each of the somatoform disorders. Find the one(s) that seem(s) the most relevant to your situation and continue reading.

SOMATIZATION DISORDER

What is it? A *somatization disorder* is characterized by chronic pain that is widespread throughout your body.[1] Over the course of several years, the pains typically affect multiple parts of your body, such as your joints, head, back, stomach, feet, and elsewhere. It's also very probable that your sexual functioning has been affected, particularly your sexual activity, performance, or enjoyment. Unusual menstruation or erectile problems are also common. You also probably have some kind of problem with your digestive system, such as stomach pain, digestion problems, diarrhea, nausea, vomiting, or bloating.[1] It's also likely that you've experienced at least one other inexplicable health problem during the illness, such as problems swallowing, seeing, hearing, feeling, walking, or thinking.

Typically, a somatization disorder lasts for many years.[1] However, if the problem is not as severe or pervasive as described above, but it has lasted for at least six months, a diagnosis of an undifferentiated somatoform disorder might be made.[1]

Who is affected? Rates of somatization disorder range from almost 1 to 2 percent for women and appear to be even less for men.[1, 3] There's some evidence suggesting that your chances of developing somatization disorder are increased if someone in your family also has this problem,[1] and the disorder typically begins before the age of thirty.[1] Estimated rates for undifferentiated somatoform disorder, however, are much higher and range from approximately 10 percent (in a study of hospital patients)[3] to almost 20 percent (in a study of the general population of Germany).[7]

What can you do about it? Group cognitive behavioral therapy, including problem solving, assertiveness training, relaxation training, and emotional expression, has been shown to be an effective treatment for somatization disorder.[8, 9] Similarly, successful results have been found using individual cognitive behavioral therapy for the treatment of undifferentiated somatoform disorder. A study of seventy-nine patients who received six to sixteen sessions of therapy led to 73 percent of the patients being rated as recovered or improved after treatment.[10]

In addition, the use of Saint-John's-wort, an herbal remedy, has been shown to relieve symptoms of anxiety, depression, and overall discomfort related to somatoform disorders, including somatization disorder.[11]

Recommended treatments for somatization disorder include:

· Cognitive behavioral therapy, see page 136

· Saint-John's-wort

CONVERSION DISORDER

What is it? A *conversion disorder* is characterized by problems moving a part of your body or using one of your senses.[1] For example, if you have conversion disorder, you might have problems keeping your balance when you walk or moving one of your arms because it's paralyzed. Or, maybe you have difficulties speaking, swallowing, or using one of your senses. It's also possible that you have a loss of feeling in a part of your body or muscle weakness. Some people experience hallucinations, dizziness, confusion, and seizures. As with all somatoform disorders, there's no known medical cause for these very serious problems. However, the symptoms do appear to increase in frequency or severity because of factors such as stress, and so they're thought to have psychological influences and possibly origins.

Who is affected? The prevalence of conversion disorder appears to be rare in the general population, less than 1 percent.[1] However, it's been reported in larger percentages of specific populations, such as mental-health clinic patients and surgical patients.[1] Conversion disorders typically develop between the ages of ten and thirty-five, but later development is not uncommon.[1]

What can you do about it? In one study of conversion disorder, patients with trouble walking were helped to make small improvements in their range of motion by using cognitive behavioral and stress-management therapies.[12] Improvements were seen in as few as twelve days and were still maintained two years later. Hypnotherapy[13] and family therapy[14] have also proved effective. Furthermore, successes have also been achieved using biofeedback,[15] a form of treatment that helps you to monitor and alter your muscle tension, heartbeat, blood pressure, and body temperature.

Recommended treatments for conversion disorder include:

· Cognitive behavioral therapy, see page 136

· Hypnotherapy, see page 152

· Family therapy, see page 146

· Biofeedback

PAIN DISORDER

What is it? A *pain disorder* is characterized by severe pain in any part of your body that causes great disturbances in your life.[1] There are two kinds of pain disorders, those that begin without any known cause and those that follow a trauma, such as a car accident. Unlike pain that eventually stops within weeks or months after a bad accident, the physical discomfort associated with a pain disorder continues for a longer period of time and it is sometimes greater than what would be expected.

Many people who seek treatment for a pain disorder are suffering from very real, very severe illnesses and problems, such as cancer, arthritis, back pain, headaches, reflex sympathetic dystrophy syndrome (now called complex regional pain syndrome), carpal tunnel syndrome, nerve damage, shingles, sports injuries, and osteoporosis. Because they often are unable to find a satisfactory medical treatment for their pain, people suffering with these conditions frequently seek help from a mental health professional.

Or, the aid of a mental health professional might be added to your treatment as part of a multiteam approach to treating your pain, which can often include the services of a medical doctor, physical therapist, acupuncturist, massage therapist, and others. When you're treated by a mental health professional, the diagnosis of a pain disorder will be given, since this will be the focus of your treatment.

Who is affected? The prevalence of pain disorder in the general population is unknown.[1] However, millions of people struggle with short- and long-term pain issues on a daily basis. Based on one survey of 3,600 adults, almost half of the general population struggles with chronic pain.[16, 17] In another study of over 5,000 patients, 40 percent of them visited their primary care physicians for pain-related issues—mostly pains occurring in their backs and heads.[18] In fact, it's estimated that 59 percent of adults experience back pain during their lives,[19] and as many as 10 million adults suffer with migraine headaches in the United States alone.[20] Many people with pain issues also frequently suffer with depression and anxiety,[21, 22] which is another reason why they are often referred to mental health professionals for treatment.

What can you do about it? Cognitive behavioral therapy has been shown to be an effective treatment for relieving the physical discomfort associated with pain disorder,[23-26] as has acceptance and commitment therapy.[27, 28] In a study using a version of acceptance and commitment therapy, the participants increased their daily functioning levels and experienced reductions in both their pain and related symptoms of depression.[29] Biofeedback is also an effective treatment for pain;[30-32] it can teach you how to monitor and control your muscle tension, heartbeat, and body temperature.

Additional pain relief treatments include acupuncture,[33-35] hypnotherapy,[36-38] exercise,[39] mindfulness-based stress reduction therapy,[40, 41] Tai Chi, concentrated breathing exercises, guided imagery, and yoga.[42] A variety of pain-relief medications is often used in conjunction with many of the above treatments. These medications may include nonsteroidal anti-inflammatory drugs (NSAIDs) such as ibuprofen (Advil/Motrin) and naproxen (Naprosyn); acetaminophen (Tylenol); anticonvulsants such as gabapentin (Neurontin); opioid analgesics such as morphine, oxycodone (OxyContin), fentanyl, and acetaminophen/hydrocodone (Vicodin); tricyclic antidepressants such as nortriptyline (Pamelor); and newer antidepressant medications such as duloxetine (Cymbalta) and venlafaxine (Effexor).[43, 44]

Recommended treatments for pain disorder include:

· Cognitive behavioral therapy, see page 136

· Acceptance and commitment therapy, see page 129

· Hypnotherapy, see page 152

· Mindfulness-based stress reduction therapy, see page 165

· Biofeedback

· Acupuncture

· Exercise / Tai Chi / yoga

· Pain relief medication

HYPOCHONDRIASIS

What is it? Hypochondriasis is, perhaps, the most widely known of the somatoform disorders, and perhaps the most misunderstood. A person with hypochondriasis, known as a *hypochondriac*, is not faking an illness. Those who pretend to be in pain in order to avoid something, such as jury duty or military service, are referred to as *malingerers*. Those who pretend to be sick or who make themselves sick for no apparent reason are said to suffer from a *factitious disorder*.

If you have *hypochondriasis*, you are genuinely concerned that you have an illness or disease, despite repeated medical examinations that can find no cause for your alarm. Chances are that you've seen many doctors looking for the one who will help you with your problems. As a result, you've probably been diagnosed with many different ailments or told that there's nothing wrong with you, despite how bad you feel. In some cases, there's a real medical problem that's being overlooked. In other cases, there might be factors that are causing you to perceive the problem to be worse than it really is. For this reason, people with hypochondriasis are often referred to mental health professionals for additional treatment.

Who is affected? The rates of hypochondriasis range from approximately 1 to 5 percent in the general population, to almost 7 percent in certain medical facilities.[1, 3] Although hypochondriasis can begin at any age, it's typically thought to begin in a person's twenties or thirties.[1]

What can you do about it? In one study of hypochondriasis, cognitive behavioral therapy was administered over the course of four months.[45] At the end of treatment, 76 percent of the people reported improvements in the severity of their symptoms. Relief for hypochondriasis has also been found using stress-management therapies, which incorporate relaxation training and problem-solving skills.[46] In addition, the use of certain kinds of antidepressants, such as fluvoxamine (Luvox), fluoxetine (Prozac), nefazodone (Serzone), and citalopram (Celexa), has been shown to be effective.[47]

Recommended treatments for hypochondriasis include:

. Cognitive behavioral therapy, see page 136

. Stress-reduction and relaxation techniques

. Antidepressant medications, see page 155

A Final Word About Making Sense of Your Problem

Hopefully, this chapter has given you a good description of the disorders with which you're struggling. Now, if you need to, review what the recommended treatments are for those disorders and write them down. Then continue to chapter 3, Making Sense of the Treatments, where you'll find comprehensive descriptions of most of the treatments mentioned in this book.

CHAPTER 3

MAKING SENSE OF THE TREATMENTS

*For the meaning of life differs from man to man, from day to day
and from hour to hour. What matters, therefore, is not the meaning
of life in general but rather the specific meaning of a person's life at a
given moment.*

—Viktor Frankl*

How to Use This Chapter

This chapter includes information about twenty-one different types of psychotherapies. It also includes a brief description of the medications used to treat mental health
problems. All of the treatments are listed in alphabetical order. Find the ones that
were recommended for your problem in chapter 2. Then, as you read the descriptions
of your recommended treatments, mark the one that sounds the most effective and
appropriate for the problems you're struggling with. This is the type of treatment
you'll want to find in your community. When you get to chapter 5, Making Sense of
the Process, you'll be given instructions on how to find the best mental health care
professional who provides the treatment you're looking for. If you're struggling with
several disorders, try to find a recommended treatment that is effective for all of them.
If there isn't a single form of therapy, you might have to start treatment for your most
distressing problem first, and then, later, get a referral for another mental health care
professional who provides a different type of treatment for your other problem.

Sometimes, people do get treated for multiple problems at the same time, for
example, attending family therapy for family problems and cognitive behavioral

* From *Man's Search for Meaning*. 1946. New York: Simon & Schuster, Inc. p. 113.

therapy for anxiety, or getting substance abuse treatment for alcohol addiction while taking medication that was prescribed for depression.

But before you begin reading this chapter, let me make some final points about mental health treatments in general. The recommended treatments found in the description of your disorder were emphasized because research has shown them to be effective. Some treatments, such as cognitive behavioral therapy and medications, appear for almost every problem because they have been frequently researched. Other treatments, such as existential therapy, have had little or no research done on them. As a result, existential therapy does not appear in any recommended treatment section. But treatments like these are still included in this chapter because many people have found them to be effective for their problems despite the lack of supportive research. Treatments with limited research support also have been included because many of them are popular, such as psychoanalysis, or because many of them show great promise for future research success, like acceptance and commitment therapy and positive psychology.

Also, depending on where you live and what your financial resources are, you might not have a choice about the type of treatment you get. If you live in a small town where there is only one psychotherapist, and she practices humanistic psychotherapy, for example, you might have to see her for the treatment of your snake phobia, despite the fact that her approach isn't a recommended treatment. Or, perhaps because of your insurance coverage, you'll find yourself with a brief psychodynamic therapist for the treatment of your bipolar disorder. Again, this isn't a recommended treatment. But, if these are your only options, you should certainly try them. Then, you should use the skills taught in chapter 5, the final chapter, Making Sense of the Process, to determine whether the treatment is working for you. If it isn't, somehow you'll need to find a new treatment. Maybe it will mean having to drive farther away from home, or seeing your psychotherapist only once or twice a month. But it's important that you get the right help for your problem, even if it's inconvenient.

Finally, be aware that some of your treatment's success depends as much on the mental health professional you're working with as it does on the treatment he or she provides to you. That is, the person who is helping you is often just as important as the scientific process that is carried out in the session. So, after you find the correct treatment for your problem, do your best to find the best match for your personality. You might have to interview a few mental health professionals before you pick one to work with, or perhaps you'll have to switch professionals once your treatment has started. This might be a hassle, but if finding the right person to work with also means that you're going to be more motivated to attend your sessions—and do the work—it will be worth the effort.

You'll be given more information about how to find the right person to work with in chapter 4, Making Sense of the Mental Health Care Professionals.

ACCEPTANCE AND COMMITMENT THERAPY

Acceptance and commitment therapy (ACT) is a relatively new form of psychotherapy that incorporates elements of behavior therapy, meditation and mindfulness practices, as well as scientific research on how humans learn.[1] ACT is based on the principle that many psychological problems are caused by efforts to control, avoid, or get rid of undesirable emotions and thoughts. Often, people try to get rid of feelings and thoughts that make them sad or anxious, just as they get rid of other things they don't like, such as old clothes. However, ACT points out that feelings and thoughts can't be controlled in the same way.

In fact, the harder you try to control your thoughts and feelings, the more powerful they become and the longer they stick around. This point can be made by imagining a picture of a pink elephant and then forcing yourself to forget about it. The harder you try not to think about it, the more you actually do. The same is true for your thoughts and emotions.

Many people are taught by their parents or society that sad and anxious thoughts or emotions are "bad," "negative," or "undesirable." Ultimately, these beliefs become rules by which you live your life. Then, when sadness or anxiety appears, you do your best to suppress the emotion, avoid it, or control it. To do this, you might try many different methods. For example, you can try not to think about how situations affect you, you can refuse to discuss your feelings, or maybe you use drugs and alcohol to help you forget. Unfortunately, however, these coping strategies only make your situation worse. Either they interfere with your relationships or they cause you to become more anxious and depressed.

One of your initial tasks in ACT is to figure out all the strategies you've used to cope with your problems. Your ACT psychotherapist will acknowledge that you've worked very hard at solving your problems in the best ways you knew how, and that you've come for treatment only after you've exhausted all your other options. After exploring your unsuccessful attempts to handle your problem, you'll be encouraged to acknowledge the fact that your coping strategies don't work. In ACT, this acknowledgement is called *creative hopelessness*,[1] and its purpose is to make you receptive to new, unexplored possibilities.

To make changes in your life, your ACT psychotherapist will help you explore your personal values. This is an important step because it steers your treatment toward a genuine purpose. ACT's ultimate goal isn't to eliminate all the pain in your life, which is impossible. The goal is to make your life more meaningful and fulfilling, while accepting the fact that sometimes life also includes sadness and anxiety.[2]

One of the initial steps toward change is to develop *self-observational skills*. This means that you'll be asked to pay attention to how your thoughts and feelings affect each other in the present moment. ACT places a large emphasis on the here and now of life. To become better aware of this, you might be instructed in some form of meditation that will help you focus on the present moment. Then, after you've developed self-observational skills, your ACT psychotherapist will help you learn to *defuse* from your thoughts. This means that you will be taught how to observe your self-critical thoughts without becoming entangled in them. These skills often include watching thoughts float past in your imagination and learning to treat your mind as a separate entity that produces thoughts without your control.

In a similar way, you'll also learn how to accept your sad and anxious thoughts, without trying to control or avoid them. Finally, your ACT psychotherapist will also help you explore the steps that need to be taken in order to live a more fulfilling life, based on your values, and help you overcome obstacles that stand in the way of those achievements.

For more information, visit the Web site of:

· Acceptance and Commitment therapy:
  www.contextualpsychology.org/act

ANALYTICAL PSYCHOTHERAPY/ JUNGIAN PSYCHOTHERAPY

Analytical psychotherapy, or Jungian psychotherapy, was developed by Carl Jung (1875–1961), a Swiss medical doctor. Originally, Jung was a close friend of Sigmund Freud and a practitioner of Freud's psychoanalysis. However, after a series of disagreements, the two friends parted company and Jung went on to develop his own form of psychotherapy, which shares some basic theories and practices with psychoanalysis.[1]

Like psychoanalysis, *analytical psychotherapy* uses the relationship between you and your psychotherapist as a method of examining your relationship problems. Analytical psychotherapy also believes in conscious and unconscious thoughts that influence your health and behaviors. However, Jung also believed that your soul, or psyche, is equally as important as unconscious and conscious thoughts, and it's the awareness of all three elements that helps you make sense of your life and the world at large.

One of the main unique principles of analytical psychotherapy is a belief in a collective unconscious that is shared by all of humanity.[2] The *collective unconscious* is much like a spiritual library that holds universal patterns of personality and ideas, a library from which you frequently receive knowledge without knowing that you're doing so. Jung studied art from many parts of the world and, through his studies, he recognized that different cultures share similar symbols and myths, a similarity that he believed is due to more than mere coincidence. Jung believed that what he called "the collective unconscious" greatly influences the lives of people across the boundaries of distance and time.

From the collective unconscious, humans often borrow universal personality patterns called *archetypes*, which influence how we act as well as how we make choices. Among these patterns are popular roles that we take on, roles that are often found in many cultures' mythologies and stories, such as the Hero, the Earth Mother, the Trickster, and the Outcast. These universal archetypes also include certain significant situations in life, such as the Quest, the Initiation, and the Journey. An analytical psychotherapist will often reframe your life using one of these archetypes. This is done to help you figure out the expectations and obstacles that you might be encountering, and the various ways in which these obstacles might be overcome.

Analytical psychotherapy is also based on the principle of balancing opposites, such as illness and health. Jung believed that symptoms of illness also hold clues that will help you recover. For example, one of the ways this occurs is through an awareness of the shadow. The *shadow* is that part of yourself that you don't want to acknowledge or recognize, like the belief that you're capable of hurting or killing another person.

However, when you deny that your shadow-self exists, you push it farther into the unconscious part of your mind, where it eventually finds a way of manifesting itself as a problem. For example, if you don't admit that you're capable of cheating, you may be constantly afraid that other people are trying to cheat you. Analytical psychotherapy believes that for this fear to subside, you must recognize your shadow, i.e., the capacity to cheat that lies within yourself.

This doesn't mean that you need to engage in cheating behaviors, but you do need to acknowledge that part of yourself that is being denied. Clues about the shadow-self can often be found in your dreams, which are an important element of treatment in analytical psychotherapy.[3] Dreams often contain hidden symbolism and archetypes that can help you solve your problems.

Analytical psychotherapy tries to help you find balance in other aspects of your life, too. This includes recognizing the male and female roles that we all take on, no matter what our gender. It also includes finding a balance in the way you interact with other people. Jung believed that we use four modes for taking in information: thinking, feeling, sensing, and being intuitive. He also believed that everyone is naturally inclined toward being introverted or extroverted. An analytical psychotherapist will help you examine these aspects of your life and, ultimately, help you find a healthy balance between them.

In practice, analytical psychotherapy can be a very creative process. Some analytical psychotherapists help their clients learn to use their imagination through writing, visualization, painting, and storytelling. Sometimes, this creative process also includes making elaborate scenes in sandboxes using different figures, symbols, and representations.

Finally, analytical psychotherapy also puts a great emphasis on helping you examine your future, not just your past. Jung recognized that it wasn't enough for some of his clients just to solve their immediate problems. Many of them wanted to continue forming a deeper understanding of themselves and their goals in life.

For more information, visit the Web sites of:

· The C.G. Jung Institute of San Francisco: www.sfjung.org

· The International Association for Analytical Psychology: www.iaap.org

BEHAVIOR THERAPY

Behavior therapy focuses on the way dysfunctional behaviors lead to mental health problems. One of the main beliefs of this treatment is that your actions and reactions are largely learned. Some behaviors are actively reinforced and rewarded with things like food and money, while other behaviors are learned by watching and imitating other people.[1] Unlike cognitive behavioral therapy, a psychotherapist working from a strictly behavioral model is not interested in the way your thoughts affect your actions and emotions. However, today, a more lenient behavior therapist will often be indistinguishable from a cognitive behavioral therapist.

Behavior therapy has gone through many changes. Early behavioral theory, at the beginning of the twentieth century, was largely influenced by the work of Ivan Pavlov (1849–1936), a Russian physiologist. Pavlov discovered that the dogs used in his research experiments salivated both when they saw their food and when they heard the ringing of a bell that announced the arrival of their food. In the dog's brain, the association of the food and the bell had become the same, and they both elicited the same response. Later, in the 1950s, American psychologist B. F. Skinner (1904–1990) brought behavioral theory to the forefront of psychology. Skinner used reinforcement such as food and punishment to guide the behavior of animals, and later humans.[2] Both of these discoveries greatly influenced the learning theories of what later became behavior therapy.

Behavior therapy focuses on actions that can be observed. Things that are unobservable, such as unconscious thoughts, are unimportant to the treatment. The focus of the treatment is also on the here and now, and what can be done to help you solve your problems. Behavior therapists aren't concerned with helping you figure out what factors caused your problems. In some ways, behavior therapy is like a medical treatment. For example, your primary care physician isn't going to be concerned with how you broke your leg; the focus is on what you can do to fix it.

Behavior therapy is based on scientific research that tests different procedures to find the most effective treatment. As a result, the treatment of one mental health problem, such as depression, is different than the treatment for another, such as phobias. The treatments are also structured and usually time-limited. Due to this systematic, step-by-step treatment method, behavior therapy has been called "cold" and "mechanistic" by its critics. However, there's a wealth of research to support the effectiveness of behavior therapy, and the truth is that it's often a much more interactive and collaborative form of treatment than many other types of psychotherapy. Throughout the length of your treatment, your behavior therapist will ask you questions, provide you with feedback, and be an active partner in your recovery.

Your behavior therapist will most likely begin treatment by asking you many specific questions about your problem, such as how long you've had the problem, how long it lasts each time it happens, and what seems to trigger the problem when it occurs. When the nature of the problem becomes clear, your psychotherapist will suggest a treatment plan and ask you to agree to it. He or she might even ask you to sign a treatment contract outlining what will happen in session.

Among the many goals of treatment, behavior therapists often teach you new problem-solving skills and new ways to change long-standing, dysfunctional habits. You will also be asked to do many activities outside of your fifty-minute session, such as recording your behaviors during the week. This is very different from other forms of psychotherapy, where the majority of the work is done in session. Also, in behavior therapy, you will be required to play the role of a participant-observer by running little experiments in your daily life.

The methods used in behavior therapy often include relaxation exercises, training in assertive communication skills, and role-playing to learn new social skills. Your psychotherapist might also ask you to engage in activities that often seem very hard, such as *systematic desensitization*[3] or *exposure and response prevention*.[4] These methods, which are often used to treat phobias and obsessive-compulsive disorder, require you to make a list of your feared situations, marking each situation with the level of fear you feel about it. Then, in a safe, systematic way, you'll be asked to expose yourself to the feared events, beginning with the least fearful situation.

You'll need to use the relaxation skills you previously learned, and you'll be required to expose yourself to fears in your daily life. But, again, these types of challenging activities are usually approached gradually, in a progressive way, so you can build up successes before taking on situations that seem impossible. In fact, your behavior therapist might even ask you to begin imagining yourself doing something difficult before you do it in real life. However, in some situations, your behavior therapist might expose you to the most feared situation on your list. This technique is called *flooding*.

For more information, visit the Web sites of:

· The Association for Behavioral and Cognitive Therapies: www.abct.org

· The National Association of Cognitive-Behavioral Therapists:
www.nacbt.org

BRIEF PSYCHODYNAMIC THERAPY

Brief psychodynamic therapy is a form of treatment largely based on psychoanalysis. However, as the name of this therapy suggests, the length of the treatment is much shorter than traditional psychoanalysis. Typically, the number of sessions will range from five to forty. The session limit will be discussed before treatment begins, and it's likely that your psychotherapist will often remind you of the termination date.

The term *brief psychodynamic therapy* actually includes a number of different treatments, each with a slightly different focus.[1] Some of them concentrate on making connections between your past childhood experiences and your current problems.[2] Others closely examine your thoughts and feelings about your psychotherapist, or discuss what it feels like to end treatment so soon.[3] Most of these elements are also explored in traditional psychoanalysis. However, you can expect your brief psychodynamic therapist to be more interactive with you in session. He or she will also provide you with more feedback than you'd normally get in psychoanalysis. The basic goal for most of these brief psychodynamic therapies is to focus on resolving one or two major problems in your life. For this reason, brief psychodynamic therapy might be a good treatment for you if you already have some insight about your problem and you're open to talking about it.

One of the brief psychodynamic therapies that has received some research support is time-limited dynamic psychotherapy (TLDP), which also incorporates elements of interpersonal therapy and cognitive behavioral therapy.[4, 5] Unlike traditional psychoanalysis, TLDP sets clear goals for treatment. One of the objectives of TLDP is to identify repetitive problems and long-standing bad habits that get in the way of creating healthy, fulfilling relationships. Your psychotherapist will briefly help you explore your past relationships and traumas to determine the origin of these patterns and habits, but most of the time will be spent helping you to resolve those issues by focusing on new ways of behaving in relationships.[6]

The relationship between you and your psychotherapist will even be used as an opportunity to help you practice your new skills. You should expect your TLDP therapist to direct your attention to how you act in session and to how you treat him or her. By engaging in this process, the ultimate goal of TLDP is to provide you with a new and improved relational experience, so that you can begin thinking of yourself in a healthier way and begin engaging in more fulfilling relationships.

COGNITIVE BEHAVIORAL THERAPY

Cognitive behavioral therapy (CBT) is a form of treatment that combines elements of both behavior therapy and cognitive therapy. Together, these two forms of treatment concentrate on the way your thoughts, behaviors, and emotions all influence each other and contribute to your mental health. CBT has proved to be a successful treatment for a number of mental health problems, especially anxiety and depression, and it's supported by a vast amount of clinical research.[1]

Behavior therapy began at the turn of the twentieth century. It focuses on the way dysfunctional behaviors lead to mental health problems. One of the core beliefs of this treatment is that your actions and reactions are largely learned. Some behaviors are actively reinforced and rewarded with things like food and money, while other behaviors are learned by watching and imitating other people.

In comparison, *cognitive therapy* examines the way your thoughts about yourself and others contribute to your mental health problems. Cognitive therapy was largely developed by Aaron Beck, an American psychiatrist, in the 1960s and 70s. While doing research on depression, he discovered that certain kinds of cognitive distortions often fueled people's mental health problems.[2] Among the common distortions that Beck identified are the following:[3]

- **Overgeneralization:** Making broad negative conclusions about life based on limited situations.

- **Black-and-white thinking:** Seeing things as either one way or another with no room for compromise.

- **Fortune telling:** Always anticipating that the worst will happen.

- **Discounting the positive:** Failing to recognize anything good that happens.

- **Emotional reasoning:** Thinking something is true just because you feel it is true.

- **Mind reading:** Assuming that other people are always thinking bad things about you.

- **Using "should" or "must" statements:** Setting unfair rules for yourself.

In addition, Beck also recognized that people who are depressed often have very pessimistic ideas about themselves, others, and the world; and they often underestimate their abilities to cope with problems.[2] In the 1980s, CBT coalesced when clinicians began using elements of both behavior and cognitive therapies together.

Today, CBT is often used when short-term therapy is the best option, such as when a client has only fifteen to twenty-five weeks available for treatment or when insurance will pay for only a limited number of sessions.[2] However, longer-term treatment using CBT is also possible. CBT is largely based on research that has determined effective treatment protocols to remedy specific mental health problems.

As a result, the treatment for one problem, such as depression, is different than the treatment for another problem, such as phobias. Due to this manualized, step-by-step method of treatment, CBT has often been called "cold" and "mechanistic" by its critics. However, there's a wealth of research to support its effectiveness, and the truth is that it's often a much more interactive and collaborative form of treatment than many other types of psychotherapy. Throughout the length of your treatment, your CBT therapist will ask you questions, provide you with feedback, and be an active partner in your recovery.

When beginning treatment, your CBT therapist will ask you many specific questions about your problem, such as how long you have had it, how long it lasts each time, and what seems to trigger the problem when it occurs. When the nature of the problem becomes clear, your psychotherapist will suggest a treatment and ask you to agree to it. He or she might even ask you to sign a treatment contract outlining the process that will be undertaken. CBT is a very interactive and collaborative process.

During treatment, your psychotherapist will ask you many questions and guide you through many activities in session. Homework will also be assigned on a weekly basis. This is very different from other forms of psychotherapy, where the majority of the work is done in the sessions. In CBT, you will be required to play the role of a participant-observer by running experiments in your daily life and recording the results. CBT is also different from some other forms of treatment because it focuses on the present instead of the past. Your CBT therapist might help you briefly explore the origins of your problem, but the focus will always return to how the past is affecting your life right now.

CBT therapists often teach their clients new problem-solving and coping methods, such as assertive communication skills, relaxation skills, and social communication skills. Often these are accomplished by means of role-playing in session. For problems like phobias and obsessive-compulsive disorder, a form of treatment called *exposure and response prevention* will most likely be used. This will require you to make a list of your feared situations, marking each situation with the level of fear you experience, and then in a safe, systematic way, you will be asked to expose yourself to the feared events, beginning with the least fearful one.

All of these techniques are also used in behavior therapy. The difference is that a CBT therapist will also help you to challenge the validity of your dysfunctional thoughts. One of the goals of CBT is to help you examine how negative thinking interferes with your emotions, behaviors, and life. To accomplish this, your CBT therapist will help you recognize the cognitive distortions that you are using and help you to modify or correct them. This is often accomplished by examining the evidence that supports and refutes the distortions.

He or she will also help you identify repetitive automatic thoughts. These are the critical thoughts you think and say to yourself, which sabotage your success and happiness. Two examples of automatic thoughts could be "I don't deserve anything good happening to me," or "Why bother trying? I'm just going to fail." These thoughts are often charged with sad and anxious emotions; automatic thoughts can occur consciously or without you even being aware that they are going through your mind.

CBT will also help you explore the deeply rooted core beliefs that you have about yourself and the world. These beliefs, called *schemas*, often develop in childhood and can be either positive or negative in nature. Schemas are very resistant to change, no matter how painful they are to your life. When negative schemas like "I'm unlovable" dominate your life, problems like depression and anxiety can naturally develop, and these problems rarely correct themselves without treatment.

However, with the help of a CBT therapist, you can run therapeutic experiments to test your beliefs about yourself and the world. For example, if you have a schema that says, "I'm not worthy," one experiment might be to ask a friend for a favor in order to determine if he's really going to reject or criticize you. The goal of these types of experiments is to help you have positive experiences that contradict your negative schema. In this experiment, for example, hopefully your friend will do you the favor without question, and thus contradict your feelings of unworthiness.

Then, after building a history of positive experimental results, the next goal will be to help you modify your negative beliefs—or to create new, healthier beliefs—ones that will help you lead a more fulfilling life.

For more information, visit the Web sites of:

- The Association for Behavioral and Cognitive Therapies: www.abct.org

- The International Association for Cognitive Psychotherapy: www.cognitivetherapyassociation.org

- The National Association of Cognitive-Behavioral Therapists: www.nacbt.org

COUPLES THERAPY

Couples therapy focuses on treating problems between two people in a relationship. Like many of the other treatment modalities found in this book, couples therapy isn't one specific treatment. Rather, it's a category of related therapies that focus on many of the same principles. In general, these treatments concentrate on your relationship as an arrangement of interdependent people whose actions affect each other. Many types of couples therapy use treatment models based on the psychotherapies found elsewhere in this book. Traditionally, this type of treatment is also referred to as "marital therapy," but due to the modern abundance of nonmarried couples who often seek help, "couples therapy" is a more accurate description.

Cognitive behavioral couples therapy looks at the way your actions and thoughts affect your partner's actions and thoughts, and vice versa. One of the principles of this treatment states that if a partner's behaviors are rewarded through some positive feedback from the other person, those behaviors will be repeated. However, if the person's feedback is negative, that behavior won't be repeated.[1] Not surprisingly, it's been observed that couples with fewer problems treat their partners in a more positive way.[2] In comparison, couples with more problems have greater communication difficulties[3] and communicate in more hostile ways.[2]

Variations of this treatment, such as *behavioral marital therapy*, focus more on creating behavioral changes rather than changing patterns of thoughts.[4] *Integrative behavioral couples therapy* seeks to help you and your partner understand why you both act the way you do, and, with that understanding, to build deeper compassion for and emotional acceptance of each other.[5]

Cognitive behavioral couples therapists will often explore new ways to handle distressing emotions, like anger and pain, which can interfere with effective communication and problem solving.[6] Some researchers have found that couples with problems often don't pay full attention to each other,[7] or they make pessimistic predictions about their relationships.[8] In couples therapy, you might be invited to participate in role-playing scenarios, in order to figure out new ways of communicating, listening, and solving problems. Another common intervention is to initiate special days on which you and your partner make extra efforts to increase positive communications and actions that are normally overlooked in your daily life.[4, 9]

Psychoanalytic or *psychodynamic couples therapy* explores the early relationships of both you and your partner, and assesses how those relationships influence your current relationship. According to this theory, the way you learn to relate to others in early relationships, such as with your parents, serves as a model, or pattern, for relating to other people when you are an adult. Many of these patterns, according to psychoanalysis, are unconscious. Therefore, part of the treatment involves helping each of you to become aware of your patterns. These insights can then help both of you to make conscious adjustments to your relationship.[10]

Emotion-focused marital therapy is a type of psychodynamic couples therapy.[11] In this treatment, early unsuccessful relationships are discussed. Then you and your partner identify how the fears and weaknesses that resulted from those relationships are interfering with your current relationship. One of the treatment goals is to help you both understand why the other person behaves in a certain way. Again, from this understanding, greater acceptance and compassion for the other person can be gained.

Systems theory explores the way you and your partner, and possibly your whole family, form a structured unit in which the actions of one member affect all of the other members.[12] In systems theory, problems are addressed as cyclical patterns of behavior. One of the commonly held beliefs in systems theory is that the partnership, or family system, generally wants to remain the same, even if the relationships are problematic. One intervention that is often used is reframing.

Reframing redefines a problem in a new way, which can lead to better understanding and greater odds for successful change. For example, maybe you hold back all of your feelings in your relationship, which then causes your partner to spend more time with friends. In this case, the psychotherapist might help both of you understand the cyclical nature of this problem, and create a new framework for conceptualizing it. This can then help the two of you to work toward making positive changes in a new way.

These are just a few examples of different couples therapies. It's probably possible to find a couples therapist who operates from any one of the modalities found in this book. Many couples therapists also use techniques described in family therapy (see page 146), as the two are often related.

For more information, visit the Web site of:

· The American Association for Marriage and Family Therapy:
www.aamft.org

DIALECTICAL BEHAVIOR THERAPY

Dialectical behavior therapy (DBT) is a treatment created in the early 1990s for people suffering with emotion dysregulation, which is also known as "borderline personality disorder."[1, 2] More recently, however, the treatment has also been suggested as a therapy for depression, anxiety, eating disorders, drug and alcohol problems, attention-deficit/hyperactivity disorder, and other personality problems.[3]

DBT is a form of cognitive behavioral therapy. Both types of treatment examine the way your thoughts, feelings, and behaviors interact and affect each other. However, a psychotherapist who uses DBT is especially interested in how your thoughts can create disruptive behaviors and emotions that interfere with your life and relationships. After examining these interactions, your DBT therapist will help you modify those thoughts, feelings, and behaviors, using different types of skills training.

The initial and most important goal of DBT is to help you eliminate suicidal and self-harming behaviors.[1] You'll also be provided with specific sets of skills to help you solve problems, improve your relationships, improve your control of your behaviors and emotions, and help you tolerate emotional discomfort. DBT also aims to help you reduce painful symptoms that arise because of trauma, since so many people with emotion dysregulation problems have also been the victims of sexual abuse. This part of the treatment might involve helping you safely and systematically confront feared situations that are currently being avoided. Your DBT therapist might also require you to join a supportive group therapy program, along with other people who are receiving DBT treatment.

DBT is largely influenced by Zen Buddhism, which emphasizes the acceptance of contradictory thoughts at the same time. The term *dialectic* refers to the examination of opposing thoughts and behaviors that takes place in DBT. For example, one of the fundamental techniques of the treatment is to teach you how to accept yourself, with all of your problems, while simultaneously acknowledging that some basic changes need to be made if your life is going to improve. Acceptance and change are two key concepts that are repeatedly balanced in DBT. Mindfulness skills based on Buddhist meditation are also taught. These skills can help you observe your actions, thoughts, emotions, and environment without making any judgmental responses.

Overall, DBT is a very active treatment. For it to be effective, you will be expected to implement and practice all of these new skills in your life outside of the therapy office. That's where most of the improvements in your life will take place. Initially, your DBT therapist may require you to agree on the goals of the treatment, especially the goals of not engaging in suicidal, self-harm, or other behaviors that interfere with the treatment process. And, as previously stated, you'll also be expected to participate in any other individual therapy or group therapy sessions that your DBT therapist requires.

For more information, visit the Web sites of:

- The Behavioral Research and Therapy Clinics: www.brtc.psych.washington.edu

- The Association for Behavioral and Cognitive Therapies: www.abct.org

EXISTENTIAL PSYCHOTHERAPY

Existential psychotherapy took hold in Europe after the destruction caused by World War II, and later it became popular in the United States. More so than other forms of psychotherapy, *existential psychotherapy* is largely influenced by philosophy, especially the writings of European existentialists such as Kierkegaard, Nietzsche, and Heidegger. The name of the psychotherapy comes from the same root as the word "exist." This form of treatment, therefore, focuses on your existence and how it influences your view of life and the world.

The aim of existential psychotherapy is to examine you as a whole person, rather than as a composite of impulses. It's built on the principle that there is no one truth to explain history or life, because each person's view of the world is unique. There is no standard technique used in existential psychotherapy; instead, it offers a set of guidelines for looking at yourself and your problems in a unique way.

Existential psychotherapy emphasizes living a fuller, more meaningful life despite the fact that many situations in modern society can feel depressing and without substance. The task is to examine the way you give meaning to the elements of your life, such as love, illness, relationships, and your personal self.[1] According to existential psychotherapy, anxiety problems develop when you are confronted with large issues that threaten you. Typically, the most disturbing issues are death, isolation, a loss of meaning, and freedom.[2]

The first three issues all seem like obvious ones with which to be concerned. However, freedom requires you to take responsibility for your actions, and it requires you to make choices that can change your world and possibly affect others. This responsibility frequently makes people nervous. Therefore, part of a treatment plan might be to help you take responsibility for making changes that have been avoided, to learn to tolerate being alone, and to find meaning in life by participating in new activities.

Existential psychotherapy does share some similarities with psychoanalysis, such as the belief in unconscious and conscious thoughts that can contribute to anxiety. Part of the goal of existential psychotherapy is to find out what those thoughts are and to examine how they're impeding your life. However, existential psychotherapy is more concerned with your present problem and future goals, rather than the task of uncovering the past roots of your problem, as you would do in psychoanalysis.

For more information, visit the Web site of:

- The International Society for Existential Psychology and Psychotherapy: www.existentialpsychology.org

EYE-MOVEMENT DESENSITIZATION AND REPROCESSING

Eye-movement desensitization and reprocessing (EMDR) was created at the turn of the twenty-first century to help people who'd experienced traumas.[1] However, there is now some research to support the claim that EMDR successfully treats other mental health problems as well.[2] EMDR was once publicized in the media to be a one-time cure for trauma. Yet, even the founder of the treatment says that this is not an accurate statement.[2, 3] EMDR, like other treatments for trauma, can take weeks, months, or years to reduce your symptoms, depending on the severity of your trauma, and it won't work for everyone.

To someone who is unfamiliar with the treatment, the methods used in EMDR might look very strange when compared with other talk-based psychotherapies. To put it simply, in EMDR you'll be asked to recall a memory that sums up your traumatic event. Then you will be told to focus on your psychotherapist's fingers, as he or she moves them from right to left, in a steady rhythm, for approximately thirty seconds at a time. Then the process is repeated. Although this may seem odd, research supporting EMDR has shown that side-to-side eye movements produce a calming effect.[4, 5] The treatment also works through a process called *desensitizing*, which means that the pain associated with your memory decreases as you continuously recall the image throughout the treatment.

Another supporting theory suggests that EMDR helps your brain to process disturbing information. Memories of a trauma are usually so upsetting that people don't want to think about them, and so the information remains unprocessed.[1] In this raw form, the memory can be very distressing, especially if it makes you think that you're to blame for what happened. EMDR supporters believe that desensitization of the memory allows the brain to process the traumatizing information and "file" it away.[6]

In actuality, the treatment is more involved than simply watching your psychotherapist's fingers move back and forth. In the initial stages, your psychotherapist will help you learn to relax and imagine a safe, special place for yourself, just in case the process of recalling the trauma becomes too overwhelming. The psychotherapist will also help you select an image from the trauma that encapsulates your experience, and then help you explore how that memory makes you think of yourself. In the next phase, you'll hold that snapshot in your memory for a few seconds, and then watch the fingers of your psychotherapist move from side to side. But once the movement starts, you'll be instructed to let that memory go and just pay attention to other images and feelings that arise.

After every set of finger movements, you'll be asked to describe the memories and feelings that came up. Then the movements begin again. Periodically, your EMDR therapist will ask you about the original memory of the trauma. The process continues until your emotional reaction to that memory is minimally disturbing. Finally, in the last stages of treatment, your EMDR therapist will help you implant a positive thought about yourself, instead of the painful one that resulted from the trauma.

In addition to using side-to-side eye movements, this treatment is also effective by using other alternating techniques, such as tapping your left knee and then your right, or snapping your fingers near your left ear and then your right. Another treatment similar to EMDR is the eye-movement technique (EMT).[7, 8] EMT is a simpler technique that also uses side-to-side eye movements, at the rate of one cycle per second for thirty seconds. This also seems to reduce the anxiety of traumatic memories. You can follow your psychotherapist's finger, focus on points on the wall, tap alternating knees, or close your eyes and move them back and forth. However, unlike EMDR, EMT requires you to hold on to the disturbing memory while you're moving your eyes. The result is that the memory breaks up and becomes harder to recall, thereby reducing the anxiety related to the memory.

For more information, visit the Web sites of:

· The EMDR Institute, Inc.: www.emdr.com

· The EMDR International Association: www.emdria.org

FAMILY THERAPY

Family therapy focuses on the relationships and interactions between family members. This treatment is often used to address problems between family members and couples, but it can also be helpful when the problem appears to be with a single member of the family, such as a depressed parent or a difficult child. Yet, even in these cases, your family therapist will address the problem as a symptom of a nonfunctional family system.[1]

Like many of the other therapies discussed in this book, *family therapy* isn't a single type of treatment. Instead, it's a category of related therapies that focus on many of the same principles. In general, they all focus on the family as an arrangement of interdependent people whose actions affect each other. The family is also regarded as a system that's out of balance and resistant to change. Problems often arise when family members use habitual modes of communication that don't work. However, the goal isn't to figure out which person is at fault or worthy of blame. Difficulties between family members are viewed as part of a cycle, and the goal is to figure out how to interrupt that cycle and solve the identified problems more effectively.

Your family therapist will want to explore the different kinds of interactions that occur between members of your family, including how the members communicate with each other and how problems are addressed during times of conflict. Your psychotherapist will also want to explore the roles that each member fills in your family system. Sometimes the role a person takes on isn't the role that is usually expected, such as a young child taking care of the parent. Often, a role-reversal like this is enough to cause many problems. Gender and cultural roles that members take on are also important and need to be explored, in order to identify their potential impact on the problem that brought the family into treatment.[2]

One of the common models of family therapy focuses on the way your family is structured.[3] Using this approach, your psychotherapist will want to examine who makes the decisions for your family, the alliances that are formed within the family, and the boundaries that exist or don't between family members and people outside your family. Family members who are too involved with each other are commonly called *enmeshed*, whereas members who don't interact are *disengaged*. Other models of family therapy are not as focused on structure as they are in the way your family interacts. Some of these forms of treatment find it useful to use seemingly strange interventions to restructure the way a family relates.[4] For example, a child who lights fires might be instructed to light more fires under the guidance of his or her parents. The goal of such an intervention is to make the child grow bored with the task and eventually stop.

Narrative family therapy examines the way family members tell the stories of their lives.[5] Your narrative family therapist will help you discover the various stories that make up your family as a whole. This often helps to redefine the family in some ways and gives each member the opportunity to create new, alternative outcomes for their lives. In narrative therapy, your family will also be instructed to think of the presenting problem as something outside of the family, instead of as a problem with just one individual member. For example, if the presenting problem is a child with a behavioral problem, your narrative therapist will encourage your family to think of the behavioral problem as an external issue that is burdening the child and the family. In this way, your family can unite with the child in addressing the issue, instead of blaming the child for the problem.

Many forms of family therapy use different methods of role-playing to examine communication styles and problem-solving skills, as well as to model new ways for family members to interact. Some family therapists might also ask you to create a family *genogram*, which is a generational map of relationships and difficulties. This can often be helpful because patterns sometimes become clearer and the genogram can display problems that have been repeated throughout multiple generations of a family.[1]

For more information, visit the Web sites of:

· The American Association for Marriage and Family Therapy: www.aamft.org

· The American Family Therapy Academy: www.afta.org

GESTALT PSYCHOTHERAPY

The form of gestalt psychotherapy popular today was largely created in the 1950s and 60s by Frederick "Fritz" Perls (1893–1970), a German medical doctor. The word "gestalt" means a whole that is greater than the sum of its individual parts. Similarly, *gestalt psychotherapy* views you as a whole being who's not separate from your surroundings, friends, family, memories, or past. Thus, in order to understand your problem, your gestalt therapist must help you understand all of those elements and how they interact in your life.[1]

However, despite the connection you have to your past, gestalt psychotherapy is primarily concerned with the here and now.[2] The goal of the treatment is to help you become more fully aware of what is happening to you in the present moment. To achieve this, your gestalt therapist might engage you in some very interactive experiences to highlight new ways of thinking, feeling, and acting.

For example, one technique involves having you talk to an empty chair in the room, as if you were talking to someone from your life with whom you have difficulty communicating. Talking to the empty chair allows you to say all the things that you always wanted to, but never did. Alternatively, you might write a letter to that person (which is never sent), and then write a response letter back from that person, imagining what he or she would say to you in return.

In other cases, you might use visualization techniques to imagine new reactions to troubling situations, or your gestalt therapist might help you focus your attention on your body posture and breathing habits.[3] Yet, despite these commonly used techniques, there is no official form of gestalt psychotherapy. Rather, there's a common philosophy that guides the treatment and places an emphasis on helping you experiment with whatever means are necessary to move you toward health and wholeness.

Because this form of treatment is so interactive, it's very important that you and your gestalt therapist develop a trusting, cooperative, and therapeutic relationship. Relationships in general are a very important focus of gestalt psychotherapy, but in session, it's exceptionally important that you trust your psychotherapist enough to engage in experimentation. To foster this trust, a gestalt therapist might share stories from his or her own life in order to illustrate a point or to help you when you're struggling. In contrast, your gestalt therapist might also openly challenge your stories and reported feelings. But, even this is done with the best of intentions. This type of challenge can help reveal an underlying thought, emotion, or behavior of which you are unaware. It can also help you understand how you affect other people. Or, it can help you learn to react to a challenge in a new, healthier way.

Other basic principles of gestalt psychotherapy include the belief that people naturally seek balance in their lives and want to improve their health. However, people sometimes get stuck using old habits that worked in the past but which no longer help in the present. For example, when you were a child, perhaps you tried to please everyone to get attention, but, as an adult, that same strategy leads only to continual emotional and physical exhaustion. In gestalt psychotherapy, you would experiment with new, healthier ways of dealing with those situations. Gestalt psychotherapy is similar to existential psychotherapy in that it's also interested in how you make sense of some of the larger issues in life, such as death, freedom, and isolation.

For more information, visit the Web sites of:

· The Association for the Advancement of Gestalt Therapy: www.aagt.org

· The Gestalt Therapy Network: www.gestalttherapy.net

HUMANISTIC/CLIENT-CENTERED THERAPY/ PERSON-CENTERED THERAPY

Humanistic psychotherapy, also known as client-centered therapy or person-centered therapy, was largely developed by American psychologist Carl Rogers (1902–1987) in the 1940s. *Humanistic psychotherapy* is a nondirective form of treatment, meaning that your humanistic therapist will follow your lead in session and regard you as the expert of your own experience. As such, your psychotherapist's job will be to follow the direction that you want to go in, instead of leading you toward some purpose or goal of treatment.[1] Your humanistic therapist trusts that you will speak naturally about what you need to do in the therapy session, without his or her guidance, and eventually you will figure out the key to your problem. He or she also trusts that you will know how often you need to come in for treatment and for how long a period of time. So, you will make these decisions as well.

Humanistic therapy takes an optimistic view of the human experience. One of the foundations of the therapy is that people naturally move toward their own growth and the fulfillment of their true potential in life. Mental health problems occur when you develop a rigid way of viewing yourself and the world and, therefore, stop growing. The aim of a humanistic therapist is to provide you with a supportive environment in which you can figure out your problem and continue growing toward self-fulfillment.

In order to facilitate this growth, your humanistic therapist will seek to embody three characteristics: to be genuine, to show you unconditional positive regard, and to be sincerely empathetic.[2] To be *genuine* means that your psychotherapist will behave as a real person who doesn't act in a phony or authoritarian way. *Unconditional positive regard* means that your psychotherapist should treat you in a completely nonjudgmental way, and accept whatever you do or say no matter what, even if your opinion differs greatly from his or her own opinion.

Empathy requires your psychotherapist to act and respond to you in a genuine, warm, and caring way, and to check in with you in order to verify that he or she has understood you correctly.

By using these techniques, your humanistic therapist seeks to help you in a number of ways. It's hoped that you will improve your self-esteem; develop a sense of control that comes from within yourself rather than from some outside source; become more open to experiencing new possibilities in your life; and develop more flexible coping styles and attitudes.[3]

Traditionally, humanistic therapy treats all patients the same, regardless of the presenting problem. It's also common that a humanistic therapist won't take a history of your problem and won't put a focus on your diagnosis. Again, the treatment is more concerned with you as a whole person, rather than just with your problems.

For more information, visit the Web site of:

. The Association for Humanistic Psychology: www.ahpweb.org

HYPNOTHERAPY

Hypnosis has been used to treat mental health problems for over 200 years. Its utilization began in late eighteenth-century France, where patients were mesmerized and relieved of their symptoms using magnets and the power of suggestion. Later, in the 1840s, James Braid, a Scottish medical doctor, used the technique as an anesthesia for his patients, but he realized that the magnets were unnecessary for the method to work. He then renamed the treatment hypnosis, from the Greek word *hypnos*, meaning "sleep." The technique was even used by Sigmund Freud to treat patients,[1] before he created psychoanalysis.

Unfortunately, hypnosis has suffered much at the hands of the popular media. Today, it's largely thought of for its entertainment value. However, *hypnotherapy*—the psychotherapeutic form of hypnosis—is officially recognized by both the American Psychological Association and the American Medical Association as an effective treatment for certain conditions. It's been shown to be effective for reducing symptoms of chronic pain,[2-4] relieving symptoms of phobias,[5] improving sports performance,[6, 7] easing childbirth,[8] and in some cases, helping to stop cigarette smoking.[9-11] Many other uses for hypnotherapy have also been successfully applied,[12] and research has shown that hypnosis has a direct, observable effect on the brain.[13, 14]

Many people expect to be put into a sleep-like trance when they undergo hypnotherapy. However, this is another misconception. Hypnosis is a state of deep relaxation in which you become more receptive to suggestions made by your hypnotherapist. Unlike the movies, your hypnotherapist will probably not use a swinging pendulum to induce your hypnotic state. Instead, you will probably be asked to concentrate on the sound of your hypnotherapist's voice, as he or she guides you into a state of deep relaxation. This can be done with guided visualization, in which you imagine a peaceful scene, or you might be asked to imagine different parts of your body becoming heavy and tired.

After being led through a few sessions of hypnosis, your hypnotherapist might ask you to try self-hypnotic techniques on your own, perhaps with the use of a tape-recorded session. This additional work can strengthen the effects of your hypnotherapy. However, despite the benefits of hypnotherapy, it should be noted that not everyone will benefit from the treatment. People who believe that hypnotism might work on them tend to be the ones for whom it's more effective.[16] But, according to research and estimates, 10 percent of the general population can't be easily hypnotized.[15]

For more information, visit the Web sites of:

- The American Association of Professional Hypnotherapists: www.aaph.org

- The American Society of Clinical Hynosis: www.asch.net

INTERPERSONAL THERAPY

Interpersonal therapy is a treatment that has been revised since its original creation in the 1940s. As its name implies, this form of treatment focuses on how you interact with other people, including your psychotherapist. One of the fundamental beliefs of interpersonal therapy is that dysfunctional relationships can be both the cause and the result of a mental health problem, so your relationships need to be examined in order to bring relief to your problem.

The original founder of interpersonal theory, Harry Stack Sullivan, an American psychiatrist, thought that the major cause of most people's problems was the anxiety that arose from interacting with other people.[1] He also believed that, as humans mature from childhood to adulthood, they pass through different stages of development in which they acquire new interpersonal skills.[1]

First, children learn how to speak and then get along with others. Next, teenagers develop close friendships and sexual relationships. Finally, adults mature into intimate relationships with those whom they love. Sullivan believed that problems occur when a person becomes stuck in one of those stages and doesn't learn the necessary skills before prematurely moving on to the next stage of development.

More recently, in the 1970s, *interpersonal therapy* (IPT) was redeveloped as a short-term, structured treatment for depression.[2] In some cases, IPT treatment may last for only twelve to sixteen sessions. However, longer treatment is often necessary. Much like the original form of interpersonal therapy, IPT focuses on how your mental health problems affect your relationships, and how those relationships contribute to your mental health problems.

Relationships with romantic partners, family members, friends, and coworkers are all equally important in IPT and need to be examined. It might also be necessary to explore what was happening in your life when your problem developed. But because of the time-limited nature of IPT, little emphasis is placed on exploring your past, beyond how it might be currently affecting your relationships.

In general, IPT focuses on four causes of typical relationship problems.[2] Fights and disagreements often cause many problems, such as those that take place between you and your partner or friends. Other problems can be caused by the death or loss of someone close to you. Changes in roles can also cause difficulties in your life, such as a divorce, the birth of a child, or acquiring new responsibilities at work. Finally, dissatisfying or difficult relationships can also cause troubles.

In order to resolve these issues, IPT focuses on developing skills to improve your relationships. This can often be accomplished by developing new methods of communicating, such as assertive communication skills, while also exploring your feelings and thoughts about the relationship. It might also be necessary to redefine what your role is and what your expectations are in a relationship. Often, you and your psychotherapist will role-play and rehearse interactions based on your relationships.

For more information, visit the Web site of:

- The International Society for Interpersonal Psychotherapy: www.interpersonalpsychotherapy.org

MEDICATIONS

Medications are often used to treat mental health illnesses either alone or in conjunction with some form of psychotherapy. A full description of medications is beyond the scope of this book. So, for a more detailed description of medications, please refer to books such as the *Handbook of Clinical Psychopharmacology for Therapists.*[1]

This section will discuss only *psychotropic medications*, which are used to treat mental health problems. It must be stressed that these medications are not cures in the way that antibiotics kill germs and cause an illness to disappear. Psychotropic medications can remove the observable symptoms of an illness, but most often, the illness will return if you stop taking your medications. *You should never stop taking medications of any kind without the instructions of your doctor or medical professional. Stopping your medications by yourself can be dangerous and potentially deadly.* Only medically trained professionals such as your primary care physician, psychiatrist, or nurse practitioner can prescribe medication for you, and in some states, such as Louisiana and New Mexico, specially trained psychologists can now prescribe psychotropic medications as well.

How do you know if you need medication?

This is a very difficult question to respond to, and there is no single correct answer. Some medical professionals will tell you that medications should always be your first treatment, while some psychotherapists will tell you that you should try medications only after psychotherapy has failed. The truth lies somewhere in the middle. For some biologically caused illnesses, like bipolar disorder and schizophrenia, medication is the primary treatment. But for other illnesses, like depression and anxiety, the decision to use medication can become more complicated.

If you're so depressed that you are suicidal, bedridden, or a danger to yourself or others, medication will be the best initial treatment, followed up with psychotherapy soon thereafter. However, let's suppose that your depression is being caused by a failing relationship. Although medication might help you feel a little better, your overall health will most likely improve only after you've dealt with the relationship problems. This is where psychotherapy might be able to help.

However, perhaps you're so depressed you need antidepressants just to begin dealing with your problems. Again, there is no clear answer about who should take medications. Research generally shows that, in many cases, a combination of psychotherapy and medication is the most effective treatment for many mental health illnesses.

Your decision to use medication can be made by discussing the issue with your primary care physician, psychiatrist, nurse practitioner, psychotherapist, family, and friends. You can also do your own research using the Internet by getting information from trusted, reputable sources, such as the National Institute of Mental Health (www.nimh.nih.gov) and the U.S. Food and Drug Administration (FDA; www.fda. gov).

The decision to use medication can be further complicated by the side effects that accompany many of them. However, these side effects are often less troublesome than the illnesses the medications are meant to treat. *And, again, it needs to be stressed that no matter how awful the side effects of any medication are, you should never stop taking it without first talking with your medical doctor.* If the side effects become unbearable, talk to your provider about adjusting the dosage or trying a different medication.

Unfortunately, another factor affecting the use of medication is cost. Some people without health insurance find both psychotherapy and medication to be beyond their budgets.

If you do consider taking medications, you'll need to consult a medical doctor. Most people initially seek help from their primary care physician.[2, 3] However, you might also consider consulting a psychiatrist. Although many primary care physicians are excellent general clinicians, psychiatrists specialize in the treatment of mental health problems and are usually more up-to-date about current treatment options. If you're already working with a psychotherapist, ask him or her for a recommendation. Often, your psychotherapist will know professionals in the community to whom they can refer you.

In order to get an effective medication you'll need to provide your medical doctor or psychiatrist with important information. First, you will need to be clear about how you are feeling and why you are seeking medication. During your initial visits, your medical doctor or psychiatrist will want to know:

- What are the symptoms or problems you've been experiencing?

- How long do they last?

- How bad do the symptoms get?

- What seems to bring on the symptoms? Are there any preceding factors?

- How long have you been experiencing these symptoms?

- Have you experienced this problem in the past?

- Does anyone else in your family have a problem like yours?

- Are you currently being treated for any other physical or mental health problems?

- Are you currently taking any other medications or herbal supplements? If yes, what are they and what are the dosages?

Again, if you're already working with a psychotherapist, he or she can help you organize this information. Your psychotherapist can also contact your medical doctor and provide him or her with important diagnostic information. It's very important that you bring a list of any medications you're already taking, including any herbal supplements, such as Saint-John's-wort and vitamins. Many substances like these can interfere with the effects of psychotropic medications and must be avoided. Make sure you also tell your doctor about any physical or mental illnesses you currently have or have suffered with in the past, including allergies. Finally, if someone else in your family is receiving medication for a problem similar to yours, tell your doctor. If the medication is working for a related family member, that medication might also work for you.

However, even with all of this information and an expert psychiatrist, there is still no guarantee that the recommended medications will help you. Prescribing the most effective medication is as much an art as it is a science. Some medications that work for some people might not work for you, and there is no way to predict the exact outcome. Also, don't be surprised if your doctor prescribes you more than one medication. Often, medications are prescribed together to make them more effective and tolerable.

If you receive medication from your medical doctor, make sure you ask how long it usually takes before you should begin feeling its beneficial effects. Many medications require a few weeks to a few months to begin working. So, don't expect to feel better right away. Give the medication time to start working. If you don't notice any effects after the date the medications are supposed to start working, contact your doctor and ask him or her for advice. Your doctor might change your dosage or ask you to try a different medication. Sometimes finding the one that will work for you is done by trial and error.

It's common to have questions about medication.[4] Make sure you bring a list of your questions for your medical doctor or psychiatrist. Often people want to know how long they're going to need to take their medication, what the potential side effects are, and what their diagnosis is. Other people want to know whether taking psychotropic medication means they're abnormal or crazy. The truth is that millions of Americans take prescription medication for mental health problems. According to a large popular-magazine poll,[5] more than 25 percent of American adults, almost 59 million people, sought treatment for a mental health problem between 2002 and 2004, and more than 80 percent took some kind of medication as a part of their treatment.

Recently, however, the news in the media about psychotropic medications has been confusing. In 2004, the FDA began requiring drug manufacturers to print special warnings on prescription packages after reports suggested that antidepressants might cause an increased risk for suicide in children and adolescents.[6] This decision in the United States came after the United Kingdom's Medicines and Healthcare Products Regulatory Agency also declared in 2003 that certain antidepressants weren't suitable for people under the age of eighteen.[7] However, in 2006, a study determined that the use of antidepressants did not increase the number of suicide attempts in adolescents, although the risk is generally greater for adolescents who take antidepressants when compared with adults who also take antidepressants.[8] In fact, the study found that the greatest risk for suicide attempts occurred in the month before the patients began taking their medications.

So, what should you do?

Despite the more recent reassurances, the information can still be confusing.

However, for the many people who have benefited from the use of psychotropic medications, the benefits have clearly outweighed the risks. And for many people who were suicidal before taking antidepressants, medications saved their lives. Ultimately, it's up to you to make the final decision about whether or not to use medication, but it's strongly suggested that you listen to the advice of the mental health professional(s) with whom you're working.

Sometimes psychotropic medications are the best first step in a successful treatment plan, and other times they provide added benefits to a psychotherapy treatment that has already begun. Become an educated consumer and ask questions of your primary care physician, psychiatrist, psychologist, and any other health care professional with whom you are working in order to make the best decision for yourself.

Although it is clearly beyond the scope of this short section to provide you with all of the information on psychotropic medications, the following is a brief summary of the major groups of those medications, including the names of some commonly used medications, what they're generally used for, and some possible side effects.

ANTI-ANXIETY MEDICATIONS

Three commonly used groups of medications are used to treat anxiety: benzodiazepines, buspirone (BuSpar), and antidepressants. Barbiturates, such as phenobarbital, were once commonly used to treat anxiety, but because of their highly addictive and dangerous nature, their usage is more limited now.

Benzodiazepines are minor tranquilizers that induce sleep and relax muscles by increasing the effects of *gamma-aminobutyric acid (GABA)*, a neurotransmitter that inhibits the responsiveness of the central nervous system (CNS). The use of benzodiazepines must be monitored because sometimes they can lead to both physical and psychological dependence as well as to an increased tolerance of their effects. The risk of overdosing on benzodiazepines is not as great as that of barbiturates. However, benzodiazepines still can be deadly when used simultaneously with alcohol or barbiturates. Benzodiazepines generally start working thirty minutes to four hours after taking them.[9]

Among the more commonly experienced side effects are drowsiness, decreased mental functioning, and decreased coordination. Benzodiazepine usage should never be stopped abruptly. Doing so may lead to withdrawal symptoms, such as difficulty sleeping, nervousness, headaches, ringing in your ears, restlessness, depression, and sensory confusion.[10] For that reason, you should always consult the medical professional who prescribed your medication before stopping your use.

Among the more common benzodiazepines are the following: alprazolam (Xanax), chlordiazepoxide (Librium, Mitran, Libritabs), clonazepam (Klonopin), clorazepate (Tranxene), diazepam (Valium), flurazepam (Dalmane), halazepam (Paxipam), lorazepam (Ativan), oxazepam (Serax), prazepam (Centrax), quazepam (Doral), temazepam (Restoril), and triazolam (Halcion).

Buspirone (BuSpar) is an atypical anti-anxiety medication. This means that it decreases your anxiety level without inducing sleep and muscle relaxation, as do barbiturates and benzodiazepines. Although it's not clear exactly how buspirone works, one theory holds that it affects the neurotransmitters serotonin[11] and dopamine.[9] One of the main advantages of buspirone is that it isn't physically or psychologically addictive. In addition, it poses little danger of overdosing and it has few interactions with other medications, although alcohol should still be avoided when taking it. Common side effects include dizziness and headaches, and the full effects of buspirone usually take three to six weeks to begin.

Among the more commonly used antidepressant medications used to treat anxiety and anxiety disorders (such as obsessive-compulsive disorder, panic disorder, and posttraumatic stress disorder) are citalopram (Celexa), clomipramine (Anafranil), escitalopram (Lexapro), fluoxetine (Prozac), fluvoxamine (Luvox), paroxetine (Paxil), sertraline (Zoloft), and venlafaxine (Effexor). These will be discussed in more detail below.

ANTIDEPRESSANT MEDICATIONS

There are four groups of medications used to treat depression: selective serotonin reuptake inhibitors, atypical antidepressants, tricyclic antidepressants, and monoamine oxidase inhibitors.

Selective serotonin reuptake inhibitors (SSRIs) are the most popular choices of antidepressants on the market,[9] and are considered to be the first-line of treatment. They were developed in the 1980s. As their name suggests, SSRIs increase the levels of the neurotransmitter serotonin. For some SSRIs, like fluoxetine (Prozac), the full benefits of the medication may take as long as six to eight weeks to be experienced. Although the risk of overdosing on SSRIs is very low, there are a number of other possible side effects. These include headaches, dizziness, stomach problems, nervousness, sleep problems, weight gain, and sexual performance problems.

Another potentially fatal, but rare, problem is *serotonin syndrome*, caused by an excessive amount of serotonin in your body. This is sometimes caused by taking SSRIs in conjunction with other serotonin-increasing medications, such as other prescriptions or the herb Saint-John's-wort. The symptoms include increased heart rate, headaches, agitation, excessive perspiration, confusion, excessive elation, and abnormally high body temperature. Immediate medical attention is always needed to treat serotonin syndrome.

SSRI use should not be stopped abruptly. Doing so may lead to headaches, agitation, upset stomach, dizziness, inability to sleep, visual problems, problems with moving, and upset mood.[12] Among the more common SSRIs are: citalopram (Celexa), escitalopram (Lexapro), fluoxetine (Prozac), fluvoxamine (Luvox), paroxetine (Paxil), and sertraline (Zoloft).

Atypical antidepressants are newer medications that work in unique ways. Venlafaxine (Effexor) and duloxetine (Cymbalta) increase the levels of the neurotransmitters serotonin and norepinephrine. Some reports found that venlafaxine can act quickly,[13, 14] but it usually takes two or more weeks to begin working. Side effects, however, such as severe nausea, are possible. An extended release version of venlafaxine is now available, which lessens some of the side effects and makes once-a-day dosing possible. Other possible side effects include dry mouth, perspiration, sleepiness, dizziness, and constipation.

Bupropion (Wellbutrin) is another atypical antidepressant that is thought to increase the levels of the neurotransmitters norepinephrine and dopamine.[15] It's not recommended for people with a history of seizures or eating disorders, because excessively high dosages can result in seizures and an excessively fast heart rate. However, bupropion is sometimes used as an aid to quit smoking. Common side effects include irritability, headaches, upset stomach, and an inability to sleep. Related sexual performance problems and weight gain problems are often lower with bupropion than with other antidepressants. Extended-release and sustained-release versions make once-a-day and twice-a-day dosing possible.

Mirtazapine (Remeron) is another atypical antidepressant that increases the levels of serotonin and norepinephrine. Like nefazodone, mirtazapine may also increase restful sleep and decrease anxiety. Possible side effects include weight gain, an increase in appetite, sleepiness, and dizziness. As a rule, mirtazapine lacks the sexual side effects of some other antidepressants. Once-a-day dosages are possible, but the full effects of the medication may take several weeks to experience, as with most of the other antidepressants.

Tricyclic antidepressants (TCAs) are often used after multiple attempts to use SSRIs and atypical antidepressants have failed. TCAs were developed in the late 1950s and the name refers to their chemical structure. Like SSRIs, TCAs are a family of related antidepressants. TCAs increase the levels of the neurotransmitter serotonin and/or norepinephrine, but they aren't used as a first-line treatment for depression because they also create a number of serious side effects.

Commonly called *anticholinergic effects*, these side effects typically include dry mouth, visual problems, constipation, urination problems, heart problems, and light-headedness, especially when getting out of bed or getting up from a seated position. Other possible side effects include drowsiness, nervousness, confusion, irritability, inability to sleep, hallucinations, and nightmares.

TCAs also pose a danger for overdosing, which can be deadly. TCAs should not be stopped abruptly, as this may cause stomach problems, headaches, chills, and perspiration. Many other medications have dangerous interactions with TCAs, so make sure you speak with your medical doctor before taking anything you haven't already asked about, and also be aware that TCAs typically take four to six weeks to take effect.

Some of the common TCAs include: amitriptyline (Elavil), clomipramine (Anafranil), desipramine (Norpramin), doxepin (Sinequan, Triadapin), imipramine (Tofranil), nortriptyline (Aventyl, Pamelor), protriptyline (Triptil, Vivactil), and trimipramine (Surmontil).

Finally, the last group of antidepressants are the oldest group, *monoamine oxidase inhibitors* (MAOIs). MAOIs were developed in the 1950s, and they too help increase the levels of serotonin, norepinephrine, and dopamine. Although they can be effective at treating some types of difficult depression, the potential side effects of MAOIs, coupled with their necessary dietary restrictions, often outweigh the benefits of their use. They also pose a danger for overdosing, which can be deadly. As with the other antidepressants, the response time can be ten days to four weeks from the time you take your first dose.

Possible side effects include anticholinergic effects, such as dry mouth, visual problems, constipation, urination problems, heart problems, and low blood pressure. In addition, other possible effects include nervousness, inability to sleep, excessive elation, and agitation. Many other medications have dangerous interactions with MAOIs, so make sure you speak with your medical doctor before taking anything you haven't already asked about. Foods that are rich in tyramine also need to be avoided.

Tyramine is a naturally occurring chemical that can raise your blood pressure. Eating foods with tyramine can lead to elevated blood pressure and strokes. These foods include certain kinds of alcohol, aged cheese (blue, Brie, cheddar, mozzarella), sour cream, yogurt, chicken liver, certain meats like salami and sausage, caffeine (tea, coffee, colas), chocolate, and more. If you're prescribed MAOIs, make sure you understand your doctor's instructions about what foods are allowed. He or she should give you a list of foods to avoid. Make sure you follow it carefully. Among the more commonly prescribed MAOIs are: moclobemide (Manerix), phenelzine (Nardil), selegiline (Eldepryl), and tranylcypromine (Parnate).

ANTIMANIA MEDICATIONS

Antimania medications are often called "mood stabilizers." The most common is lithium (Eskalith, Lithobid), a naturally occurring substance. It's not exactly clear how it reduces mood swings, but lithium generally begins to lessen symptoms of mania within one to three weeks, although it may take longer to fully control your mania. It's reported to be effective in as many as 60 to 80 percent of the patients treated.[9, 16] People taking lithium, however, must have their blood monitored regularly. This is done to avoid high, toxic levels of lithium.

Hand tremors are one of the most common side effects of lithium. Other possible side effects include weight gain, fatigue, nausea, general weakness, excessive thirst, or excessive urination. However, many of these lessen in severity, disappear, or are treatable with additional medication. Lithium can also affect thyroid functioning, although problems occur rarely,[16] so this needs to be monitored as well.

Someone taking lithium also needs to be cautious of substances and activities that may lower the level of salt in the body, and therefore raise the level of lithium to a potentially toxic amount. These potentially dangerous activities include lowering the amount of salt you usually use in your diet, sweating excessively from too much exercise, having a fever, spending an excessive amount of time in a hot climate, taking certain medications, and becoming dehydrated from excessive vomiting or diarrhea.

Be sure to talk with your medical provider about the specific details of these circumstances, and if you experience symptoms of lithium overdose, get immediate medical attention. These symptoms include vomiting, nausea, excessive tremors, dizziness, blurry vision, confusion, fatigue, irregular heartbeat, and seizures.[17] Women who are pregnant or planning to get pregnant should discuss the use of lithium with their doctors. Some evidence suggests that the use of lithium during pregnancy can result in certain birth defects and complications,[9, 16, 17] although this happens very rarely.

Valproic acid (Depakene) and divalproex sodium (Depakote) are medications used to treat seizures that are also approved by the FDA to treat mania and are reported to be well-tolerated.[18, 19] Possible side effects include tiredness, nausea, vomiting, weight gain, and tremors. However, these can often be reversed or controlled with a change in dosage. A smaller number of patients may also experience temporary hair loss or increased appetite.

Valproic acid is often used to treat patients when lithium has proven ineffective. Women who are pregnant or planning to become pregnant should talk to their doctors about possible birth defects associated with the use of this medication.[20] In addition, young women should speak with their doctors about the potential dangers of polycystic ovary syndrome as a possible result of using valproic acid.[21]

Carbamazepine (Equetro, Tegretol) is another antiseizure medication that has proven effective for the treatment of mania.[22] Typical side effects include nausea, vomiting, sleepiness, dizziness, difficulty moving, and difficulties with vision.[23]

ANTIPSYCHOTIC MEDICATIONS

The medications used to treat schizophrenia and other psychoses can be divided into two groups: traditional and atypical medications. *Antipsychotic medications* are also known as "neuroleptics" or "major tranquilizers" because they have a very calming effect on people who take them. The medications often cause sleepiness, emotional soothing, and a lessening of agitation. Both classes of medication reduce the level of the neurotransmitter dopamine, and some atypicals also reduce the level of serotonin.

Both traditional and atypical medications lessen the severity of hallucinations, lessen delusions, and calm disturbed thinking. The newer atypical medications may also improve symptoms such as low energy, lack of emotion, lack of expression, and lack of interest. The time it takes the medications to begin working varies from person to person and from medication to medication. Generally, improvements can be seen in as little as a few weeks to a few months.[17]

But, remember, you need to continue taking your medications even after your symptoms improve in order to control your illness. A very common problem with all antipsychotic medications is that patients often stop taking them, because of side effects or other reasons,[24] which often leads to a relapse of symptoms. One alternative might be *depot* medications, which are injectable medications that can be taken once every few weeks, instead of oral medications that need to be taken every day.

Medication is the most important treatment for schizophrenia,[25] and it's often very effective despite the unpleasant side effects. A long-term study comparing the effectiveness of one traditional and one atypical medication found that almost 75 percent of the patients using either medication experienced clinical improvements, some within only three weeks.[26]

Among the more commonly prescribed traditional antipsychotic medications are: chlorpromazine (Thorazine), fluphenazine (Prolixin, Permitil), haloperidol (Haldol), loxapine (Loxitane), mesoridazine (Serentil), molindone (Moban), prochlorperazine (Compazine), perphenazine (Trilafon), thioridazine (Mellaril), thiothixene (Navane), and trifluoperazine (Stelazine). The dosage of these medications needs to be carefully monitored because they can cause *extrapyramidal* side effects, which include involuntary muscle spasms, difficulty moving, fidgeting, shaking that resembles Parkinson's disease, and *tardive dyskinesia*, an involuntary movement of the face, mouth, tongue, arms, and legs. If you experience signs of tardive dyskinesia, you should contact the medical professional who prescribed your medication as soon as possible. These symptoms can be controlled with early changes to your medication.

Among the more commonly prescribed atypical antipsychotic medications are: aripiprazole (Abilify), clozapine (Clozaril), olanzapine (Zyprexa), quetiapine (Seroquel), risperidone (Risperdal), and ziprasidone (Geodon). These medications pose less risk for extrapyramidal side effects and tardive dyskinesia, but some of them do pose a risk for anticholinergic effects, such as dry mouth, visual problems, constipation, urination problems, heart problems, and low blood pressure. Weight gain and sexual performance problems are also possible. People taking clozapine also need to have their blood monitored regularly to prevent *agranulocytosis*, a decrease of white blood cells that can lead to fatal infections.

All antipsychotic medications, but particularly traditional medications, pose an additional risk for a potentially lethal condition called *neuroleptic malignant syndrome*. If you experience either muscle rigidity or tremors and a high fever, with possible confusion, especially within the first few weeks of taking your medication, seek immediate medical attention and make the attending professionals aware of your medication. Also, be aware that many other medications interfere with the effectiveness of antipsychotic medications, so be sure to check with your medical provider before taking anything additional.

For more information, visit the Web sites of:

. The American Psychiatric Association: www.psych.org and www.healthyminds.org

MINDFULNESS THERAPY

Mindfulness therapy uses meditation and other techniques to help you focus your attention and build greater acceptance of yourself.[1] This type of treatment borrows much of its philosophy and methods from Buddhist traditions, which use meditative practices to cultivate awareness, insight, and freedom from suffering.[2] From a Western perspective, mindfulness techniques can also help you let go of thoughts and feelings that cause pain.[3]

Meditation helps focus your attention on what you're experiencing and thinking in the present moment.[1] By doing that, it also helps you become more aware of your immediate thoughts, feelings, and actions. This type of concentration takes practice, but it can have many benefits. Focusing on the present moment allows you to disengage from repetitious and painful thoughts about the past and future.[3] It also gives you space to step back from your experience and understand what's really happening in a clearer way. This insight can then help you make a choice about how to act in the immediate moment instead of relying on automatic, habitual reactions.

There are two popular forms of mindfulness therapy. The first is *mindfulness-based stress reduction*.[4, 5] This treatment was originally designed to help hospital patients reduce their levels of stress and pain by using meditation techniques and yoga. It's usually taught in an eight- to ten-week course, but you'll also be expected to practice the techniques on a daily basis at home, by yourself. The techniques used in this treatment focus on your breathing and the feelings in your body. When distractions arise, you'll be instructed to notice the distractions without getting hooked into them or forming any opinions about them. You'll also be instructed not to judge yourself for becoming distracted.

A similar treatment is called *mindfulness-based cognitive therapy*,[6] which also incorporates elements of cognitive behavioral therapy to help you observe your experiences, thoughts, and emotions. And again, one of the key goals is to help you observe your experiences without making judgments about them.

Of the many results that are possible, mindfulness techniques like these often lead to a greater tolerance of distressing situations, greater relaxation, a change in thinking styles, the development of less judgmental views of yourself and your experiences, and an increase in skills to cope with difficult situations.[7] In studies, mindfulness therapy has resulted in positive effects on the immune system;[8] reduced chronic pain;[9, 10] decreased binge eating;[11] lessened stress in cancer patients;[12, 13] decreased repetitive, sad thinking in depressed patients;[14] and reduced odds of having another major depressive episode.[15]

For more information, visit the Web site of:

· The Center for Mindfulness: www.umassmed.edu/cfm

POSITIVE PSYCHOLOGY

Positive psychology is a relatively new form of psychotherapy that focuses on a person's strengths and virtues.[1] It's meant to complement and balance other types of psychotherapy that largely focus on the treatment of problems and deficits.[2] One of the goals of positive psychology is to help you create a happier, more fulfilling life, and to reach your greatest potential. Another goal is to explore how focusing on positive strengths in your life can help you maintain psychological health and possibly prevent mental health problems like depression and anxiety.

In an attempt to create a cross-cultural list of virtues, one group of positive psychologists studied the values of ancient philosophies from both Asia and the West.[3] Among the common virtues found were wisdom, courage, humanity, justice, temperance, and transcendence, which refers to beliefs and actions that help explain the meaning of life. By exploring these qualities with you, a psychotherapist using positive psychology hopes to help you build strengths and skills, such as creativity, hope, love, bravery, fairness, humor, kindness, forgiveness, gratitude, and authenticity.[1]

There's been some evidence that cultivating these strengths may be good for your health as well. For example, research has suggested that higher levels of hope,[4] altruism,[5] and optimism[6, 7] can improve both your physical and mental health. In addition, happiness[8, 9] and the expression of positive emotions[10, 11] have been associated with longer, healthier, and more fulfilling lives.

Studies of positive psychology techniques have demonstrated that simple treatment exercises can have dramatic effects. One study found that activities such as utilizing your strengths on a daily basis, delivering a letter to thank someone, and recording three good things that happened to you each day can increase happiness and decrease symptoms of depression for as long as six months.[12] Other techniques used in positive psychology include writing, meditation, and getting out into nature.[2]

For more information, visit the Web site of:

· The Positive Psychology Center: www.ppc.sas.upenn.edu

PSYCHOANALYSIS/PSYCHODYNAMIC THERAPY

Psychoanalysis was the first form of psychotherapy, originally created in the late nineteenth century by Sigmund Freud (1856–1939), an Austrian medical doctor and biological researcher. Freud based his treatment on what he found to be helpful for his clients, and like all good scientists, he consistently revised his theories when he was presented with new evidence that didn't fit with his older ideas. As a result, psychoanalysis is a treatment that has undergone much revision, by both Freud and his later followers. It's also a theory that is defined differently by the different mental health care professionals who practice it. As a result, there's no single explanation of what psychoanalytic treatment is.

Mental health care professionals who use this form of treatment are called *psychoanalysts*. Some of them have abandoned a number of Freud's earlier ideas, such as the *Oedipus complex* (the belief that a child sexually desires their opposite-sex parent), while other professionals have retained some of those ideas. Today it's common for many mental health professionals to refer to the treatment they use as "psychodynamic therapy," in order to differentiate themselves from some of the earlier forms of psychoanalysis. But, regardless of the debate over the differences between psychoanalysis and psychodynamic treatments, it's probably sufficient for someone entering one of these treatments to know the basic principles on which both are based.

One widely held principle emphasizes the key role of the unconscious mind. According to psychoanalysis, your thoughts, beliefs, and awareness work in a multilayered way. Some thoughts are fully within your awareness and are called conscious thoughts. Those thoughts that are almost within your awareness are called preconscious thoughts. And some thoughts are beyond your awareness; they are called your unconscious thoughts.

Many psychoanalysts also believe that the mind is organized according to the roles it plays in problem solving. This is famously known as the id, ego, and superego division.[1] The *id* represents your instinctual needs and impulses. The *superego* is often thought of as the parental rule-maker, which imposes morality and standards. And the *ego* is left to make decisions based on the needs of both the id and the superego, while also dealing with the requirements of your conscious reality.

According to one of Freud's later theories,[2] anxiety arises when an unpleasant thought or idea attempts to rise from the level of unconsciousness to the conscious level of your awareness. At this point, the ego employs a series of defenses to keep the thought hidden, and thus avoid conflict. Among the more commonly used defenses is *repression*, which keeps a thought blocked in your unconscious. For example, suppose a woman unconsciously wants a divorce, even though she won't consciously admit it. As a result, each time someone mentions "divorce" she unknowingly represses the thought and changes the subject, or perhaps she completely forgets entire conversations that focus on the issue.

Another principle of this treatment states that the origin of mental health problems often lies in childhood. According to psychoanalysis, children pass through unique developmental phases that are related to different biological functions, such as breastfeeding and toilet training. It's believed that if you experience difficulties during one of these phases, and have problems getting your needs met, you'll later develop problems related to that phase. Equally damaging can be the way you are mistreated in childhood by a parent, family member, or other person.

Many psychoanalysts believe in the influence of unconscious drives or instincts that also guide your life. One of the most common is the drive to seek pleasure, called the *libido*. Other psychoanalysts believe that all of your thoughts, feelings, and actions are determined by your past experiences. Nothing happens by accident, according to this belief, and if you look hard enough, with the help of a psychoanalyst, you can figure out what happened in your past that caused you to act the way you do in the present.

Psychoanalysts also use specific methods of treatment in session. Some clients are surprised when they enter psychoanalysis because their analyst is very quiet and doesn't say much or offer any advice on how to fix their problem. Instead, most psychoanalysts will allow you to talk in a very free and unguided way. This is called *free association*. Later, when the psychoanalyst has heard enough information to make an informed observation, he or she will then interpret what is happening in your life. By doing this, the psychoanalyst is trying to help you become aware of your unconscious thoughts and the defenses you are using to avoid resolving conflicts.

It's also common for psychoanalysts to talk about the relationship you have with them, in order to examine the problems you may have in your other personal relationships. For example, a client will often treat the psychoanalyst in the same way that the client treated a parent. This is called *transference*. When this occurs, your psychoanalyst will inform you in order to help you resolve the unsettled conflict that you might have had with your parent.

Many psychoanalysts will also frequently ask their patients to discuss their dreams. Early in his career, Freud stated that the best way to discover the unconscious thoughts of a client, and possibly the origin of the client's problem, was to investigate the client's dreams, because that is where Freud believed unconscious desires are most freely expressed.[3]

In addition to psychoanalysis and psychodynamic therapy, many related treatments share similar principles but focus on different elements. For example, *object relations therapy* emphasizes the relationships a person has and how those relationships are internalized and handled. And *control mastery therapy* believes that people want to solve their problems and have unconscious plans to do so that need to be discovered.[4]

For more information, visit the Web sites of:

- The American Psychoanalytic Association: www.apsa.org

- The National Association for the Advancement of Psychoanalysis: www.naap.org

- San Francisco Control Mastery Research Group: www.controlmastery.org

RATIONAL EMOTIVE BEHAVIOR THERAPY

Rational emotive behavior therapy (REBT) was created in the 1950s by American psychologist Albert Ellis. REBT is regarded as one of the first forms of cognitive therapy because it examines how your thoughts affect your emotions and behaviors. According to REBT, rational thoughts are healthy thoughts that help you live a more gratifying life, while irrational thoughts get in the way of your growth and happiness.[1]

REBT will help you focus on the present moments of your life. It's acknowledged that your self-defeating, irrational thoughts were formed in the past, but the aim of the treatment is to change how those thoughts are affecting you now. As a memory aid, Ellis developed an "ABCDE" approach to mental health.[2] "A" stands for the actions and activities in your life, which lead to "C," behavioral and emotional consequences or results. However, what determines how you react to those events is "B," your beliefs. Take, for example, the action of a presidential election. The consequence of the election, and your reaction to the results, are determined by your belief about who would make a better leader. If the person you like wins, you're happy. If not, you're disappointed.

To make changes in your life, an REBT therapist will help you dispute ("D") your negative thoughts and rules by looking for evidence that contradicts your irrational beliefs.[2] For example, if you believe, "I'm never going to be any good," your REBT therapist will help you to look for and examine events in your life in which you were successful. An REBT therapist might also help you examine your emotional reactions to a situation, to determine if they're 100 percent accurate. For example, if you're convinced that you're "going to die" if you give a presentation in front of your colleagues, your psychotherapist might help you reexamine that situation, and relabel your emotional experience in a more accurate way. Maybe the presentation invokes a certain degree of fear and nervousness that's absolutely normal and understandable. Such relabeling of your emotions can lead to a new experience ("E") of the event.[2]

In addition to these techniques, REBT utilizes other active treatments such as visualization methods, assertiveness skills training, risk-taking training, and role-playing.

REBT believes that all humans have the same basic goals. These are to maintain their lives, to live in a way that's free from suffering, and to be at least moderately happy. When the results of an activity bring about one of these goals for you, you try to repeat the activity. When consequences of actions lead to pain or dissatisfaction, you try to avoid those actions in the future. Most people experience minor obstacles when trying to achieve their goals. As a result, they feel sad or frustrated.

However, according to REBT, some barriers can cause serious problems in your life if you follow strict rules about how your life is supposed to operate. For example, if you fail a test and you have a rule that says "I should never fail a test," you're going to react to that situation in a severely negative way. Perhaps you will become depressed, sad, or anxious about the next test. Equally damaging are the irrational beliefs that people have about themselves, such as "I'm never going to be any good." This kind of negative thought can lead you from one failure to the next in your life, until the thought is altered.

For more information, visit the Web site of:

· The Albert Ellis Institute: www.rebt.org

SCHEMA-FOCUSED THERAPY

Schema-focused therapy examines the repetitive, dysfunctional patterns of thoughts and relationships that interfere with your life. A *schema* is a strongly held positive or negative belief that you have about yourself, and it is accepted as true, even if a negative schema causes harm or difficulties in your life.[1] The creator of schema-focused therapy, American psychologist Jeffrey Young, has defined some common maladaptive schemas that develop in childhood and persist into adulthood.[1] (See Schema-Focused Relationship Problems, page 104, for detailed descriptions of each individual schema.)

The overall goals of schema-focused therapy are to reduce the strength of your negative schemas, to develop healthier thoughts and feelings about yourself, and to help you engage in healthier behaviors.[2] Schema-focused therapy generally includes two stages of treatment, starting with an exploratory stage. In this beginning phase, you and your psychotherapist will examine your problems and identify the schemas that have been interfering with your life. This may include having you fill out a detailed questionnaire of some common schema problems. Your schema-focused therapist will also help you understand how your early childhood experiences created those beliefs, help you recognize any feelings associated with those beliefs, and assist you in identifying how you've coped with those distressing thoughts and feelings in the past.

Generally, people deal with schema-related problems in three different ways. They avoid the problem, they maintain the problem, or they overcompensate and do the exact opposite of what their schemas tell them to do.[2] Unfortunately, all of these actions only serve to make the schema stronger, and the associated problems worse.

The second phase of treatment focuses on changing the schema and its related behaviors. This includes examining the evidence in your life that supports and refutes your schema. Usually, more evidence can be found to disprove your negative thoughts about yourself, rather than finding evidence that supports them. So, part of treatment also involves creating new, positive thoughts about yourself based on the new evidence.

Schema-focused therapy will also help you get in touch with any childhood pain that might have been caused by these negative thoughts. Part of your treatment might include the use of imaginational exercises to heal those old wounds. You'll also investigate how your schemas affect your current relationships, including your relationship with your psychotherapist. Instead of relying on dysfunctional methods of coping with your schema, your psychotherapist will help you initiate healthier behavioral changes to counteract your old schema patterns. This might include learning new communication skills and relaxation skills, which you'll need to practice in your daily life. Homework is a regular part of schema-focused therapy.

For more information, visit the Web site of:

. The Schema Therapy Institute: www.schematherapy.com

SOMATIC PSYCHOTHERAPIES

Somatic psychotherapies are a category of treatments that emphasize the connection between your body, mind, and emotions. These treatments focus on healing the body in order to provide relief from physical, mental, and emotional pain. *Soma* means "body" in Greek, and often these types of treatments are referred to as body-oriented psychotherapies.

Many of these treatments share the underlying belief that hidden emotions can be experienced and released through body movements and adjustments. This is often accomplished through techniques like massage or deep tissue manipulations, such as *Rolfing*. However, many forms of somatic psychotherapy combine these or similar techniques with general principles of psychotherapy. Often, somatic psychotherapy will include general massage, light physical touch, deep tissue manipulation, relaxation techniques, movement, or exercise.

Like many types of somatic psychotherapies, the *Rosen Method* uses gentle touch to release muscle tension. This process often causes old memories and feelings to reemerge. It's often used to treat pain and frequently used in conjunction with many of the other forms of psychotherapy found in this book. *Hakomi experiential psychotherapy* uses mindfulness techniques to focus your attention on your physical habits and expressions, and then explores painful memories that are often attached to them. *Process-oriented psychology* is based on many principles from Jungian psychotherapy. In addition to focusing on the connection between your mind and body, it also examines your dreams and how they influence your life.

For more information, visit the Web sites of:

· The Rosen Institute: www.rosenmethod.org

· The Hakomi Institute: www.hakomiinstitute.com

· The Process Work Institute: www.processwork.org

TRANSPERSONAL PSYCHOLOGY

Transpersonal psychology is a treatment that combines psychotherapy with spiritual principles and beliefs. However, this treatment is different than religious counseling, which emphasizes the doctrine of one particular faith. A transpersonal psychologist will often borrow spiritual and religious teachings from many faiths, including Buddhism, Christianity, Judaism, Sufism, Hinduism, and even agnosticism.

Transpersonal means to go beyond individual experience and existence. This includes recognizing the connection between all people, all things, and ultimately the connection between you and the divine, or you and God.[1] To do this, according to transpersonal psychology, you must move beyond traditional conscious experiences and traditional ways of knowing. Transpersonal psychology respects many nontraditional means of gaining information, such as intuition, psychic phenomena, and spiritual, religious, or mystical experiences. Among the goals many transpersonal therapists share is the goal of helping you find the purpose of your life, as well as the purposes of events that appeared to happen to you accidentally.[2]

Another goal is to help you find a connection between your body, mind, and spirit. Many transpersonal psychologists believe that the psychological, spiritual, and emotional development of each person is part of the bigger evolution of the human species and the universe as a whole.[3] And, according to at least one influential transpersonal theorist, spiritual development is the ultimate purpose of life and the true aim of transpersonal psychology.[2]

As with other models of psychotherapy highlighted in this book, there isn't just one form of transpersonal psychology. Many transpersonal psychotherapists utilize meditation techniques and methods of prayer, but they may also use techniques from other types of psychotherapy.

For more information, visit the Web site of:

. The Association for Transpersonal Psychology: www.atpweb.org

A Final Word About Making Sense of the Treatment

Whatever form of psychotherapy or medication you decide to use, it's important that you give the process a reasonable amount of time to start working. This holds true whether you're using a treatment that's been recommended in this book, or whether you're using a treatment that just sounds interesting to you. Change takes time. Later, in chapter 5, Making Sense of the Process, you'll be told how to evaluate if your treatment is working for you, and what to do if it's not. But, for now, just be aware that your treatment might take longer than you'd like it to, but also remember that you've already taken the first steps by reading this book. Now, turn to the next chapter, Making Sense of the Mental Health Care Professionals, to learn more about the different clinicians you might be contacting in the future.

CHAPTER 4

MAKING SENSE OF THE MENTAL HEALTH CARE PROFESSIONALS

The good life is a process, not a state of being. It is a direction not a destination.

—Carl Rogers*

Who Are They?

Mental health care professionals are the people you'll meet when you seek treatment for your mental health problem. In general, they can be categorized into a few groups. Medical doctors and psychiatrists are medically trained professionals who can prescribe medications. Psychologists are nonmedical doctors trained in psychotherapy and psychological testing. Master's level counselors also provide psychotherapy but have less training than psychologists. Social workers can also provide psychotherapy but, traditionally, they use a case management style to enlist support for a person. Advanced practice nurses, such as nurse practitioners, can also prescribe medications in some states and some of them, who specialize in the treatment of mental health problems, also provide psychotherapy. And, finally, there are a number of other treatment providers whose help you might seek in the treatment of your problem, such as a hypnotherapist or spiritual counselor.

All of these professionals who specialize in the treatment of mental health problems can call themselves *psychotherapists*. This is a general term and it shouldn't be confused with psychologist, psychiatrist, or others. Also, be aware that many of these

---

*   From *On Becoming a Person*. 1961. Boston: Houghton Mifflin.

professionals often work together when treating someone. For example, you might have a psychiatrist who prescribes your medication and a psychologist who provides your psychotherapy. Or, you might have a nurse practitioner who treats your physical health problem, a social worker who helps you with a substance abuse issue, and a marriage and family therapist who provides your family with counseling. These types of situations are common, and the fact that you're working with one of these professionals doesn't exclude the possibility that you also can work with another.

MEDICAL DOCTORS/PSYCHIATRISTS (MD, DO)

Medical doctors (MD) and *doctors of osteopathy* (DO) are medically trained professionals who treat health problems and can prescribe medications. Often, people will consult their primary care provider for the treatment of their mental health problem. As a rule, this is a good place to start. Your *primary care provider* (PCP) is a general clinician who is trained to recognize and diagnose mental health problems, and he or she can prescribe medications for their treatment.

However, *psychiatrists* are medical doctors who specialize in the treatment of mental health problems and they are often more up-to-date about the best medications available for complex problems. It is likely that your PCP will refer you to a psychiatrist for more specialized treatment, or you can ask your PCP for a referral. Some psychiatrists also offer psychotherapy as part of their treatment, but often they are more costly than visits with psychologists or master's level counselors. Other psychiatrists offer only medications and will sometimes refer to themselves as *psychopharmacologists*. If you're seeing your psychiatrist solely for medications, you should expect to see him or her as seldom as once every few months to monitor your prescription. You should also expect that during those follow-up visits, your psychiatrist may spend as little as twenty minutes with you, checking on your progress.

In general, you should seek help from a medical doctor or psychiatrist if:

- You're considering the use of medications to treat your mental health problem, or you're currently on medication and it needs to be adjusted, due to side effects or the fact that it isn't working.

- You're looking for a referral to a specialist, such as a psychiatrist, psychologist, or other mental health care professional.

- You have a medical problem that you suspect is causing your mental health problem or interacting with it. For example, perhaps you have a thyroid condition and you're experiencing symptoms of depression or bipolar disorder, or you have a heart condition and you are experiencing panic attacks.

- You need to be admitted to a hospital for the treatment of your mental health problem, either due to its severity or because you are a danger to yourself or others.

- You want a general checkup to rule out any undiagnosed physical problems. For anyone experiencing any kind of physical or mental health problem, this is always a good place to start.

PSYCHOLOGISTS (PH.D., PSY.D., ED.D.)

Psychologists are nonmedically trained doctors who are experts in psychotherapy and can diagnose mental health problems, often by using psychological testing. Psychologists cannot prescribe medications—with the exception of specially trained psychologists in Louisiana and New Mexico, who gain this privilege by receiving additional training in psychopharmacology.

Psychologists earn doctoral degrees in philosophy (Ph.D.), psychology (Psy.D.), and education (Ed.D.), but the differences between the degrees are minimal for the sake of this summary. All of these professionals receive extensive training in graduate school and supervised clinical internships in which they learn to recognize, diagnose, and treat mental health problems using one or more forms of psychotherapy.

Psychologists commonly treat individuals, couples, and families. However, many psychologists specialize in the use of one of the modalities found in this resource, such as cognitive behavioral therapy and they may also specialize in the treatment of a particular problem, such as depression. You can find a psychologist who specializes in a treatment and a specific mental health problem by contacting your state or county psychological association, some of which are listed in the appendix in the back of this book.

Psychologists are also the only professionals qualified to perform psychological testing called *assessments*. These tests are often performed when a person has a complex problem that is difficult to diagnose. Other neuropsychological tests are performed when a person has a head injury and the extent of the impairment needs to be diagnosed. Most psychologists who provide psychotherapy see their clients on a regular basis, such as once a week, and most sessions last an average of fifty minutes. Psychologists who provide testing see their clients for one or more sessions lasting a few hours each.

In general, you should seek help from a psychologist if:

- You're seeking psychotherapy for any mental health problem, especially complex ones, such as depression, anxiety, trauma, substance abuse, and obsessive-compulsive disorder.

- You're seeking an expert in a particular type of psychotherapy, such as cognitive behavioral therapy or dialectical behavior therapy.

- You're seeking psychological testing to determine the nature of your problem.

- You're seeking neuropsychological testing to determine the extent of impairment from an injury.

- You're seeking a mental health care professional who specializes in the treatment of a particular population, such as a *geropsychologist* who assists the elderly, a sports psychologist who treats athletes, or a health psychologist who specializes in treating people with medical problems.

MASTER'S LEVEL COUNSELORS (MFT, MA)

Master's level counselors are psychotherapists who specialize in the treatment of relationships. For example, marriage and family therapists (MFT) receive specialized training in graduate school for working with couples and families. Most of these professionals, however, also treat individuals. Many MFTs have private practices and, more commonly, they're being hired to work in hospitals. Other professionals with master's degrees (MA) in psychology can also provide counseling, but in limited settings such as schools and social services. Most master's level counselors have not received the amount of specialized training that psychologists have received, nor can they administer psychological testing in most cases. However, master's level counselors generally charge less than psychologists and psychiatrists for their services.

In general, you should seek help from a master's level counselor if:

- You're seeking couples or family counseling.

- You're seeking individual counseling and you need competent, affordable help, or you have a nonspecific problem and need to talk to someone about your feelings.

SOCIAL WORKERS (MSW, LCSW)

Social workers can provide psychotherapy but, generally, their training focuses on case management skills to help people gather social and economic support. People with master's degrees in social work (MSW) and licensed clinical social work (LCSW) are often experts in how issues like poverty, physical abuse, substance abuse, domestic violence, illness, unemployment, educational problems, disability, and other stressors affect individuals, families, and communities. Social workers can treat families and individuals in private practice, hospitals, clinics, community programs, social services, schools, and other institutions.

In general, you should seek help from a social worker if:

- You're in need of gathering resources or social support to treat your problem.

- You're seeking family therapy.

- You're seeking individual counseling and need competent, affordable help, or you have a nonspecific problem and need to talk to someone about your feelings.

- You're already receiving support through a community program or social service.

ADVANCED PRACTICE NURSES

Advanced practice nurses, such as nurse practitioners (NP), can often serve as your primary care provider (PCP) in both private practice and hospital settings. They are registered nurses (RN) who have completed master's degrees and can diagnose, treat, and often prescribe medication for all of your health care needs. Like an MD, an NP might be the first person you seek help from for your mental health problem. In many cases, your advanced practice nurse will provide you with a referral for specialized treatment. However, all advanced practice nurses are trained to recognize and treat many common mental health problems, and some specialize in treating more complicated mental health problems by providing psychotherapy in addition to medications.

In general, you should seek help from an advanced practice nurse if:

· You're already working with one as your PCP and you need continuing help.

· You need a referral to a specialist, such as a psychiatrist, psychologist, or other mental health care provider.

· You're considering the use of medications to treat your mental health problem, and your advanced practice nurse can prescribe medications.

· You have a medical problem that you suspect is either causing your mental health problem or interacting with it.

· You want a general checkup to rule out any undiagnosed physical problems.

OTHER COUNSELING OPTIONS

Despite the large number of licensed health care professionals, many people often seek help from other nonlicensed counselors. This is sometimes done because a counselor comes highly recommended or because of personal beliefs. Either way, you should always be cautious when seeking help for a serious mental health problem from someone with limited training in the treatment of that problem. Always ask the counselor about his or her training and experience with your problem, and if you aren't satisfied with the answer, seek help from a professional.

Among the most common people who are sought for advice are *spiritual counselors*. In general, you should seek help from a counselor from your spiritual tradition if:

- You're hoping to use your tradition or religion as a framework for your problem.

- You're hoping to use principles from your tradition to guide your decisions and clarify your values.

Hypnotherapists are also popular choices for some treatments. Many hypnotherapists are also licensed professionals with some other degree, such as a Ph.D. in psychology. However, some hypnotherapists are merely laypeople who have taken a training course. In general, hypnotherapists are not licensed by any state licensing board; some are certified only by the programs in which they trained. Again, be sure to ask about the person's professional qualifications and experience treating problems such as yours. In general, you should seek help from a hypnotherapist if:

- Research suggests that your problem might be improved with the use of hypnotherapy.

Life coaches are also becoming increasingly popular. These are nonlicensed and often noncertified tutors who can help you explore your goals in life and increase your motivation. However, they do not treat mental health problems. In general, you should seek help from a life coach if:

- You're seeking help changing careers or looking for motivation in your life.

A Final Word About Choosing a Mental Health
Care Professional

Many people in times of need seek help from their friends and family for support, advice, and shared experiences. Although this can often be helpful, it will benefit you to be aware of your friends' limitations, expectations, and biases, and for you to recognize when you should seek help from someone more qualified to treat your problem. Seeking help for a mental health issue can be a major commitment. So, to make the best use of your time, money, and other resources, use the guidelines in this chapter to help you choose the most appropriate type of mental health care professional. Then, in chapter 5, you'll learn how to find the professional you're looking for and how to interview that person, so that you can be sure that he or she is the best match for your needs.

CHAPTER 5

MAKING SENSE OF THE PROCESS

Anyone who has never made a mistake has never tried anything new.
—Attributed to Albert Einstein

By this point, hopefully, you have a better, more educated understanding about the mental health problem you're struggling with, and you have been able to make a decision about the kind of treatment you'd like to pursue. Now, you need to find the right mental health care professional to help you. The following questions and answers will guide you in finding the best help for your mental health needs.

What Is Your Diagnosis and What Do You Do with It?

Your diagnosis is the guide for your treatment. For example, if you're suffering with depression, the treatment you receive is going to be different than if you're dealing with panic attacks. Your diagnosis also allows one professional, such as your psychologist, to talk with another professional, such as your psychiatrist, in order to convey accurate information about your condition and treatment.

Now that you've used the self-assessment checklist in chapter 1, Making Sense of Your Symptoms, you probably have a better idea about the nature of your problem. However, don't be too quick to label yourself with a diagnosis before seeking the help of a mental health care professional; only he or she can give you the benefit of a professional evaluation.

Chapter 2, Making Sense of Your Problem, gave you suggestions for effective treatments for your problem. By this point, you should have read through the description of those specific treatments in chapter 3, Making Sense of the Treatments, and the descriptions of the different treatment providers in chapter 4, Making Sense of the Mental Health Care Professionals. Being educated about these three elements—diagnosis, treatment, and professional resources—will help you find the best treatment for your problem. With that information you'll be able to make an informed decision about the type of treatment and professional you're going to look for.

You're nearly ready to make your first phone call.

How Do You Find the Right Mental Health Care Professional?

If you don't already have a recommendation for a mental health care provider who offers the type of treatment you're looking for, you can get a referral by:

- Asking your primary care provider.

- Contacting your insurance company.

- Contacting the national, state, or county association that governs the type of professional you're looking for, such as the Alameda County Psychological Association or the California Association of Marriage and Family Therapists. (Check your phone book, the Internet, or appendix B, Additional Contact Information, in the back of this book for some phone numbers.) Contacting an association of professionals who provide the type of treatment that you're looking for, such as the Association for Behavioral and Cognitive Therapies or the EMDR International Association, can also be helpful. (Check the treatment descriptions in chapter 3, Making Sense of the Treatments, for Internet contact information.)

What to Ask When You Call a Mental Health Care Professional the First Time

When you speak with a mental health care professional for the first time, you should briefly explain the nature of your problem and why you're calling. Then, ask a few basic questions, such as:

- "Do you have experience treating problems like mine?"

If the answer is no, ask the person for a referral to someone who does have experience treating your problem.

- "What kinds of treatments do you usually suggest for problems like mine?"

If the suggested treatment is one that you're not familiar with from reading this book, ask the person to give you an idea of what it might involve. If the treatment doesn't sound like something you want to try, ask for a referral to someone else. In addition, if the answer is vague and unfocused, ask for specific steps of the treatment. If the psychotherapist can't describe the treatment very well, he or she may not know it very well. Again, ask for a referral to someone else.

If you are satisfied with the answers to these questions, you should also ask:

· "How much will the treatment cost?" and

· "Do you accept my insurance?"

Most professionals charge per session, and prices vary as much by specialty as they do by state. If you are satisfied with the answers you get, ask to make an appointment.

Do not expect to spend too much time on the phone with the person. You simply want to find out if the mental health care provider has the specific skills you're looking for to treat your problem.

What to Expect in Your First Sessions

Your first session with a psychotherapist or psychiatrist will largely be spent gathering information. Typical sessions last fifty minutes, but some initial sessions can be longer or shorter. Your mental health professional will want to gather as much detailed information as possible about your problem. Afterward, he or she might offer you a diagnosis in the first session or in the next, but if one is not offered, you should ask. You want to know what the person will be treating you for so that you can educate yourself about your problem.

Perhaps your mental health care provider will disagree with the diagnosis you found in this book. If this is the case, ask what information the new diagnosis is based on. Do not be afraid to question the people who are treating you.

After a diagnosis has been made, your mental health care provider should offer and discuss preliminary treatment plans with you. Again, if he or she does not, ask about a treatment plan. Some psychotherapists, such as cognitive behavioral therapists, might even ask you to agree to a treatment plan and sign a contract outlining that plan. This is done so that you are fully prepared for the steps of treatment. However, many other psychotherapists might not offer you a treatment plan unless you ask for one.

In addition to this information-gathering, another very important process takes place during the first sessions of a treatment. This second development is the building of a relationship. Psychotherapy is a very intimate process in which you'll be revealing many aspects of your life to someone you've never met before. If you don't feel comfortable with the person you're working with, the process isn't going to work very well. So, in the first session or two, in addition to assessing the qualifications of the mental health care professional, you should also pay attention to how you feel in the room with that person.

Again, the relationship between you and the mental health care professional is exceptionally important—some would say it's the most important aspect of your treatment. If you don't feel comfortable for some reason, ask the person for a referral to someone else who is qualified to treat your problem. Do your best to be honest. If you can ask for a referral while you're seeing your provider, that's great. But if you feel embarrassed and have to ask over the phone, that's okay too. Just do the best you can. Remember, you deserve to be treated by someone you feel comfortable with and you should never feel forced to stay in a treatment that feels unpleasant.

What Will You Talk About with Your Mental Health Care Professional?

After the initial sessions are spent gathering information, it's quite possible that you and your psychotherapist will talk about anything related to your problem. Depending on the modality of treatment you're working in, you might spend time talking about your early life, your beliefs, your relationships, the activities you do on a regular basis, traumas you've survived, your thoughts about the world, and just about anything else. The goal of all the treatment modalities is to help you solve the problem that brought you into psychotherapy. However, the path you follow to get to that solution can often take you through many different topics, memories, experiences, thoughts, and beliefs.

What Else Will You Do in the Sessions?

Psychotherapy is much more than just talking. All of the forms of psychotherapy outlined in this book use conversation to explore your problem with the goal of helping you come to some resolution. In addition to this, some modalities of treatment, such as interpersonal therapy and cognitive behavioral therapy, will also teach you specific skills to help you change your life. These might include new social skills, communication skills, and coping skills. Moreover, treatments like cognitive behavioral therapy also will require you to do homework on a regular basis. This will help you to monitor your thoughts, feelings, and behaviors outside of session and help you make quicker, more effective changes in your life.

How Do You Know If Your Treatment Is Working?

Every few weeks you should reevaluate the effectiveness of your treatment, whether it's psychotherapy or medications, or a combination of both. If your mental health care provider doesn't suggest this, you should. Make a plan with him or her to reevaluate what's happening after the first eight weeks of treatment. (For medications, this might need to be a little longer.) Collaboratively, decide on a reasonable goal to achieve by that time. Then, if you're not satisfied with your progress in eight weeks, discuss your concerns. Maybe your medications need to be adjusted, or perhaps the form of psychotherapy being used is not the right one for you.

However, be fair in your evaluation. You cannot expect complicated problems to disappear completely in only a matter of weeks. Consider how old you are, how long the problem has been occurring, how deeply ingrained the problem is, and then assume that the treatment will take significant effort to counteract your old patterns. Also, be aware that you can judge the treatment accurately only if you've been attending your sessions regularly and doing what you and your mental health care professional have agreed upon. If you're not doing those things, you're just wasting your time and money. But, if you have been following the treatment and you're still not satisfied, ask your mental health care provider for his or her opinion about what's happening. Again, maybe the treatment needs to be adjusted, or your goals need to be adjusted, or maybe you need to find a different form of treatment.

How Long Do You Need to Stay in Treatment?

Unfortunately, for most mental health problems, there is no simple answer to this question. In general, a good basic rule to follow is this: If you don't notice improvements after six to twelve months in treatment, you should consider an alternate form of treatment or, at least, get a second opinion. But, remember, different problems take different amounts of time to treat, and complex problems can take even longer. Moreover, each person responds differently to both medications and psychotherapy, and some forms of treatment, like psychoanalysis, have no set time limit; whereas cognitive behavioral therapy often uses treatment protocols that specify an eight- to sixteen-week process. Therefore, you need to be your own best judge.

Set goals for yourself with your mental health care provider and when you reach those goals, reevaluate if you want to commit to further treatment. If your goal is to be able to make a public speech without having a panic attack, and you reach that goal, maybe you'll stop treatment. However, perhaps your goal is to treat your post-traumatic stress disorder (PTSD) so that you can sleep at night and stop having nightmares about the automobile accident that caused your PTSD. But when that's accomplished, you might decide that you also want to start driving again, so you may possibly set a new goal.

Ninety-nine percent of the progress and change that takes place in mental health treatment happens slowly, and progress comes in small accomplishments, like dropping coins into a large jar. Those nickels and dimes might not look like much to begin with, but after a few months, you can save enough money to buy yourself something nice.

For some problems, however, the answer to the question about when to stop treatment is different. Chronic biological problems, like schizophrenia and bipolar disorder, require you to continue treatment for the rest of your life. Illnesses such as these demand that you follow a lifelong regimen of medications to control the symptoms. Currently, that is the most effective treatment. As difficult as this might sound, consider that without treatment, the lives of those who have these illnesses are unfulfilling at best, and very painful at worst. However, even the treatment of these illnesses must be modified over time; your prescriptions may have to be adjusted, and your psychotherapy may have to be modified. Again, inform your medical doctor and psychotherapist about how your treatment is working and don't be afraid to ask questions.

What Do You Do If You Think You're Not Getting Better?

If you are not improving, you need to ask yourself some questions:

- Have you have done everything that you and your mental health care professional agreed upon, such as taking your medications regularly, attending sessions regularly, and doing your homework when asked to?

- Has a reasonable amount of time elapsed for the treatment to start working?

- Has the time you set to achieve your treatment goals passed?

Remember, the changes you're trying to make in your life are going to take time. Remember, too, that each person and problem is different, so no one can give you a definite time frame for your improvement. Some changes take months, others take years. But, if you have been making sincere efforts, and you're still not improving, you might need to try something different. Maybe you need to set new goals in treatment. The goals you were aiming for might be too big for you right now. Maybe you need to set smaller, more manageable goals for yourself.

For example, instead of making your goal "Get a new job," how about "Look in the want ads." Instead of "Get rid of my depression," how about "Get out of the house more." As the old adage goes, you need to know how to walk before you can run. And every big goal has many small steps toward its achievement. If you're feeling defeated, talk to your mental health care provider about restating your goals.

If you still think that your treatment isn't working even after you've tried restating your goals, it might be time to try a new form of treatment. If you're using medications, maybe you need to talk to your psychiatrist about trying a new drug. Or, maybe you need to find a new psychiatrist. If you are trying one form of psychotherapy, perhaps it is time to try another. Go back and read through the descriptions of your problem in chapter 2, Making Sense of Your Problem. Take note of the treatments recommended for your problem. See if there's something that you haven't tried yet. If you've been trying psychotherapy and it hasn't been working, perhaps it's time to try some type of medication or a medical procedure. Or, if there's nothing new that's left to try, see whether there's a form of treatment that appeals to you in chapter 3, Making Sense of the Treatments.

Sometimes, the treatment that works best is the one that you believe will help you. But, remember, if you switch forms of psychotherapy, you might also have to switch psychotherapists. Most psychotherapists specialize in just one or two forms of treatment. Changing the person you're working with might be hard for you to do, but it may be necessary. Explain the situation to your psychotherapist; most professionals will understand. Many people see several different psychotherapists over the course of their lifetimes. Finding the right psychotherapist for your problem can be like buying a used car: you have to take it for a test drive before you decide to buy it. And, ethically, your psychotherapist even has an obligation to stop your treatment if it becomes clear to him or her that it isn't working for you. Thus, he or she might be glad to give you a referral to someone who provides the type of treatment you're looking for.

What Are the Ethical Guidelines for Your Treatment?

Each profession (psychiatrist, psychologist, medical doctor, marriage and family therapist, etc.) has its own set of ethical guidelines that governs the treatments provided to you. These guidelines protect you as a consumer of mental health treatment. In general, these ethical principles dictate that patients should be treated fairly by their providers, without discrimination. Mental health care providers should always do their best to help you, while also doing their best not to harm you.

Sexual relationships between mental health care providers and patients are forbidden. In fact, *dual* relationships in general are discouraged, unless they are unavoidable. For instance, it would be frowned upon for a psychologist to provide services to someone he or she knows, because the personal relationship could interfere with the professional relationship. Likewise, social relationships between provider and patient are also not approved.

Professionals are also required to provide only treatments and services for which they have been trained; when a problem requires a treatment they are not qualified to give, they are required to refer you to another professional. They are also required to continue studying in their fields in order to stay current about the newest treatments.

At the beginning of your treatment, your mental health care provider should also give you information about how treatment works, fee information, and have you sign a consent form to begin treatment. In addition, all of your records are to be protected and kept confidential, unless you make a request that they be shared.

What Are Your Rights to Confidentiality?

One of the most important ethical obligations your mental health care professional has is to keep all of your information confidential. This includes your personal information as well as everything you say in session. Your provider should discuss confidentiality and its limits with you, or provide you with information about it, in the first or second session. In general, the information you disclose in session cannot be revealed to anyone without your permission, including your spouse, partner, children, boss, parents, or spiritual leader. If asked, your mental health care professional can't even verify to someone else that you are a patient.

Before your confidential information can be released to anyone, for whatever reason, you will have to sign a release form. For example, this might happen if you're switching psychotherapists and you want your records transferred. In addition, your mental health care provider must make reasonable efforts to keep your confidential records safe and secure.

When Is Your Mental Health Care Professional Required to Break Your Confidentiality?

Although your mental health care provider has an important obligation to keep all of your information private, there are a few instances in which he or she may be forced by law to break your confidentiality. These laws vary from state to state, so be sure to check with your treatment provider about the specific circumstances. In general, however, your mental health care provider may break your confidentiality if:

- You say you're going to kill yourself and you have a plan to do it. Your provider must inform the police to stop you.

- You say that you're going to harm someone else. Your provider must take steps to protect that person, including calling the police and the person.

- You say that you know of a child or adolescent under the age of eighteen who's being harmed. In some states, this also includes certain sexual activities between minors and between minors and adults. In both cases, your provider must notify child protective services.

- You say that you know of a dependent adult who's being harmed, such as someone who is mentally or physically challenged. Your provider must notify family protective services.

- You say that you know of an elderly adult who's being harmed. Your provider must notify adult protective services.

- You're a minor under the age of eighteen. In some cases, your mental health care provider may reveal information to your parents.

- You're seeing a mental health care provider hired by a company to screen you for a job. The provider will make a report to the company.

- You're seeing a mental health care provider hired by a court to screen you for legal reasons, such as child custody. The provider will make a report to the judge.

- Your mental health care provider is ordered by a judge to reveal information about you in court. The provider must oblige.

- Your treatment is being paid for by your insurance. Your provider will send regular reports about your treatment to the insurance company in order to be reimbursed.

Furthermore, since the Patriot Act was passed after September 11, 2001, the federal government has the right to inspect your files if you are suspected of being a threat to national security. And, even if your mental health care provider is aware of your file being inspected, he or she cannot tell you.

What Do You Do If There's Been a Breach of Ethics in Your Treatment?

If your mental health care provider has violated the legal or ethical guidelines that govern your treatment, you should contact your state's governing board for that profession, such as your state's medical or psychological board. Such ethical violations include having sex with your current or former mental health care provider, even if he or she tells you that it's part of your treatment, or that it's okay. No treatment of any kind should ever include sex with your doctor or counselor. If you've been the victim of any type of abusive treatment such as this, contact your state's governing board immediately.

What Are Some Methods of Psychological Testing and When Do You Need It?

There are many different forms of psychological testing, and describing them all is beyond the scope of this book. In general, psychological testing is used to assess the severity of a disorder, personality type, intelligence, neurological problems, cognitive functioning, behavioral functioning, and emotional functioning. Your mental health care provider may refer you for testing if he or she has difficulty diagnosing your problem or if your problem requires specialized treatment. Many people who are hospitalized are given assessment batteries; these are a collection of different tests, used to assess multiple aspects of their functioning.

What Is the DSM?

The descriptions of the illnesses in this book are largely adapted from the *Diagnostic and Statistical Manual of Mental Disorders* (DSM), which is published by the American Psychiatric Association. The DSM is the official handbook of diagnostic criteria used by mental health professionals in the United States and some foreign countries, and it's what your mental health care professional will use to make your diagnosis.

The DSM is arranged by categories, such as substance use disorders, mood disorders, anxiety disorders, and so forth. Each category is then subdivided into specific problems, such as depression and bipolar disorder for mood disorders, and then each problem is described according to the different associated symptoms, such as excessive sadness and hopelessness for depression. Every few years, the DSM is updated with new information to help clinicians make more accurate diagnoses. Some disorders are removed; for example, homosexuality was labeled an illness until 1973. And new disorders are added, such as post-traumatic stress disorder, which was added in 1980.

What Do You Do Now?

My hope is that this book has helped you become a more educated consumer of mental health care services. I also hope that it's helped you better understand the problems you're struggling with and the treatments that offer you the best chances for living a healthier, more fulfilling life.

What you do now might be one of the most important things you ever do in your life: that is, to get help. You may need to review this chapter a few more times before you make your first phone call. Perhaps you're scared about calling. That's understandable. So was I the first time I had to call someone to ask for help. But most of the people you'll find in the field of mental health care are compassionate and good listeners. That's why most of us entered this field in the first place, to help others.

It also might be useful to know that many people in this field have their own psychotherapists with whom they check in regularly. With the stress that comes with this type of job, it's important that professionals also have people to whom they can turn for support.

So what do you do now?

- Review what you've learned about your mental health problem in chapter 2.

- Review what you've learned about the recommended treatments in chapter 3.

- Review what type of mental health care professional you'll be looking for in chapter 4.

- Get a referral for a mental health care professional who provides the type of treatment you're looking for from your primary care provider, your insurance company, someone you trust, or from the reference information in appendix B, Additional Contact Information.

- Review the questions in this chapter that you will ask when you make your first phone call.

- Make the phone call and set up an appointment.

- After that, review the information in this chapter once again so that you can evaluate the progress of your treatment at some point in the near future.

A Final Word About Making Sense of the Process

If you've gotten this far in reading *Getting Help* it shows that you're highly motivated to improve your life, and I have high hopes that you will successfully complete your goal of living a happier, more fulfilling life. No one wants to suffer with a mental health problem. No one chooses to take on the problems that you are struggling with. But, unfortunately, you do have to make the choice to overcome those problems and actively seek help to change your life. That's where most people usually get stuck. But in completing *Getting Help*, you've already taken a major step toward your recovery, and you should feel hopeful about that. Good luck in the rest of your journey.

APPENDIX A

ADDITIONAL READING FOR TOPICS COVERED IN *GETTING HELP*

For Chapter 2: Making Sense of Your Problem

Adjustment Disorder

McKay, M., M. Davis, and P. Fanning. 1997. *Thoughts and Feelings: Taking Control of Your Moods and Your Life*. Oakland, CA: New Harbinger Publications. (Unfortunately, there is no recommended book on this specific topic, but this book covers many issues related to adjustment disorder.)

Anger Control Problems

McKay, M., and P. D. Rogers. 2000. *The Anger Control Workbook*. Oakland, CA: New Harbinger Publications.

McKay, M., P. D. Rogers, and J. McKay. 2003. *When Anger Hurts: Quieting the Storm Within*. Oakland, CA: New Harbinger Publications.

Anorexia

Heffner, M., and G. H. Eifert. 2004. *The Anorexia Workbook: How to Accept Yourself, Heal Your Suffering, and Reclaim Your Life*. Oakland, CA: New Harbinger Publications.

Antisocial Personality

Hare, R. D. 1999. *Without Conscience: The Disturbing World of the Psychopaths Among Us*. New York: The Guilford Press. (From one of the leading researchers, this is a book for family members, victims, and those who are curious.)

Attention-Deficit/Hyperactivity Disorder

Roberts, M. S., and G. J. Jansen. 1997. *Living with ADD: A Workbook for Adults with Attention Deficit Disorder.* Oakland, CA: New Harbinger Publications.

Bipolar Disorder/Manic Depression

Fast, J. A., and J. D. Preston. 2004. *Loving Someone with Bipolar Disorder.* Oakland, CA: New Harbinger Publications. (A book for family members.)

Miklowitz, D. J. 2002. *The Bipolar Disorder Survival Guide: What You and Your Family Need to Know.* New York: The Guilford Press. (A book for patients.)

Body Dysmorphic Disorder

Claiborne, J., and C. Pedrick. 2002. *The BDD Workbook: Overcome Body Dysmorphic Disorder and End Body Image Obsessions.* Oakland, CA: New Harbinger Publications.

Bulimia

McCabe, R. E., T. L. McFarlane, and M. P. Olmstead. 2004. *The Overcoming Bulimia Workbook: Your Comprehensive, Step-by-Step Guide to Recovery.* Oakland, CA: New Harbinger Publications.

Dependent Personality

Bornstein, R. F. 1993. *The Dependent Personality.* New York: The Guilford Press. (An academic review, but one of the few books on the market covering this topic.)

Depression

Burns, D. D. 1999. *Feeling Good: The New Mood Therapy.* New York: Avon Books.

Copeland, M. E. 2001. *The Depression Workbook: A Guide for Living with Depression and Manic Depression.* Oakland, CA: New Harbinger Publications.

Davis, M., E. R. Eshelman, and M. McKay. 2000. *The Relaxation and Stress Reduction Workbook.* Oakland, CA: New Harbinger Publications.

McKay, M., M. Davis, and P. Fanning. 1995. *Messages: The Communication Skills Book.* Oakland, CA: New Harbinger Publications.

McKay, M., M. Davis, and P. Fanning. 1997. *Thoughts and Feelings: Taking Control of Your Moods and Your Life.* Oakland, CA: New Harbinger Publications.

McKay, M., and P. Fanning. 2000. *Self-Esteem: A Proven Program of Cognitive Techniques for Assessing, Improving, and Maintaining Your Self-Esteem.* Oakland, CA: New Harbinger Publications.

Dissociative Disorders

A. T. W. [pseudonym] 2005. *Got Parts? An Insider's Guide to Managing Life Successfully with Dissociative Identity Disorder.* Ann Arbor, MI: Loving Healing Press.

Alderman, T., and K. Marshall. 1998. *Amongst Ourselves: A Self-Help Guide to Living with Dissociative Identity Disorder*. Oakland, CA: New Harbinger Publications.

Drug and Alcohol Addiction Problems

Fanning, P., and J. T. O'Neill. 1996. *The Addiction Workbook: A Step-By-Step Guide to Quitting Alcohol and Drugs*. Oakland, CA: New Harbinger Publications.

Shaw, B. F., P. Ritvo, and J. Irvine. 2005. *Addiction and Recovery for Dummies*. Hoboken, NJ: Wiley Publishing, Inc.

Emotion Dysregulation

Friedel, R. O. 2004. *Borderline Personality Disorder Demystified: An Essential Guide to Understanding and Living with BPD*. New York: Marlowe & Company.

Mason, P. T., and R. Kreger. 1998. *Stop Walking on Eggshells: Taking Your Life Back When Someone You Care About Has Borderline Personality Disorder*. Oakland, CA: New Harbinger Publications. (A book for family and friends of the patient.)

Extreme Suspicion of Others

Kantor, M. 2004. *Understanding Paranoia: A Guide for Professionals, Families, and Sufferers*. Westport, CT: Praeger Publishers.

Generalized Anxiety Disorder

Bourne, E. J. 2005. *The Anxiety and Phobia Workbook*. Oakland, CA: New Harbinger Publications.

Davis, M., E. R. Eshelman, and M. McKay. 2000. *The Relaxation and Stress Reduction Workbook*. Oakland, CA: New Harbinger Publications.

McKay, M., P. Fanning, and M. Davis. 1998. *Thoughts and Feelings: Taking Control of Your Moods and Your Life*. Oakland, CA: New Harbinger Publications.

Impulse Control Disorders

Bernstein, A. 2003. *How to Deal with Emotionally Explosive People*. New York: McGraw-Hill.

Claiborn, J., and C. Pedrick. 2001. *The Habit Change Workbook: How to Break Bad Habits and Form Good Ones*. Oakland, CA: New Harbinger Publications.

Grant, J., and S. W. Kim. 2003. *Stop Me Because I Can't Stop Myself: Taking Control of Impulsive Behavior*. New York: McGraw-Hill.

Keuthen, N. J., D. Stein, and G. A. Christenson. 2001. *Help for Hair Pullers: Understanding and Coping with Trichotillomania*. Oakland, CA: New Harbinger Publications.

Obsessive-Compulsive Disorder

Colas, E. 1999. *Just Checking: Scenes from the Life of an Obsessive Compulsive*. New York: Washington Square Press. (One woman's story about dealing with OCD.)

Hyman, B., and C. Pedrick. 2005. *The OCD Workbook: Your Guide to Breaking Free from Obsessive-Compulsive Disorder*. Oakland, CA: New Harbinger Publications.

Landsman, K. J., K. Rupertus, and C. Pedrick. 2005. *Loving Someone with OCD: Help for You and Your Family*. Oakland, CA: New Harbinger Publications.

Panic Disorder

Bourne, E. J. 2005. *The Anxiety and Phobia Workbook*. Oakland, CA: New Harbinger Publications.

McKay, M., P. Fanning, and M. Davis. 1998. *Thoughts and Feelings: Taking Control of Your Moods and Your Life*. Oakland, CA: New Harbinger Publications.

Phobia

Antony, M. M., and R. E. McCabe. 2005. *Overcoming Animal and Insect Phobias: How to Conquer Fear of Dogs, Snakes, Rodents, Bees, Spiders, and More*. Oakland, CA: New Harbinger Publications.

Antony, M. M., and R. P. Swinson. 2000. *The Shyness and Social Anxiety Workbook: Proven Techniques for Overcoming Your Fears*. Oakland, CA: New Harbinger Publications.

Bourne, E. J. 2005. *The Anxiety and Phobia Workbook*. Oakland, CA: New Harbinger Publications.

Brown, D. 1996. *Flying Without Fear*. Oakland, CA: New Harbinger Publications.

McKay, M., P. Fanning, and M. Davis. 1998. *Thoughts and Feelings: Taking Control of Your Moods and Your Life*. Oakland, CA: New Harbinger Publications.

Pollard, C. A., and E. Zuercher-White. 2003. *The Agoraphobia Workbook: A Comprehensive Program to End Your Fear of Symptom Attacks*. Oakland, CA: New Harbinger Publications.

Post-traumatic Stress Disorder

Matsakis, A. 1996. *I Can't Get Over It: A Handbook for Trauma Survivors*. Oakland, CA: New Harbinger Publications.

Pennebaker, J. W. 1997. *Opening Up: The Healing Power of Expressing Emotions*. New York: The Guilford Press.

Williams, M. B., and S. Poijula. 2002. *The PTSD Workbook: Simple, Effective Techniques for Overcoming Traumatic Stress Symptoms*. Oakland, CA: New Harbinger Publications.

Schema-Focused Relationship Problems

McKay, M., M. Davis, and P. Fanning. 1995. *Messages: The Communication Skills Book*. Oakland, CA: New Harbinger Publications.

McKay, M., and P. Fanning. 1991. *Prisoners of Belief: Exposing and Changing Beliefs That Control Your Life*. Oakland, CA: New Harbinger Publications.

Young, J. E., and J. S. Klosko. 1994. *Reinventing Your Life: The Breakthrough Program to End Negative Behavior … and Feel Great Again*. New York: Plume.

Schizoid Personality

Beck, A. T., A. Freeman, and D. D. Davis. 2003. *Cognitive Therapy of Personality Disorders*. New York: The Guilford Press. (A book written for professionals, but one of the few that addresses schizoid personality problems.)

Schizophrenia

Mueser, K. T. , and S. Gingerich. 2006. *The Complete Family Guide to Schizophrenia: Helping Your Loved One Get the Most Out of Life*. New York: The Guilford Press.

Temes, R. 2002. *Getting Your Life Back Together When You Have Schizophrenia*. Oakland, CA: New Harbinger Publications.

Torrey, E. F. 2001. *Surviving Schizophrenia: A Manual for Families, Consumers, and Providers*. New York: HarperCollins.

Self-Focused Personality

Beck, A. T., A. Freeman, and D. D. Davis. 2003. *Cognitive Therapy of Personality Disorders*. New York: The Guilford Press. (A book written for professionals, but one of the few that addresses self-focused personality problems.)

Brown, N. 2001. *Children of the Self-Absorbed: A Grown-Up's Guide to Getting Over Narcissistic Parents*. Oakland, CA: New Harbinger Publications.

Brown, N. 2003. *Loving the Self-Absorbed: How to Create a More Satisfying Relationship with a Narcissistic Partner*. Oakland, CA: New Harbinger Publications.

Somatoform Disorders

Asmundson, G. J. G., and S. Taylor. 2005. *It's Not All in Your Head: How Worrying About Your Health Could Be Making You Sick—and What You Can Do About It*. New York: The Guilford Press.

Caudill, M. 2001. *Managing Pain Before It Manages You*. New York: The Guilford Press.

Dahl, J., and T. Lundgren. 2006. *Living Beyond Your Pain: Using Acceptance and Commitment Therapy to Ease Chronic Pain*. Oakland, CA: New Harbinger Publications.

Davis, M., E. R. Eshelman, and M. McKay. 2000. *The Relaxation and Stress Reduction Workbook*. Oakland, CA: New Harbinger Publications.

Friedberg, F. 2006. *Fibromyalgia and Chronic Fatigue Syndrome: Seven Proven Steps to Less Pain and More Energy*. Oakland, CA: New Harbinger Publications.

For Chapter 3: Making Sense of the Treatments

Acceptance and Commitment Therapy

Hayes, S. C., and S. Smith. 2006. *Get Out of Your Mind and Into Your Life: The New Acceptance and Commitment Therapy.* Oakland, CA: New Harbinger Publications.

Analytical Psychotherapy/Jungian Psychotherapy

Cambray, J., and L. Carter, eds. 2004. *Analytical Psychology: Contemporary Perspectives in Jungian Analysis.* New York: Brunner-Routledge.

Behavior Therapy

O'Donohue, W., and L. Krasner. 1999. *Theories of Behavior Therapy: Exploring Behavior Change.* Washington, DC: American Psychological Association.

Brief Psychodynamic Therapy

Messer, S. B., and C. S. Warren. 1995. *Models of Brief Psychodynamic Therapy: A Comparative Approach.* New York: The Guilford Press.

Cognitive Behavioral Therapy

Beck, J. S. 1995. *Cognitive Therapy: Basics and Beyond.* New York: The Guilford Press.

Dobson, K. S. 2002. *Handbook of Cognitive-Behavioral Therapies.* New York: The Guilford Press.

Couples Therapy

Gurman, A. S., and N. S. Jacobson, eds. 2002. *Clinical Handbook of Couple Therapy.* New York: The Guilford Press.

Dialectical Behavior Therapy

Linehan, M. M. 1993. *Cognitive-Behavioral Treatment of Borderline Personality Disorder.* New York: The Guilford Press.

Marra, T. 2005. *Dialectical Behavior Therapy in Private Practice: A Practical and Comprehensive Guide.* Oakland, CA: New Harbinger Publications.

Existential Psychotherapy

Frankl, V. E. 1984. *Man's Search for Meaning: An Introduction to Logotherapy.* New York: Touchstone.

Yalom, I. D. 1980. *Existential Psychotherapy.* New York: Basic Books.

Eye-Movement Desensitization and Reprocessing

Shapiro, F., and M. S. Forrest. 1997. *EMDR: Eye Movement Desensitization and Reprocessing: The Breakthrough "Eye Movement" Therapy for Overcoming Anxiety, Stress, and Trauma*. New York: Basic Books.

Family Therapy

Minuchin, S. 1974. *Families and Family Therapy*. Cambridge, MA: Harvard University Press.

Gestalt Psychotherapy

Perls, F. S., R. Hefferline, and P. Goodman. 1974. *Gestalt therapy: Excitement and Growth in the Human Personality*. Gouldsboro, ME: Gestalt Journal Press.

Humanistic Psychotherapy/Client-Centered Therapy/ Person-Centered Therapy

Rogers, C. R. 1989. *On Becoming a Person: A Therapist's View of Psychotherapy*. New York: Houghton Mifflin.

Hypnotherapy

Hadley, J., and C. Straudacher. 1996. *Hypnosis for Change*. Oakland, CA: New Harbinger Publications.

Yapko, M. D. 1995. *Essentials of Hypnosis*. New York: Brunner/Mazel.

Interpersonal Therapy

Weissman, M. M., and J. C. Markowitz. 2000. *Comprehensive Guide to Interpersonal Psychotherapy*. New York: Basic Books.

Medications

Preston, J. D., J. O'Neal, and M. C. Talaga. 2004 *Handbook of Clinical Psychopharmacology for Therapists*. Oakland, CA: New Harbinger Publications.

Preston, J. D., and J. Preston. 2004. *Clinical Psychopharmacology Made Ridiculously Simple*. Miami, FL: MedMaster. (Both of these books about medications are written for professionals, but provide easy-to-understand information.)

Mindfulness Therapy

Brantley, J. 2003. *Calming Your Anxious Mind: How Mindfulness and Compassion Can Free You from Anxiety, Fear, and Panic*. Oakland, CA: New Harbinger Publications.

Kabat-Zinn, J. 2005. *Full Catastrophe Living: Using the Wisdom of Your Body and Mind to Face Stress, Pain, and Illness*. New York: Bantam Dell.

Positive Psychology

Seligman, M. 1998. *Learned Optimism: How to Change Your Mind and Your Life*. New York: Simon & Schuster, Inc.

Seligman, M. 2004. *Authentic Happiness: Using the New Positive Psychology to Realize Your Potential for Lasting Fulfillment*. New York: Free Press.

Psychoanalysis/Psychodynamic Therapy

Mitchell, S. A., and M. J. Black. 1995. *Freud and Beyond: A History of Modern Psychoanalytic Thought*. New York: Basic Books.

Rational Emotive Behavior Therapy

Ellis, A. 2001. *Overcoming Destructive Beliefs, Feelings, and Behaviors: New Directions for Rational Emotive Behavior Therapy*. Amherst, NY: Prometheus Books.

Schema-Focused Therapy

Young, J. E., J. S. Klosko, and M. E. Weishaar. 2003. *Schema Therapy: A Practitioner's Guide*. New York: The Guilford Press.

Somatic Psychotherapies

Feldenkrais, M. 1991. *Awareness Through Movement: Easy-to-Do Health Exercises to Improve Your Posture, Vision, Imagination, and Personal Awareness*. New York: HarperCollins. (A book about the Feldenkrais technique.)

Kurtz, R. 1990. *Body-Centered Psychotherapy: The Hakomi Method*. Mendocino, CA: Life Rhythm.

Mindell, A. 1998. *Dreambody: The Body's Role in Revealing the Self*. Portland, OR: Lao Tse Press. (A book about process-oriented psychotherapy.)

Rolf, I. P. 1990. *Rolfing and Physical Reality*. Rochester, VT: Inner Traditions.

Rosen, M., and S. Brenner. 2003. *Rosen Method Bodywork: Accessing the Unconscious Through Touch*. Berkeley, CA: North Atlantic Books.

Transpersonal Psychology

Scotton, B. W., A. B. Chinen, and J. R. Battista, eds. 1996. *Textbook of Transpersonal Psychiatry and Psychology*. New York: Basic Books. (An academic book, but very thorough.)

APPENDIX B

ADDITIONAL CONTACT INFORMATION

National Alliance on Mental Illness (NAMI)

"The nation's voice on mental illness." (From the NAMI Web site.) Created in 1979, NAMI supports mental health research, and advocates for people struggling with mental health problems and their families on the federal and state levels of government. All fifty states have additional state and local NAMI chapters that provide educational information and support groups. The NAMI Web site will help you locate your local chapter and it also contains helpful information about many mental health care issues.

(800)950-6264 is the toll-free information helpline and referral service.

The NAMI Web site is www.nami.org.

American Psychological Association (APA)

"APA is the largest association of psychologists worldwide." (From the APA Web site.) Founded in 1892, the APA is the national governing body of psychologists in the United States. Its goals are to advance the science of psychology, to govern the ethical conduct of psychologists, to provide education about mental health issues to the general public, to support psychological research, to improve the training of psychologists, and to promote the use of psychology in health care. The Web site provides information for the general public about mental health issues including updated information about the latest research.

(800) 374-2721 is the APA general toll-free number in the United States and Canada.

The APA Web site is www.apa.org.

The APA also provides referrals to registered psychologists in all fifty states and Canadian provinces:

(800) 964-2000 is the APA's Find a Psychologist toll-free number. This number will connect you to your state or province's local psychological association.

The Find a Psychologist Web site is http://locator.apahelpcenter.org. It will locate the nearest registered psychologist based on your zip or postal code.

Canadian Psychological Association (CPA)

Organized in 1939, the CPA provides the same services for Canada as the APA does for the United States.

(888) 472-0657 is the CPA toll-free number.

The CPA Web site is www.cpa.ca.

State and Provincial Psychological Associations

You can also get a referral for a psychologist by contacting your state or provincial psychological association directly:

Alabama Psychological Association
www.alapsych.org
(334) 262-8245

Alaska Psychological Association
www.ak-pa.org
(907) 344-8878

Alberta, Psychologists' Association of
www.psychologistsassociation.ab.ca
(780) 424-0294

Arizona Psychological Association
www.azpa.org
(480) 675-9477

Arkansas Psychological Association
www.arpapsych.org
(501) 614-6500

British Columbia Psychological Association
www.psychologists.bc.ca
(604) 730-0501

California Psychological Association
www.calpsychlink.org
(916) 286-7979

Colorado Psychological Association
www.coloradopsych.org
(303) 692-9303

Connecticut Psychological Association
www.connpsych.org
(860) 586-7522

Delaware Psychological Association
www.depsych.org
(302) 475-1574

District of Columbia Psychological Association
www.dcpsychology.org
(202) 336-5559

Florida Psychological Association
www.flapsych.com
(850) 656-2222

Georgia Psychological Association
www.gapsychology.org
(404) 634-6272

Guam Psychological Association
(671) 646-4078

Hawaii Psychological Association
www.hawaiipsych.org
(808) 521-8995

Idaho Psychological Association
www.idahopsych.org
(208) 375-0125

Illinois Psychological Association
www.illinoispsychology.org
(312) 372-7610

Indiana Psychological Association
www.indianapsychologist.org
(317) 686-5348

Iowa Psychological Association
www.iowapsychology.org
(712) 848-3595

Kansas Psychological Association
www.kspsych.org
(785) 856-9572

Kentucky Psychological Association
www.kpa.org
(502) 894-0777

Louisiana Psychological Association
www.louisianapsychologist.org
(225) 766-0185

Maine Psychological Association
www.mepa.org
(207) 621-0732

Manitoba Psychological Society, Inc.
www.mps.mb.ca
(204) 488-7398

Maryland Psychological Association
www.marylandpsychology.org
(410) 992-4258

Massachusetts Psychological Association
www.masspsych.org
(781) 263-0080

Michigan Psychological Association
www.michpsych.org
(517) 347-1885

Minnesota Psychological Association
www.mnpsych.org
(651) 203-7249

Mississippi Psychological Association
www.mpassoc.org
(601) 362-7755

Missouri Psychological Association
www.mopsych.org
(314) 259-1076

Montana Psychological Association
www.wtp.net/mpa
(406) 252-2559

Nebraska Psychological Association
www.nebpsych.org
(402) 475-0709

Nevada State Psychological Association
www.nevadapsychologists.org
(702) 454-0050

New Hampshire Psychological Association
www.nhpaonline.org
(603) 225-9925

New Jersey Psychological Association
www.psychologynj.org
(973) 243-9800

New Mexico Psychological Association
www.nmpa.com
(505) 883-7376

New York State Psychological Association
www.nyspa.org
(518) 437-1040

North Carolina Psychological Association
www.ncpsychology.com
(919) 872-1005

North Dakota Psychological Association
(701) 223-9045

Nova Scotia, Association of Psychologists of
www.apns.ca
(902) 422-9183

Ohio Psychological Association
www.ohpsych.org
(614) 224-0034

Oklahoma Psychological Association
www.okpsych.org
(405) 879-0069

Ontario Psychological Association
www.psych.on.ca
(416) 961-5552

Oregon Psychological Association
www.opa.org
(503) 253-9155

Pennsylvania Psychological Association
www.papsy.org
(717) 232-3817

Puerto Rico Association of Psychologists
www.asppr.org
(787) 751-7100

Quebec Ordre des Psychologues (Association of Psychologists)
www.ordrepsy.qc.ca
(514) 738-1881

Rhode Island Psychological Association
www.ripsych.org
(401) 736-2900

South Carolina Psychological Association
www.scpa.affiniscape.com
(877) 640-7272

South Dakota Psychological Association
www.psysd.org
(605) 336-0244

Tennessee Psychological Association
www.tpaonline.org
(901) 372-1015

Texas Psychological Association
www.texaspsyc.org
(512) 280-4099

Utah Psychological Association
www.utahpsych.org
(801) 359-5646

Vermont Psychological Association
www.vermontpsych.org
(802) 229-5447

Virginia Psychological Association
www.vapsych.org
(804) 643-7300

Virgin Islands Psychological Association
(340) 719-3870

Washington State Psychological Association
www.wapsych.org
(206) 547-4220

West Virginia Psychological Association
www.wvpsychology.org
(304) 345-5805

Wisconsin Psychological Association
www.wipsychology.org
(608) 251-1450

Wyoming Psychological Association
www.wypsych.org
(307) 745-3167

American Board of Professional Psychology (ABPP)

Created in 1947, the ABPP has established additional qualifications for psychologists who want to acquire recognition in their specialties. These psychologists can be identified by "ABPP" listed after their name and degree, which signifies their status; for example: Jane Smith, Psy.D., ABPP.

Currently, the ABPP certifies specialists in cognitive and behavioral psychology, clinical psychology, clinical child and adolescent psychology, clinical health psychology, clinical neuropsychology, counseling psychology, family psychology, forensic psychology, group psychology, organizational and business consulting psychology, psychoanalysis, rehabilitation psychology, and school psychology.

(800) 255-7792 is the ABPP toll-free number.

The ABPP Web site is www.abpp.org.

American Psychiatric Association

Created in 1844, the American Psychiatric Association is an organization of medical doctors who have chosen to specialize in the research and treatment of mental health care issues. As such, the goals of this organization are to promote mental health research and treatment, as well as to govern the ethical conduct of psychiatrists. The American Psychiatric Association has created a Web site for the general public to help promote mental health education. It has also created an Answer Center hotline to help you find a psychiatrist near you. The Web site contains free brochures about mental health problems that you can download.

(888) 35-PSYCH is the Answer Center toll-free number to find a psychiatrist in your area and for general questions.

The American Psychiatric Association's professional Web site is www.psych.org.

The American Psychiatric Association's educational Web site is www.healthyminds.org.

American Association for Marriage and Family Therapy (AAMFT)

Created in 1942, AAMFT promotes research, education, and treatment of marriage and family therapy issues. It also governs the training and ethical conduct of marriage and family therapists. Its Web site includes information on mental health issues for the general public, as well as a service to help you find a marriage and family therapist located near you.

The AAMFT phone number is (703) 838-9808.

The AAMFT Web site is www.aamft.org.

The Therapist Locator Web site is www.therapistlocator.net.

National Institute of Mental Health (NIMH)

NIMH is a part of the National Institutes of Health, which is run by the United States Department of Health and Human Services. The goal of NIMH is to support biomedical research of mental health issues. Its Web site contains helpful information about the latest research being conducted, as well as free brochures that you can download.

The NIMH Web site is www.nimh.nih.gov.

Additional Services to Locate a Psychotherapist

The *Psychology Today* Web site, including their Find a Therapist directory, is www.psychologytoday.com.

The National Register of Health Service Providers in Psychology Web site, including their Find a Psychologist directory, is www.nationalregister.org.

REFERENCES

Introduction

1. Mathew, S. J., H. B. Simpson, and B. A. Fallon. 2000. Treatment strategies for obsessive-compulsive disorder. *Psychiatric Annals* 30: 699-708.
2. Treatment for Adolescents with Depression Study Team. 2004. Fluoxetine, cognitive-behavioral therapy, and their combination for adolescents with depression: Treatment for Adolescents with Depression Study (TADS) randomized controlled trial. *Journal of the American Medical Association* 292: 807-820.
3. DeRubeis, R. J., S. D. Hollon, J. D. Amsterdam, R. C. Shelton, P. R. Young, R. M. Salomon, et al. 2005. Cognitive therapy vs medications in the treatment of moderate to severe depression. *Archives of General Psychiatry* 62: 409-416.
4. Hollon, S. D., R. B. Jarrett, A. A. Nierenberg, M. E. Thase, M. Trivedi, and A. J. Rush, et al. 2005. Psychotherapy and medication in the treatment of adult and geriatric depression: Which monotherapy or combined treatment? *Journal of Clinical Psychiatry* 66: 455-468.
5. Lam, D. H., E. R. Watkins, P. Hayward, J. Bright, K. Wright, N. Kerr, et al. 2003. A randomized controlled study of cognitive therapy for relapse prevention for bipolar affective disorder: Outcome of the first year. *Archives of General Psychiatry* 60: 145-152.
6. Wang, P. S., P. A. Berglund, M. Olfson, H. A. Pincus, K. B. Wells, and R. C. Kessler. 2005. Failure and delay in initial treatment contact after first onset of mental disorders in the National Comorbidity Survey Replication. *Archives of General Psychiatry* 62: 603-613.

Chapter 2—Adjustment Disorder

1. American Psychiatric Association. 2000. *Diagnostic and Statistical Manual of Mental Disorders.* Text revision ed. Washington, DC: American Psychiatric Association.
2. Strain, J. J., G. C. Smith, J. S. Hammer, D. P. McKenzie, M. Blumenfield, P. Muskin, et al. 1998. Adjustment disorder: A multisite study of its utilization and interventions in the consultation-liaison psychiatry setting. *General Hospital Psychiatry* 20: 139-149.
3. Jones, R., W. R. Yates, and M. H. Zhou. 2002. Readmission rates for adjustment disorders: Comparison with other mood disorders. *Journal of Affective Disorders* 71: 199-203.
4. Casey, P., C. Dowrick, and G. Wilkinson. 2001. Adjustment disorders: Fault line in the psychiatric glossary. *British Journal of Psychiatry* 179: 479-481.
5. Bronish, T. 1991. Adjustment reactions: A long-term prospective and retrospective follow-up of former patients in a crisis intervention ward. *Acta Psychiatrica Scandinavica* 84: 86-93.
6. Greenberg, W. A., D. N. Rosenfeld, and E. A. Ortega. 1995. Adjustment disorder as an admission diagnosis. *American Journal of Psychiatry* 152: 459-461.

Anger Control Problems

1. Deffenbacher, J. L., and M. McKay. 2000. *Overcoming Situational and General Anger: A Protocol for the Treatment of Anger Based on Relaxation, Cognitive Restructuring, and Coping Skills Training.* Oakland, CA: New Harbinger Publications.

2. Berkowitz, L., and E. Harmon-Jones. 2004. Toward an understanding of the determinants of anger. *Emotion* 4: 107-130.

3. Deffenbacher, J. L., E. R. Oetting, R. S. Lynch, and C. D. Morris. 1996. The expression of anger and its consequences. *Behaviour Research and Therapy* 34: 575-590.

4. Averill, J. R. 1982. *Anger and Aggression: An Essay on Emotion.* New York: Springer-Verlag.

5. Bongard, S., and M. al'Absi. 2005. Domain-specific anger expression and blood pressure in an occupational setting. *Journal of Psychosomatic Research* 58: 43-49.

6. Booth-Kewley, S., and H. S. Friedman. 1987. Psychological predictors of heart disease: A quantitative review. *Psychological Bulletin* 101: 343-362.

7. Everson, S. A., D. E. Goldberg, G. A. Kaplan, J. Julkunen, and J. T. Salonen. 1998. Anger expression and incident hypertension. *Psychosomatic Medicine* 60: 730-735.

8. Rozanski, A., J. A. Blumenthal, and J. Kaplan. 1999. Impact of psychological factors on the pathogenesis of cardiovascular disease and implications for therapy. *Circulation* 99: 2192-2217.

9. Bleil, M. E., J. M. McCaffery, M. F. Muldoon, K. Sutton-Tyrrell, and S. B. Manuck. 2004. Anger-related personality traits and carotid artery atherosclerosis in untreated hypertensive men. *Psychosomatic Medicine* 66: 633-639.

10. Raikkonen, K., K. A. Matthews, K. Sutton-Tyrrell, and L. H. Kuller. 2004. Trait anger and the metabolic syndrome predict progression of carotid atherosclerosis in healthy middle-aged women. *Psychosomatic Medicine* 66: 903-908.

11. Carson, J. W., F. J. Keefe, V. Goli, A. M. Fras, T. R. Lynch, S. R. Thorp, et al. 2005. Forgiveness and chronic low back pain: A preliminary study examining the relationship of forgiveness to pain, anger, and psychological distress. *Journal of Pain* 6: 84-91.

12. Fernandez, E., and DC Turk. 1995. The scope and significance of anger in the experience of chronic pain. *Pain* 61: 165-175.

13. Kerns, R. D., R. Rosenberg, and M. C. Jacob. 1994. Anger expression and chronic pain. *Journal of Behavioral Medicine* 17: 57-67.

14. Greenwood, K. A., R. Thurston, M. Rumble, S. J. Waters, and F. J. Keefe. 2003. Anger and persistent pain: Current status and future directions. *Pain* 103: 1-5.

15. Shin, C., J. Kim, H. Yi, H. Lee, J. Lee, and K. Shin. 2005. Relationship between trait-anger and sleep disturbances in middle-aged men and women. *Journal of Psychosomatic Research* 58: 183-189.

16. Norlander, B., and C. Eckhardt. 2005. Anger, hostility, and male perpetrators of intimate partner violence: A meta-analytic review. *Clinical Psychology Review* 25: 119-152.

17. Posternak, M. A., and M. Zimmerman. 2002. Anger and aggression in psychiatric outpatients. *Journal of Clinical Psychiatry* 63: 665-672.

18. Koh, K. B., C. H. Kim, and J. K. Park. 2002. Predominance of anger in depressive disorders compared with anxiety disorders and somatoform disorders. *Journal of Clinical Psychiatry* 63: 486-492.

19. Picardi, A., P. Morosini, P. Gaetano, M. Pasquini, and M. Biondi. 2004. Higher levels of anger and aggressiveness in major depressive disorder than in anxiety and somatoform disorders. *Journal of Clinical Psychiatry* 65: 442-443.

20. Koh, K. B., D. K. Kim, S. Y. Kim, and J. K. Park. 2005. The relation between anger expression, depression, and somatic symptoms in depressive disorders and somatoform disorders. *Journal of Clinical Psychiatry* 66: 485-491.

21. Hewig, J., D. Hagemann, J. Seifert, E. Naumann, and D. Bartussek. 2004. On the selective relation of frontal cortical asymmetry and anger-out versus anger-control. *Journal of Personality and Social Psychology* 87: 926-939.

22. Dougherty, D. D., L. M. Shin, N. M. Alpert, R. K. Pitman, S. P. Orr, M. Lasko, et al. 1999. Anger in healthy men: A PET study using script-driven imagery. *Biological Psychiatry* 46: 466-472.

23. Harmon-Jones, E. 2004. Contributions from research on anger and cognitive dissonance to understanding the motivational functions of asymmetrical frontal brain activity. *Biological Psychology* 67: 51-76.

24. Wang, X., R. Trivedi, F. Treiber, and H. Snieder. 2005. Genetic and environmental influences on anger expression, John Henryism, and stressful life events: The Georgia Cardiovascular Twin Study. *Psychosomatic Medicine* 67: 16-23.

25. Ekman, P., W. V. Friesen, M. O'Sullivan, A. Chan, I. Diacoyanni-Tarlatzis, K. Heider, et al. 1987. Universals and cultural differences in the judgments of facial expressions of emotion. *Journal of Personality and Social Psychology* 53: 712-717.

26. Ekman, P. 1992. An argument for basic emotions. *Cognition and Emotion* 6: 169-200.

27. Ekman, P. 1993. Facial expression and emotion. *American Psychologist* 48: 384-392.

28. Konwar, N., and U. Ram. 2004. Cultural differences in anger. *Psychological Studies* 49: 193-195.

29. Ohbuchi, K.-I., T. Kumagai, and E. Atsumi. 2002. Motives of and responses to anger in conflict situations: A cross-cultural analysis. *Tohoku Psychologica Folia* 61: 11-21.

30. Ohbuchi, K.-I., T. Tamura, B. M. Quigley, J. T. Tedeschi, N. Madi, M. H. Bond, et al. 2004. Anger, blame, and dimensions of perceived norm violations: Culture, gender, and relationships. *Journal of Applied Social Psychology* 34: 1587-1603.

31. Suchday, S., and K. T. Larkin. 2004. Psychophysiological responses to anger provocation among Asian, Indian, and white men. *International Journal of Behavioral Medicine* 11: 71-80.

32. Cheng, H.-L., B. Mallinckrodt, and L.-C. Wu. 2005. Anger expression toward parents and depressive symptoms among undergraduates in Taiwan. *Counseling Psychologist* 33: 72-97.

33. Kim, I. J., and N. W. S. Zane. 2004. Ethnic and cultural variations in anger regulation and attachment patterns among Korean American and European American male batterers. *Cultural Diversity and Ethnic Minority Psychology* 10: 151-168.

34. Bandura, A., D. Ross, and S. A. Ross. 1963. Vicarious reinforcement and imitative learning. *Journal of Abnormal and Social Psychology* 67: 601-607.

35. Bandura, A., D. Ross, and S. A. Ross. 1961. Transmission of aggression through imitation of aggressive models. *Journal of Abnormal and Social Psychology* 63: 575-582.

36. Clark, T. R., and V. Phares. 2004. Feelings in the family: Interparental conflict, anger, and expressiveness in families with older adolescents. *Family Journal: Counseling and Therapy for Couples and Families* 12: 129-138.

37. Kashani, J. H., L. A. Canfield, S. M. Soltys, and J. C. Reid. 1995. Psychiatric inpatient children's family perceptions and anger expression. *Journal of Emotional and Behavioral Disorders* 3: 13-18, 39.

38. Cox, R. L., N. L. Lopez, and H. G. Schneider. 2003. Anger expression: Parental and cognitive factors. *Psychological Reports* 93: 59-65.

39. Sigfusdottir, I.-D., G. Farkas, and E. Silver. 2004. The role of depressed mood and anger in the relationship between family conflict and delinquent behavior. *Journal of Youth and Adolescence* 33: 509-522.

40. Alpert, J. E., T. Petersen, P. A. Roffi, G. I. Papakostas, R. Freed, M. M. Smith, et al. 2003. Behavioral and emotional disturbances in the offspring of depressed parents with anger attacks. *Psychotherapy and Psychosomatics* 72: 102-106.

41. Meier, B. P., and M. D. Robinson. 2004. Does quick to blame mean quick to anger? The role of agreeableness in dissociating blame and anger. *Personality and Social Psychology Bulletin* 30: 856-867.

42. Kuppens, P. 2005. Interpersonal determinants of trait anger: Low agreeableness, perceived low social esteem, and the amplifying role of the importance attached to social relationships. *Personality and Individual Differences* 38: 13-23.

43. Berkowitz, L. 1990. On the formulation and regulation of anger and aggression: A cognitive-neoassociationist view. *American Psychologist* 45: 494-503.

44. Dahlen, E. R., R. C. Martin, K. Ragan, and M. M. Kuhlman. 2004. Boredom proneness in anger and aggression: Effects of impulsiveness and sensation seeking. *Personality and Individual Differences* 37: 1615-1627.

45. Lazarus, R. S. 1991. *Emotion and Adaptation*. New York: Oxford University Press.

46.	DiGiuseppe, R., and R. C. Tafrate. 2003. Anger treatment for adults: A meta-analytic review. *Clinical Psychology: Science and Practice* 10: 70-84.

47.	DiGiuseppe, R., and R. C. Tafrate. 2001. A comprehensive treatment model for anger disorders. *Psychotherapy: Theory, Research, Practice, Training* 38: 262-271.

48.	Del Vecchio, T., and K. D. O'Leary. 2004. Effectiveness of anger treatments for specific anger problems: A meta-analytic review. *Clinical Psychology Review* 24: 15-34.

49.	Sukhodolsky, D. G., H. Kassinove, and B. S. Gorman. 2004. Cognitive-behavioral therapy for anger in children and adolescents: A meta-analysis. *Aggression and Violent Behavior* 9: 247-269.

50.	Deffenbacher, J. L., L. B. Filetti, R. S. Lynch, E. R. Dahlen, and E. R. Oetting. 2002. Cognitive-behavioral treatment of high anger drivers. *Behaviour Research and Therapy* 40: 895-910.

51.	Ireland, J. L. 2004. Anger management therapy with young male offenders: An evaluation of treatment outcome. *Aggressive Behavior* 30: 174-185.

52.	Lin, W.-F., D. Mack, R. D. Enright, D. Krahn, and T. W. Baskin. 2004. Effects of forgiveness therapy on anger, mood, and vulnerability to substance use among inpatient substance-dependent clients. *Journal of Consulting and Clinical Psychology* 72: 1114-1121.

53.	Dua, J. K., and M. L. Swinden. 1992. Effectiveness of negative-thought-reduction, meditation, and placebo training treatment in reducing anger. *Scandinavian Journal of Psychology* 33: 135-146.

54.	Leifer, R. 1999. Buddhist conceptualization and treatment of anger. *Journal of Clinical Psychology* 55: 339-351.

55.	Fava, M., J. Alpert, A. A. Nierenberg, N. Ghaemi, R. O'Sullivan, J. Tedlow, et al. 1996. Fluoxetine treatment of anger attacks: A replication study. *Annals of Clinical Psychiatry* 8: 7-10.

56.	Fava, M., J. F. Rosenbaum, J. A. Pava, M. K. McCarthy, R. J. Steingard, and E. Bouffides. 1993. Anger attacks in unipolar depression: I. Clinical correlates and response to fluoxetine treatment. *American Journal of Psychiatry* 150: 1158-1163.

57.	Mischoulon, D., D. D. Dougherty, K. A. Bottonari, R. L. Gresham, S. B. Sonawalla, A. J. Fischman, et al. 2002. An open pilot study of nefazodone in depression with anger attacks: Relationships between clinical response and receptor binding. *Psychiatry Research: Neuroimaging* 116: 151-161.

Anorexia

1.	American Psychiatric Association. 2000. *Diagnostic and Statistical Manual of Mental Disorders.* Text revision ed. Washington, DC: American Psychiatric Association.

2.	Davis, C., D. K. Katzman, S. Kaptein, C. Kirsh, H. Brewer, K. Kalmbach, et al. 1997. The prevalence of high-level exercise in the eating disorders: Etiological implications. *Comprehensive Psychiatry* 38: 321-326.

3.	Keys, A., A. Henschel, and H. L. Taylor. 1947. The size and function of the human heart at rest in semistarvation and in subsequent rehabilitation. *American Journal of Physiology* 150: 153.

4.	Cooke, R. A., and J. B. Chambers. 1995. Anorexia nervosa and the heart. *British Journal of Hospital Medicine* 54: 313-317.

5.	Johnson, G. L., L. L. Humphries, P. B. Shirley, A. Mazzoleni, and J. A. Noonan. 1986. Mitral valve prolapse in patients with anorexia nervosa and bulimia. *Archives of Internal Medicine* 146: 1525-1529.

6.	Powers, P. S. 1982. Heart failure during treatment of anorexia nervosa. *American Journal of Psychiatry* 139: 1167-1170.

7.	Golden, N. H., M. S. Jacobson, J. Schebendach, M. V. Solanto, S. M. Hertz, and I. R. Shenker. 1997. Resumption of menses in anorexia nervosa. *Archive of Pediatric and Adolescent Medicine* 151: 16-21.

8.	Di Pascoli, L., A. Lion, D. Milazzo, and L. Caregaro. 2004. Acute liver damage in anorexia nervosa. *International Journal of Eating Disorders* 36: 114-117.

9.	Mehler, P. S., and M. Krantz. 2003. Anorexia nervosa medical issues. *Journal of Women's Health* 12: 331-340.

10. Steinhausen, H.-C. 2002. The outcome of anorexia nervosa in the 20th century. *American Journal of Psychiatry* 159: 1284-1293.

11. National Association of Anorexia Nervosa and Associated Disorders. 2005. Facts about eating disorders. National Association of Anorexia Nervosa and Associated Disorders 2005 [cited January 8, 2005]. Available from www.anad .org/site/anadweb/content.php?type=1andid=6982.

12. Fichter, M. M., and N. Quadflieg. 1999. Six-year course and outcome of anorexia nervosa. *International Journal of Eating Disorders* 26: 359-385.

13. Pompili, M., I. Mancinelli, P. Girardi, A. Ruberto, and R. Tatarelli. 2004. Suicide in anorexia nervosa: A meta-analysis. *International Journal of Eating Disorders* 36: 99-103.

14. Zipfel, S., B. Lowe, D. L. Reas, H. C. Deter, and W. Herzog. 2000. Long-term prognosis in anorexia nervosa: Lessons from a 21-year follow-up study. *Lancet* 355: 721-722.

15. Sullivan, P. F. 1995. Mortality in anorexia nervosa. *American Journal of Psychiatry* 152: 1073-1074.

16. American Psychiatric Association Work Group on Eating Disorders. 2000. Practice guideline for the treatment of patients with eating disorders (revision). *American Journal of Psychiatry* 157: 1-39.

17. Russell, C. J., and P. K. Keel. 2002. Homosexuality as a specific risk factor for eating disorders in men. *International Journal of Eating Disorders* 31: 300-306.

18. Crosscope-Happel, C., D. E. Hutchins, H. G. Getz, and G. L. Hayes. 2000. Male anorexia nervosa: A new focus. *Journal of Mental Health Counseling* 22: 365-370.

19. Ray, S. L. 2004. Eating disorders in adolescent males. *Professional School Counseling* 8: 98-101.

20. Patel, D. R., H. D. Pratt, and D. E. Greydanus. 2003. Treatment of adolescents with anorexia nervosa. *Journal of Adolescent Research* 18: 244-260.

21. Scheider, J. A. 1991. Gender identity issues in male bulimia nervosa. In *Psychodynamic Treatment of Anorexia Nervosa and Bulimia*, edited by C. Johnson. New York: The Guilford Press.

22. Phelps, L., and E. Bajorek. 1991. Eating disorders of the adolescent: Current issues in etiology, assessment, and treatment. *School Psychology Review* 20: 9-23.

23. McCarthy, M. 1990. The thin ideal, depression and eating disorders in women. *Behaviour Research and Therapy* 28: 205-215.

24. Williams, M. S., S. R. Thomsen, and J. K. McCoy. 2003. Looking for an accurate mirror: A model for the relationship between media use and anorexia. *Eating Behaviors* 4: 127-134.

25. Bennett, D., M. Sharpe, C. Freeman, and A. Carson. 2004. Anorexia nervosa among female secondary school students in Ghana. *British Journal of Psychiatry* 185: 312-317.

26. Surgenor, L. J., J. Horn, and S. M. Hudson. 2003. Empirical scrutiny of a familiar narrative: Sense of control in anorexia nervosa. *European Eating Disorders Review* 11: 291-305.

27. Karwautz, A., G. Nobis, M. Haidvogl, G. Wagner, A. Hafferl-Gattermayer, C. Wober-Bingol, et al. 2003. Perceptions of family relationships in adolescents with anorexia nervosa and their unaffected sisters. *European Child and Adolescent Psychiatry* 12: 128-135.

28. Hay, P. 2004. Australian and New Zealand clinical practice guidelines for the treatment of anorexia nervosa. *Australian and New Zealand Journal of Psychiatry* 38: 659-670.

29. Channon, S., P. de Silva, D. Hemsley, and R. Perkins. 1989. A controlled trial of cognitive-behavioral and behavioral treatment of anorexia nervosa. *Behavior Research and Therapy* 7: 529-535.

30. Serfaty, M., D. Turkington, M. Heap, L. Ledsham, and E. Jolley. 1999. Cognitive therapy versus dietary counseling in the outpatient treatment of anorexia nervosa: Effects of the treatment phase. *European Eating Disorders Review* 7: 334-350.

31. LeGrange, D., I. Eisler, C. Dare, and G. F. Russell. 1992. Evaluation of family treatment in adolescent anorexia nervosa: A pilot study. *International Journal of Eating Disorders* 12: 347-357.

32. Eisler, I., C. Dare, G. F. Russell, G. Szmukler, D. LeGrange, and E. Dodge. 1997. Family and individual therapy in anorexia nervosa. A 5-year follow-up. *Archives of General Psychiatry* 54: 1025-1030.

33. Russell, G. F., G. Szmukler, C. Dare, and I. Eisler. 1987. An evaluation of family therapy in anorexia nervosa and bulimia nervosa. *Archives of General Psychiatry* 44: 1047-1056.

34. Brambilla, F., A. Draisci, A. Peirone, and M. Brunetta. 1995. Combined cognitive-behavioral, psychopharmacological and nutritional therapy in bulimia nervosa. *Neuropsychobiology* 32: 68-71.

35. Kaye, W. H., T. Nagata, T. E. Weltzin, L. K. G. Hsu, M. S. Sokol, C. McConaha, et al. 2001. Double-blind placebo-controlled administration of fluoxetine in restricting- and restricting-purging-type anorexia nervosa. *Biological Psychiatry* 49: 644-652.

Antisocial Personality

1.   American Psychiatric Association. 2000. *Diagnostic and Statistical Manual of Mental Disorders.* Text revision ed. Washington, DC: American Psychiatric Association.

2.   O'Connor, L. E. 2000. Pathogenic beliefs and guilt in human evolution: Implications for psychotherapy. In *Genes on the Couch: Explorations in Evolutionary Psychology*, edited by P. Gilbert and K. G. Bailey. New York: Brunner-Routledge.

3.   Hare, R. D. 1996. Psychopathy: A clinical construct whose time has come. *Criminal Justice and Behavior* 23: 25-54.

4.   Hare, R. D. 1991. *The Hare Psychopathy Checklist-Revised.* Toronto, Canada: Multi-Health Systems.

5.   Cooke, D. J., C. Michie, S. D. Hart, and R. D. Hare. 1999. Evaluating the Screening Version of the Hare Psychopathy Checklist-Revised (PCL:SV). An item response theory analysis. *Psychological Assessment* 11: 3-13.

6.   Looman, J., J. Abracen, R. Serin, and P. Marquis. 2005. Psychopathy, treatment change, and recidivism in high-risk, high-need sexual offenders. *Journal of Interpersonal Violence* 20: 549-568.

7.   Hare, R. D. 1999. Psychopathy as a risk factor for violence. *Psychiatric Quarterly* 70: 181-197.

8.   Hare, R. D., D. Clark, M. Grann, and D. Thornton. 2000. Psychopathy and the predictive validity of the PCL-R: An international perspective. *Behavioral Sciences and the Law* 18: 623-645.

9.   Hare, R. D. 1983. Diagnosis of antisocial personality disorder in two prison populations. *American Journal of Psychiatry* 140: 887-890.

10. Cote, G., and S. Hodgins. 1990. Co-occurring mental disorders among criminal offenders. *Bulletin of the American Academy of Psychiatry and Law* 18: 271-281.

11. Bland, R. C., S. C. Newman, R. J. Dyck, and H. Orn. 1990. Prevalence of psychiatric disorders and suicide attempts in a prison population. *Canadian Journal of Psychiatry* 35: 407-413.

12. Moran, P. 1999. The epidemiology of antisocial personality disorder. *Social Psychiatry and Psychiatric Epidemiology* 34: 231-242.

13. Singleton, N., H. Meltzer, R. Gatward, J. W. Coid, and D. Deasy. 1998. *Psychiatric Morbidity Among Prisoners in England and Wales.* London: Office for National Statistics.

14. Robertson, R. G. 1987. The female offender: A Canadian study. *Canadian Journal of Psychiatry* 32: 749-755.

15. Jordan, K., W. E. Schlenger, J. A. Fairbank, and J. M. Caddell. 1996. Prevalence of psychiatric disorders among incarcerated women. II. Convicted felons entering prison. *Archives of General Psychiatry* 53: 513-519.

16. Teplin, L. A., K. M. Abram, and G. M. McClelland. 1996. Prevalence of psychiatric disorders among incarcerated women. I. Pretrial jail detainees. *Archives of General Psychiatry* 53: 505-512.

17. Martin, R. L., C. R. Cloninger, S. B. Guze, and P. J. Clayton. 1985. Mortality in a follow-up of 500 psychiatric outpatients. II. Cause specific mortality. *Archives of General Psychiatry* 42: 58-66.

18. Black, D. W., C. H. Baumgard, and C. E. Bell. 1995. A 16- to 45-year follow-up of 71 men with antisocial personality disorder. *Comprehensive Psychiatry* 36: 130-140.

19. Links, P. S., B. Gould, and R. Ratnayake. 2003. Assessing suicidal youth with antisocial, borderline, or narcissistic personality disorder. *Canadian Journal of Psychiatry* 48: 301-310.

20. Verona, E., C. J. Patrick, and T. E. Joiner. 2001. Psychopathy, antisocial personality, and suicide risk. *Journal of Abnormal Psychology* 110: 462-470.

21. Chioqueta, A. P., and T. C. Stiles. 2004. Assessing suicide risk in Cluster C personality disorders. *Crisis* 25: 128-133.

22. McDonald, A. S., and G. C. L. Davey. 1996. Psychiatric disorders and accidental injury. *Clinical Psychology Review* 16: 105-127.

23. Rydelius, P.-A. 1988. The development of antisocial behaviour and sudden violent death. *Acta Psychiatrica Scandinavica* 77: 398-403.

24. Goodwin, R. D., and S. P. Hamilton. 2003. Lifetime comorbidity of antisocial personality disorder and anxiety disorders among adults in the community. *Psychiatry Research* 117: 159-166.

25. Sareen, J., M. B. Stein, B. J. Cox, and S. T. Hassard. 2004. Understanding comorbidity of anxiety disorders with antisocial behavior: Findings from two large community surveys. *Journal of Nervous and Mental Disease* 192: 178-186.

26. Grant, B. F., D. S. Hasin, F. S. Stinson, D. A. Dawson, S. P. Chou, W. J. Ruan, et al. 2005. Co-occurrence of 12-month mood and anxiety disorders and personality disorders in the US: Results from the National Epidemiologic Survey on Alcohol and Related Conditions. *Journal of Psychiatric Research* 39: 1-9.

27. Skodol, A. E., R. L. Stout, T. H. McGlashan, C. M. Grilo, J. G. Gunderson, M. T. Shea, et al. 1999. Co-occurrence of mood and personality disorders: A report from the Collaborative Longitudinal Personality Disorders Study (CLPS). *Depression and Anxiety* 10: 175-182.

28. Grant, B. F., F. S. Stinson, D. A. Dawson, S. P. Chou, W. J. Ruan, and R. P. Pickering. 2004. Co-occurrence of 12-month alcohol and drug use disorders and personality disorders in the United States: Results from the National Epidemiologic Survey on Alcohol and Related Conditions. *Archives of General Psychiatry* 61: 361-368.

29. Slutske, W. S., S. Eisen, H. Xian, W. R. True, M. J. Lyons, J. Goldberg, et al. 2001. A twin study of the association between pathological gambling and antisocial personality disorder. *Journal of Abnormal Psychology* 110: 297-308.

30. Grant, B. F., D. S. Hasin, F. S. Stinson, D. A. Dawson, S. P. Chou, W. J. Ruan, et al. 2004. Prevalence, correlates, and disability of personality disorders in the United States: Results from the National Epidemiologic Survey on Alcohol and Related Conditions. *Journal of Clinical Psychiatry* 65: 948-958.

31. Torgersen, S., E. Kringlen, and V. Cramer. 2001. The prevalence of personality disorders in a community sample. *Archives of General Psychiatry* 58: 590-596.

32. Ekselius, L., M. Tillfors, T. Furmark, and M. Fredrikson. 2001. Personality disorders in the general population: DSM-IV and ICD-10 defined prevalence as related to sociodemographic profile. *Personality and Individual Differences* 30: 311-320.

33. Button, T. M. M., J. Scourfield, N. Martin, S. Purcell, and P. McGuffin. 2005. Family dysfunction interacts with genes in the causation of antisocial symptoms. *Behavior Genetics* 35: 115-120.

34. Beck, J. E., and D. S. Shaw. 2005. The influence of perinatal complications and environmental adversity on boys' antisocial behavior. *Journal of Child Psychology and Psychiatry* 46: 35-46.

35. Torgersen, S., S. Lygren, P. A. Oien, I. Skre, S. Onstad, J. Edvardsen, et al. 2000. A twin study of personality disorders. *Comprehensive Psychiatry* 41: 416-425.

36. Viding, E., R. J. R. Blair, T. E. Moffitt, and R. Plomin. 2005. Evidence for substantial genetic risk for psychopathy in 7-year-olds. *Journal of Child Psychology and Psychiatry* 46: 592-597.

37. Smith, C. A., and D. P. Farrington. 2004. Continuities in antisocial behavior and parenting across three generations. *Journal of Child Psychology and Psychiatry* 45: 230-247.

38. Reti, I. M., J. F. Samuels, W. W. Eaton, O. J. Bienvenu III, P. T. Costa Jr., and G. Nestadt. 2002. Adult antisocial personality traits are associated with experience of low parental care and maternal overprotection. *Acta Psychiatrica Scandinavica* 106: 126-133.

39. Caspi, A., T. E. Moffitt, J. Morgan, M. Rutter, A. Taylor, L. Arseneault, et al. 2004. Maternal expressed emotion predicts children's antisocial behavior problems: Using monozygotic-twin differences to identify environmental effects on behavioral development. *Developmental Psychology* 40: 149-161.

40. Olweus, D. 1979.   Stability of aggressive reaction patterns in males: A review. *Psychological Bulletin* 86: 852-875.

41. Roff, J. D., and R. D. Wirt. 1984. Childhood aggression and social adjustment as antecedents of delinquency. *Journal of Abnormal Child Psychology* 12: 111-126.

42. Caspi, A., T. E. Moffitt, D. L. Newman, and P. A. Silva. 1996. Behavioural observations at age 3 years predict adult psychiatric disorders. Longitudinal evidence from a birth cohort. *Archives of General Psychiatry* 53: 1033-1039.

43. Kumari, V., M. Das, S. Hodgins, E. Zachariah, I. Barkataki, M. Howlett, et al. 2005. Association between violent behaviour and impaired prepulse inhibition of the startle response in antisocial personality disorder and schizophrenia. *Behavioural Brain Research* 158: 159-166.

44. Seguin, J. R. 2004. Neurocognitive elements of antisocial behavior: Relevance of an orbito-frontal cortex account. *Brain and Cognition* 55: 185-197.

45. Raine, A., T. E. Moffitt, A. Caspi, R. Loeber, M. Stouthamer-Loeber, and D. Lynam. 2005. Neurocognitive impairments in boys on the life-course persistent antisocial path. *Journal of Abnormal Psychology* 114: 38-49.

46. Blair, R. J. R. 2004. The roles of orbital frontal cortex in the modulation of antisocial behavior. *Brain and Cognition* 55: 198-208.

47. Coolidge, F. L., L. L. Thede, and K. L. Jang. 2004. Are personality disorders psychological manifestations of executive function deficits? Bivariate heritability evidence from a twin study. *Behavior Genetics* 34: 75-84.

48. Neugebauer, R., H. W. Hoek, and E. Susser. 1999. Prenatal exposure to wartime famine and development of antisocial personality disorder in early adulthood. *Journal of the American Medical Association* 282: 455-462.

49. Simonoff, E., J. Elander, J. Holmshaw, A. Pickles, R. Murray, and M. Rutter. 2004. Predictors of antisocial personality: Continuities from childhood to adult life. *British Journal of Psychiatry* 184: 118-127.

50. Bernstein, D. P., J. A. Stein, and L. Handelsman. 1998. Predicting personality pathology among adult patients with substance use disorders: Effects of childhood maltreatment. *Addictive Behaviors* 23: 855-868.

51. Kim-Cohen, J., T. E. Moffitt, A. Taylor, S. J. Pawlby, and A. Caspi. 2005. Maternal depression and children's antisocial behavior: Nature and nurture effects. *Archives of General Psychiatry* 62: 173-181.

52. Kasen, S., P. Cohen, A. E. Skodol, J. G. Johnson, E. Smailes, and J. S. Brook. 2001. Childhood depression and adult personality disorder: Alternative pathways of continuity. *Archives of General Psychiatry* 58: 231-236.

53. Donnellan, M. B., K. H. Trzesniewski, R. W. Robins, T. E. Moffitt, and A. Caspi. 2005. Low self-esteem is related to aggression, antisocial behavior, and delinquency. *Psychological Science* 16: 328-335.

54. Eamon, M. K., and C. Mulder. 2005. Predicting antisocial behavior among Latino young adolescents: An ecological systems analysis. *American Journal of Orthopsychiatry* 75: 117-127.

55. Dishion, T. J., S. E. Nelson, C. E. Winter, and B. M. Bullock. 2004. Adolescent friendship as a dynamic system: Entropy and deviance in the etiology and course of male antisocial behavior. *Journal of Abnormal Child Psychology* 32: 651-663.

56. Rowe, R., B. Maughan, C. M. Worthman, E. J. Costello, and A. Angold. 2004. Testosterone, antisocial behavior, and social dominance in boys: Pubertal development and biosocial inter-action. *Biological Psychiatry* 55: 546-552.

57. Crits-Christoph, P., and J. P. Barber. 2002. Psychological treatments for personality disorders. In *A Guide to Treatments That Work*, edited by P. E. Nathan and J. M. Gorman. New York: Oxford University Press.

58. Quality Assurance Project. 1991. Treatment outlines for antisocial personality disorder. *Australian and New Zealand Journal of Psychiatry* 25: 541-547.

59. Beck, A. T., A. Freeman, J. Pretzer, D. D. Davis, B. Fleming, J. S. Beck, et al. 1990. *Cognitive Therapy of Personality Disorders*. New York: The Guilford Press.

60. Ladd, G. T., and N. M. Petry. 2003. Antisocial personality in treatment-seeking cocaine abusers: Psychosocial functioning and HIV risk. *Journal of Substance Abuse Treatment* 24: 323-330.

61. Davidson, K. M., and P. Tyrer. 1996. Cognitive therapy for antisocial and borderline personality disorders: Single case study series. *British Journal of Clinical Psychology* 35: 413-429.

62. Bateman, A. W., and P. Fonagy. 2000. Effectiveness of psychotherapeutic treatment of personality disorder. *British Journal of Psychiatry* 177: 138-143.

63. Leichsenring, F., and E. Leibing. 2003. The effectiveness of psychodynamic therapy and cognitive behavior therapy in the treatment of personality disorders: A meta-analysis. *American Journal of Psychiatry* 160: 1223-1232.

64. Roth, A., and P. Fonagy. 1996. Personality disorders. In *What Works for Whom? A Critical Review of Psychotherapy Research*. New York: The Guilford Press.

Attention-Deficit/Hyperactivity Disorder

1. Hesslinger, B., L. T. van Elst, E. Nyberg, P. Dykierek, H. Richter, M. Berner, et al. 2002. Psychotherapy of attention deficit hyperactivity disorder in adults: A pilot study using a structured skills training program. *European Archives of Psychiatry and Clinical Neuroscience* 252: 177-184.

2. American Psychiatric Association. 2000. *Diagnostic and Statistical Manual of Mental Disorders*. Text revision ed. Washington, DC: American Psychiatric Association.

3. Fitzgerald, M. 2001. Psychopharmacological treatment of adolescent and adult attention deficit hyperactivity disorder. *Irish Journal of Psychological Medicine* 18: 93-98.

4. Wilens, T. 1995. Attention deficit hyperactivity disorder and co-morbid substance use disorders in adults. *Psychiatric Services* 46: 761-763.

5. Montano, B. 2004. Diagnosis and treatment of ADHD in adults in primary care. *Journal of Clinical Psychiatry* 65: 18-21.

6. Faraone, S. V., J. Biederman, T. Spencer, T. Wilens, L. J. Seidman, E. Mick, et al. 2000. Attention-deficit/hyperactivity disorder in adults: An overview. *Biological Psychiatry* 48: 9-20.

7. Biederman, J., J. Newcorn, and S. Sprich. 1991. Comorbidity of attention deficit hyperactivity disorder with conduct, depressive, anxiety, and other disorders. *American Journal of Psychiatry* 148: 564-577.

8. Barkley, R. A. 1996. Attention-deficit/hyperactivity disorder. In *Child Psychopathology*, edited by E. J. Mash and R. A. Barkley. New York: The Guilford Press.

9. Wolraich, M. L., J. N. Hannah, A. Baumgaertel, and I. D. Feurer. 1998. Examination of DSM-IV criteria for attention deficit/hyperactivity disorder in a county-wide sample. *Journal of Developmental and Behavioral Pediatrics* 19: 162-168.

10. Manuzza, S., R. G. Klein, A. Bessler, P. Malloy, and M. LaPadula. 1993. Adult outcome of hyperactive boys: Educational achievement, occupational rank, and psychiatric status. *Archives of General Psychiatry* 50: 565-576.

11. Barkley, R. A. 1990. *Attention-Deficit Hyperactivity Disorder: A Handbook For Diagnosis and Treatment*. New York: The Guilford Press.

12. Gittleman, R., S. Manuzza, R. Shenker, and N. Bonagura. 1985. Hyperactive boys almost grown up. I. Psychiatric status. *Archives of General Psychiatry* 42: 937-947.

13. Weiss, G., and L. Hechtman. 1993. *Hyperactive Children Grown Up*. 2nd ed. New York: The Guilford Press.

14. Manuzza, S., R. G. Klein, N. Bonagura, P. Malloy, R. L. Giampino, and K. A. Addalli. 1991. Hyperactive boys almost grown up. V. Replication of psychiatric status. *Archives of General Psychiatry* 48: 77-83.

15. Mendelson, W., N. Johnson, and M. A. Stewart. 1971. Hyperactive children as teenagers: A follow-up study. *Journal of Nervous and Mental Disease* 163: 273-279.

16. Bellak, L., and R. B. Black. 1992. Attention-deficit hyperactivity disorder in adults. *Clinical Therapy* 14: 138-147.

17. Gorman, C., and L. Greenberg. 1997. *All You Ever Wanted to Know About Attention Deficits but Didn't Know When to Ask*. Los Alamitos, CA: Universal Attention Disorders, Inc.

18. Biederman, J., T. Wilens, T. Spencer, S. V. Faraone, E. Mick, J. S. Ablon, et al. 1996. Diagnosis and treatment of adult attention-deficit/hyperactivity disorder. In *Challenges in Clinical Practice*, edited by M. H. Pollack, M. W. Otto, and J. F. Rosenbaum. New York: The Guilford Press.

19. Murphy, K., and R. A. Barkley. 1996. Prevalence of DSM-IV symptoms of ADHD in adult licensed drivers: Implications for clinical practice. *Journal of Attention Disorders* 1: 147-161.

20. Shekim, W. O., R. F. Asarnow, E. Hess, K. Zaucha, and N. Wheeler. 1990. A clinical demographic profile of a sample of adults with attention deficit hyperactivity disorder, residual state. *Comprehensive Psychiatry* 31: 416-425.

21. Castellanos, F. X., J. N. Giedd, W. L. Marsh, S. D. Hamburger, A. C. Vaituzis, D. P. Dickstein, et al. 1996. Quantitative brain magnetic resonance imaging in attention-deficit hyperactivity disorder. *Archives of General Psychiatry* 53: 607-616.

22. Castellanos, F. X., W. S. Sharp, R. F. Gottesman, D. K. Greenstein, J. N. Giedd, and J. L. Rapoport. 2003. Anatomic brain abnormalities in monozygotic twins discordant for attention deficit hyperactivity disorder. *American Journal of Psychiatry* 160: 1693-1695.

23. Faraone, S. V. 2004. Genetics of adult attention-deficit/hyperactivity disorder. *Psychiatric Clinics of North America* 27: 303-321.

24. Faraone, S. V., and A. E. Doyle. 2001. The nature and heritability of attention-deficit/hyperactivity disorder. *Child and Adolescent Psychiatric Clinics of North America* 10: 299-316.

25. Levy, F., D. A. Hay, M. McStephen, C. Wood, and I. Waldman. 1997. Attention-deficit hyperactivity disorder: A category or a continuum? Genetic analysis of a large-scale twin study. *Journal of the American Academy of Child and Adolescent Psychiatry* 36: 737-744.

26. McGough, J. J., and R. A. Barkley. 2004. Diagnostic controversies in adult attention deficit hyperactivity disorder. *American Journal of Psychiatry* 161: 1948-1956.

27. Robison, L. M., D. A. Sclar, T. L. Skaer, and R. S. Galin. 2004. Treatment modalities among US children diagnosed with attention-deficit hyperactivity disorder: 1995–99. *International Clinical Psychopharmacology* 19: 17-22.

28. Turner, DC, A. D. Blackwell, J. H. Dowson, A. McLean, and B. J. Sahakian. 2005. Neurocognitive effects of methylphenidate in adult attention-deficit/hyperactivity disorder. *Psychopharmacology* 178: 286-295.

29. Spencer, T. 2004. ADHD treatment across the life cycle. *Journal of Clinical Psychiatry* 65: 22-26.

30. Wilens, T., T. Spencer, and J. Biederman. 2000. Pharmacotherapy of attention-deficit/hyperactivity disorder. In *Attention-Deficit Disorders and Comorbidities in Children, Adolescents, and Adults*, edited by T. E. Brown. Washington, DC: American Psychiatric Press.

31. Weiss, M. D., and C. Murray. 2003. Assessment and management of attention-deficit hyperactivity disorder in adults. *Canadian Medical Association Journal* 168: 715-722.

32. Ramsay, J. R., and A. L. Rostain. 2003. A cognitive therapy approach for adult attention deficit/hyperactivity disorder. *Journal of Cognitive Psychotherapy* 17: 319-334.

33. McDermott, S. P. 2000. Cognitive therapy for adults with attention-deficit/hyperactivity disorder. In *Attention-Deficit Disorders and Comorbidities in Children, Adolescents, and Adults*, edited by T. E. Brown. Washington, DC: American Psychiatric Press.

34. Ramsay, J. R., and A. L. Rostain. 2005. Adapting psychotherapy to meet the needs of adults with attention-deficit/hyperactivity disorder. *Psychotherapy: Theory, Research, Practice, Training* 42: 72-84.

35. Wiggins, D., K. Singh, H. G. Getz, and D. E. Hutchins. 1999. Effects of brief group intervention for adults with attention deficit/hyperactivity disorder. *Journal of Mental Health Counseling* 21: 82-92.

36. Wilens, T., S. P. McDermott, J. Biederman, A. Abrantes, A. Hahesy, and T. J. Spencer. 1999. Cognitive therapy in the treatment of adults with ADHD: A systematic chart review of 26 cases. *Journal of Cognitive Psychotherapy* 13: 215-226.

37. Stevenson, C. S., S. Whitmont, L. Bornholt, D. Livesey, and R. J. Stevenson. 2002. A cognitive remediation programme for adults with Attention Deficit Hyperactivity Disorder. *Australian and New Zealand Journal of Psychiatry* 36: 610-616.

38. Safren, S. A., S. Sprich, S. Chulvick, and M. W. Otto. 2004. Psychosocial treatments for adults with attention-deficit/hyperactivity disorder. *Psychiatric Clinics of North America* 27: 349-360.

Bipolar Disorder/Manic Depression

1.   American Psychiatric Association. 2000. *Diagnostic and Statistical Manual of Mental Disorders.* Text revision ed. Washington, DC: American Psychiatric Association.

2.   Kessler, R. C., K. A. McGonagle, S. Zhao, C. B. Nelson, M. Hughes, S. Eshleman, et al. 1994. Lifetime and 12-month prevalence of DSM-III-R psychiatric disorders in the United States. *Archives of General Psychiatry* 51: 8-19.

3.   Angst, J., and R. Selloro. 2000. Historical perspectives and natural history of bipolar disorder. *Biological Psychiatry* 48: 445-457.

4.   U.S. Department of Health and Human Services. 1999. *Mental Health: A Report of the Surgeon General.* Rockville, MD: U.S. Department of Health and Human Services, Substance Abuse and Mental Health Services Administration, Center for Mental Health Services, National Institutes of Health, National Insitute of Mental Health.

5.   National Institute of Mental Health. 2002. *Bipolar Disorder.* In NIH Publication No. 02-3679. Bethesda, MD: National Institute of Mental Health, National Institutes of Health, US Department of Health and Human Services.

6.   Fagiolini, A., D. J. Kupfer, P. Rucci, J. A. Scott, D. M. Novick, and E. Frank. 2004. Suicide attempts and ideation in patients with bipolar I disorder. *Journal of Clinical Psychiatry* 65: 509-514.

7.   Goodwin, F. K., and K. R. Jamison. 1990. Suicide. In *Manic-Depressive Illness*, edited by F. K. Goodwin and K. R. Jamison. New York: Oxford University Press.

8.   Chen, Y.-W., and S. C. Dilsaver. 1996. Lifetime rates of suicide attempts among subjects with bipolar and unipolar disorders relative to subjects with other axis I disorders. *Biological Psychiatry* 39: 896-899.

9.   Guze, S. B., and E. Robins. 1970. Suicide and primary affective disorders. *British Journal of Psychiatry* 117: 437-438.

10. CPG Team for Bipolar Disorder. 2004. Australian and New Zealand clinical practice guidelines for the treatment of bipolar disorder. *Australian and New Zealand Journal of Psychiatry* 38: 280-305.

11. Harris, E. C., and B. Barraclough. 1997. Suicide as an outcome for mental disorders: a meta-analysis. *British Journal of Psychiatry* 170: 205-228.

12. Kessler, R. C., W. T. Chiu, O. Demler, and E. E. Walters. 2005. Prevalence, severity, and comorbidity of 12-month DSM-IV disorders in the National Comorbidity Survey Replication. *Archives of General Psychiatry* 62: 617-627.

13. Camacho, A. 2004. Are some forms of substance abuse related to the bipolar spectrum? Hypothetical considerations and therapeutic implications. *Primary Psychiatry* 11: 42-46.

14. McElroy, S. L., L. L. Altschuler, T. Suppes, P. E. Keck Jr., M. A. Frye, K. D. Denicoff, et al. 2001. Axis I psychiatric comorbidity and its relationship to historical illness variables in 288 patients with bipolar disorder. *American Journal of Psychiatry* 158: 420-426.

15. Grant, B. F., F. S. Stinson, D. A. Dawson, P. Chou, M. C. Dufour, W. Compton, et al. 2004. Prevalence and co-occurrence of substance use disorders and independent mood and anxiety disorders: Results from the National Epidemiologic Survey on Alcohol and Related Conditions. *Archives of General Psychiatry* 61: 807-816.

16. Dalton, E. J., T. D. Cate-Carter, E. Mundo, S. V. Parikh, and J. L. Kennedy. 2003. Suicide risk in bipolar patients: The role of co-morbid substance use disorders. *Bipolar Disorders* 5: 58-61.

17. Simpson, S. G., and K. R. Jamison. 1999. The risk of suicide in patients with bipolar disorders. *Journal of Clinical Psychiatry* 60: 53-56.

18. Simon, N. M., M. W. Otto, S. R. Wisniewski, M. Fossey, K. Sagduyu, E. Frank, et al. 2004. Anxiety disorder comorbidity in bipolar disorder patients: Data from the first 500 participants in the Systematic Treatment Enhancement Program for Bipolar Disorder (STEP-BD). *American Journal of Psychiatry* 161: 2222-2229.

19. Bauer, M. S., L. Altshuler, D. R. Evans, T. Beresford, W. O. Williford, and R. Hauger. 2005. Prevalence and distinct correlates of anxiety, substance, and combined comorbidity in a multi-site public sector sample with bipolar disorder. *Journal of Affective Disorders* 85: 301-315.

20. Pini, S., G. B. Cassano, E. Simonini, M. Savino, A. Russo, and S. A. Montgomery. 1997. Prevalence of anxiety disorders comorbidity in bipolar depression, unipolar depression and dysthymia. *Journal of Affective Disorders* 42: 145-153.

21. Skodol, A. E., R. L. Stout, T. H. McGlashan, C. M. Grilo, J. G. Gunderson, M. T. Shea, et al. 1999. Co-occurrence of mood and personality disorders: A report from the Collaborative Longitudinal Personality Disorders Study (CLPS). *Depression and Anxiety* 10: 175-182.

22. Grant, B. F., D. S. Hasin, F. S. Stinson, D. A. Dawson, S. P. Chou, W. J. Ruan, et al. 2005. Co-occurrence of 12-month mood and anxiety disorders and personality disorders in the US: Results from the national epidemiologic survey on alcohol and related conditions. *Journal of Psychiatric Research* 39: 1-9.

23. McElroy, S. L., R. Kotwal, and S. Malhotra. 2004. Comorbidity of bipolar disorder and eating disorders: What can the clinician do? *Primary Psychiatry* 11: 36-41.

24. Murray, C. J. L., and A. D. Lopez, eds. 1996. *Summary: The Global Burden of Disease: A Comprehensive Assessment of Mortality and Disability from Diseases, Injuries, and Risk Factors In 1990 and Projected to 2020.* Cambridge, MA: Published by the Harvard School of Public Health on behalf of the World Health Organization and the World Bank: Harvard University Press.

25. Kessler, R. C., P. A. Berglund, O. Demler, R. Jin, and E. E. Walters. 2005. Lifetime prevalence and age-of-onset distributions of DSM-IV disorders in the National Comorbidity Survey Replication. *Archives of General Psychiatry* 62: 593-602.

26. Narrow, W. E. 1998. *One-year prevalence of depressive disorders among adults 18 and over in the U.S.: NIMH ECA prospective data. Population estimates based on U.S. census estimated residential population age 18 and over on July 1, 1998.* Unpublished table.

27. Coryell, W., J. Endicott, and M. Keller. 1992. Rapidly cycling affective disorder. Demographics, diagnosis, family history, and course. *Archives of General Psychiatry* 49: 126-131.

28. Blehar, M. C., J. R. DePaulo, E. S. Gershon, T. Reich, S. G. Simpson, and J. I. Nurnberger. 1998. Women with bipolar disorder: Findings from the NIMH Genetics Initiative sample. *Psychopharmacology Bulletin* 34: 239-243.

29. National Institute of Mental Health. 1998. *Genetics and Mental Disorders.* In NIH Publication No. 98-4268. Rockville, MD: National Institute of Mental Health.

30. Ackenheil, M. 2001. Neurotransmitters and signal transduction processes in bipolar affective disorders: A synopsis. *Journal of Affective Disorders* 62: 101-111.

31. Mahmood, T., and T. Silverstone. 2001. Serotonin and bipolar disorder. *Journal of Affective Disorders* 66: 1-11.

32. Miklowitz, D. J. 2001. Bipolar disorder. In *Clinical Handbook of Psychological Disorders: A Step-by-Step Treatment Manual*, edited by D. H. Barlow. New York: The Guilford Press.

33. Miklowitz, D. J., and M. J. Goldstein. 1997. *Bipolar Disorder: A Family-Focused Treatment Approach.* New York: The Guilford Press.

34. Malkoff-Schwartz, S., E. Frank, B. Anderson, J. T. Sherrill, L. Siegel, D. Patterson, et al. 1998. Stressful life events and social rhythm disruption in the onset of manic and depressive bipolar episodes: A preliminary investigation. *Archives of General Psychiatry* 55: 702-707.

35. Wang, P. S., M. Lane, M. Olfson, H. A. Pincus, K. B. Wells, and R. C. Kessler. 2005. Twelve-month use of mental health services in the United States. Results from the National Comorbidity Survey Replication. *Archives of General Psychiatry* 62: 629-640.

36. Wang, P. S., P. A. Berglund, M. Olfson, H. A. Pincus, K. B. Wells, and R. C. Kessler. 2005. Failure and delay in initial treatment contact after first onset of mental disorders in the National Comorbidity Survey Replication. *Archives of General Psychiatry* 62: 603-613.

37. Chou, J. C.-Y. 2004. Review and update of the American Psychiatric Association Practice Guideline for Bipolar Disorder. *Primary Psychiatry* 11: 73-84.

38. Goodwin, F. K., B. Fireman, G. E. Simon, E. M. Hunkeler, J. Lee, and D. Revicki. 2003. Suicide risk in bipolar disorder during treatment with lithium and divalproex. *Journal of the American Medical Association* 290: 1467-1473.

39. Anderson, T. R., J. F. Goldberg, and M. Harrow. 2004. A review of medication side effects and treatment adherence in bipolar disorder. *Primary Psychiatry* 11: 48-54.

40. Johnson, R. E., and B. H. McFarland. 1996. Lithium use and discontinuation in a health maintenance organization. *American Journal of Psychiatry* 153: 993-1000.

41. Lingam, R., and J. Scott. 2002. Treatment non-adherence in affective disorders. *Acta Psychiatrica Scandinavica* 105: 164-172.

42. Craighead, W. E., D. J. Miklowitz, E. Frank, and F. C. Vajk. 2002. Psychosocial treatments for bipolar disorder. In *A Guide to Treatments That Work,* edited by P. E. Nathan and J. M. Gorman. New York: Oxford University Press.

43. Scott, J. 2001. Cognitive therapy as an adjunct to medication in bipolar disorder. *British Journal of Psychiatry* 178: s164-s168.

44. Chor, P. N., M. A. Mercier, and I. S. Halper. 1988. Use of cognitive therapy for treatment of a patient suffering from a bipolar affective disorder. *Journal of Cognitive Psychotherapy* 2: 51-58.

45. Zaretsky, A. E., Z. V. Segal, and M. Gemar. 1999. Cognitive therapy for bipolar depression: A pilot study. *Canadian Journal of Psychiatry* 44: 491-494.

46. Lam, D. H., E. R. Watkins, P. Hayward, J. Bright, K. Wright, N. Kerr, et al. 2003. A randomized controlled study of cognitive therapy for relapse prevention for bipolar affective disorder: Outcome of the first year. *Archives of General Psychiatry* 60: 145-152.

47. Lam, D. H., J. Bright, S. Jones, P. Hayward, N. Schuck, D. Chisholm, et al. 2000. Cognitive therapy for bipolar illness—a pilot study of relapse prevention. *Cognitive Therapy and Research* 24: 503-520.

48. Palmer, A. G., H. Williams, and M. Adams. 1995. CBT in a group format for bi-polar affective disorder. *Behavioural and Cognitive Psychotherapy* 23: 153-168.

49. Patelis-Siotis, I., L. T. Young, J. C. Robb, M. Marriott, P. J. Bieling, L. C. Cox, et al. 2001. Group cognitive behavioral therapy for bipolar disorder: A feasibility and effectiveness study. *Journal of Affective Disorders* 65: 145-153.

50. Miklowitz, D. J., T. L. Simoneau, E. L. George, J. A. Richards, A. Kalbag, N. Sachs-Ericsson, et al. 2000. Family-focused treatment of bipolar disorder: 1-year effects of a psychoeducational program in conjunction with pharmacotherapy. *Biological Psychiatry* 48: 582-592.

51. Clarkin, J. F., I. D. Glick, G. L. Haas, J. H. Spencer, A. B. Lewis, J. Peyser, et al. 1990. A randomized clinical trial of inpatient family intervention. V. Results for affective disorders. *Journal of Affective Disorders* 18: 17-28.

52. Frank, E., D. J. Kupfer, C. L. Ehlers, T. H. Monk, C. Cornes, S. Carter, et al. 1994. Interpersonal and social rhythm therapy for bipolar disorder: Integrating interpersonal and behavioural approaches. *Behaviour Therapy* 17: 153-166.

53. Klerman, G. L. 1988. Principles of interpersonal psychotherapy for depression. In *Depression and Mania*, edited by A. Georgotas and R. Cancro. New York: Elsevier.

54. Bauer, M., and R. McBride. 1997. *Structured Group Psychotherapy for Bipolar Disorder.* New York: Springer.

55. Colom, F., E. Vieta, A. Martinez-Arn, M. Reinares, J. M. Goikolea, A. Benabarre, et al. 2003. A randomized trial on the efficacy of group psychoeducation in the prophylaxis of recurrences in bipolar patients whose disease is in remission. *Archives of General Psychiatry* 60: 402-407.

56. Kahn, D. A. 1993. The use of psychodynamic psychotherapy in manic-depressive illness. *Journal of the American Academy of Psychoanalysis and Dynamic Psychiatry* 21: 441-455.

57. Perry, A., N. Tarrier, R. Morriss, E. McCarthy, and K. Limb. 1999. Randomized controlled trial of efficacy of teaching patients with bipolar disorder to identify early symptoms of relapse and obtain treatment. *British Medical Journal* 318: 149-153.

58. Osher, Y., Y. Bersudsky, and R. H. Belmaker. 2005. Omega-3 eicosapentaenoic acid in bipolar depression: Report of a small open-label study. *Journal of Clinical Psychiatry* 66: 726-729.

59. Stoll, A. L., C. A. Locke, L. B. Marangell, and W. E. Severus. 1999. Omega-3 fatty acids and bipolar disorder: A review. *Prostaglandins, Leukotrienes, and Essential Fatty Acids* 60: 329-337.

60. Stoll, A. L., E. Severus, M. P. Freeman, S. Rueter, H. A. Zboyan, E. Diamond, et al. 1999. Omega 3 fatty acids in bipolar disorder: A preliminary double-blind, placebo-controlled trial. *Archives of General Psychiatry* 56: 407-412.

Body Dysmorphic Disorder

1. American Psychiatric Association. 2000. *Diagnostic and Statistical Manual of Mental Disorders.* Text revision ed. Washington, DC: American Psychiatric Association.
2. Veale, D., and S. Riley. 2001. Mirror, mirror on the wall, who is the ugliest of them all? The psychopathology of mirror gazing in body dysmorphic disorder. *Behaviour Research and Therapy* 39: 1381-1393.
3. Phillips, K. A. 1991. Body dysmorphic disorder: The distress of imagined ugliness. *American Journal of Psychiatry* 148: 1138-1149.
4. Neziroglu, F., and S. Khemlani-Patel. 2003. Therapeutic approaches to body dysmorphic disorder. *Brief Treatment and Crisis Intervention* 3: 307-322.
5. Phillips, K. A., J. Grant, J. Siniscalchi, and R. S. Albertini. 2001. Surgical and nonpsychiatric medical treatment of patients with body dysmorphic disorder. *Psychosomatics* 42: 504-510.
6. Phillips, K. A., J. M. Siniscalchi, and S. L. McElroy. 2004. Depression, anxiety, anger, and somatic symptoms in patients with body dysmorphic disorder. *Psychiatric Quarterly* 75: 309-320.
7. Gunstad, J., and K. A. Phillips. 2003. Axis I comorbidity in body dysmorphic disorder. *Comprehensive Psychiatry* 44: 270-276.
8. Simeon, D., E. Hollander, D. J. Stein, L. Cohen, and B. Aronowitz. 1995. Body dysmorphic disorder in the DSM-IV field trial for obsessive-compulsive disorder. *American Journal of Psychiatry* 152: 1207-1209.
9. Eisen, S. V., J. A. Shaul, H. S. Leff, V. Stringfellow, B. R. Clarridge, and P. D. Cleary. 2001. Toward a national consumer survey: Evaluation of the CABHS and MHSIP instruments. *Journal of Behavioral Health Services and Research* 28: 347-369.
10. Frare, F., G. Perugi, G. Ruffolo, and C. Toni. 2004. Obsessive-compulsive disorder and body dysmorphic disorder: A comparison of clinical features. *European Psychiatry* 19: 292-298.
11. Rauch, S. L., K. A. Phillips, E. Segal, N. Makris, L. M. Shin, P. J. Whalen, et al. 2003. A preliminary morphometric magnetic resonance imaging study of regional brain volumes in body dysmorphic disorder. *Psychiatry Research: Neuroimaging* 122: 13-19.
12. Jolanta, J. R.-J., and M. S. Tomasz. 2000. The links between body dysmorphic disorder and eating disorders. *European Psychiatry* 15: 302-305.
13. Grant, J. E., S. W. Kim, and E. D. Eckert. 2002. Body dysmorphic disorder in patients with anorexia nervosa: Prevalence, clinical features and delusionality of body image. *International Journal of Eating Disorders* 32: 291-300.
14. Phillips, K. A., and S. F. Diaz. 1997. Gender differences in body dysmorphic disorder. *Journal of Nervous and Mental Disease* 185: 570-577.
15. Faravelli, C., S. Salvatori, F. Galassi, L. Aiazzi, C. Drei, and P. Cabras. 1997. Epidemiology of somatoform disorders: A community survey in Florence. *Social Psychiatry and Psychiatric Epidemiology* 32: 24-29.
16. Otto, M. W., S. Wilhelm, L. S. Cohen, and B. L. Harlow. 2001. Prevalence of body dysmorphic disorder in a community sample of women. *American Journal of Psychiatry* 158: 2061-2063.
17. Bienvenu, O. J., J. F. Samuels, M. A. Riddle, R. Hoehn-Saric, K. Liang, B. A. M. Cullen, et al. 2000. The relationship of obsessive-compulsive disorder to possible spectrum disorders: Results from a family study. *Biological Psychiatry* 48: 287-293.
18. Bilby, E. L. 1998. The relationship between body dysmorphic disorder and depression, self-esteem, somatization, and obsessive-compulsive disorder. *Journal of Clinical Psychology* 54: 489-499.
19. Neziroglu, F., M. C. Anderson, and J. A. Yaryura-Tobias. 1999. An in-depth review of obsessive-compulsive disorder, body dysmorphic disorder, hypochondriasis, and trichotillomania: Therapeutic issues and current research. *Crisis Intervention* 5: 59-94.
20. Carroll, D. H., L. Scahill, and K. A. Phillips. 2002. Current concepts in body dysmorphic disorder. *Archives of Psychiatric Nursing* 16: 72-79.
21. Gabbay, V., M. A. O'Dowd, A. J. Weiss, and G. M. Asnis. 2002. Body dysmorphic disorder triggered by medical illness? *American Journal of Psychiatry* 159: 493.

22. Hausmann, A., B. Mangweth, T. Walch, C. I. Rupp, and H. G. Pope Jr. 2004. Body-image dissatisfaction in gay versus heterosexual men: Is there really a difference? *Journal of Clinical Psychiatry* 65: 1555-1558.

23. Andrist, L. C. 2003. Media images, body dissatisfaction, and disordered eating in adolescent women. *American Journal of Maternity and Child Nursing* 28: 119-123.

24. Pope, H. G., Jr., K. A. Phillips, and R. Olivardia. 2000. *The Adonis Complex: The Secret Crisis of Male Body Obsession.* New York: Free Press.

25. Harris, D. L., and A. T. Carr. 2001. Prevalence of concern about physical appearance in the general population. *British Journal of Plastic Surgery* 54: 223-226.

26. Gruber, A. J., H. G. Pope Jr., J. K. Lalonde, and J. I. Hudson. 2001. Why do young women diet? The roles of body fat, body perception, and body ideal. *Journal of Clinical Psychiatry* 62: 609-611.

27. Mangweth, B., A. Hausmann, T. Walch, A. Hotter, C. I. Rupp, W. Biebl, et al. 2004. Body fat perception in eating-disordered men. *International Journal of Eating Disorders* 35: 102-108.

28. Eisen, J. L., K. A. Phillips, M. E. Coles, and S. A. Rasmussen. 2004. Insight in obsessive compulsive disorder and body dysmorphic disorder. *Comprehensive Psychiatry* 45: 10-15.

29. Veale, D., M. Ennis, and C. Lambrou. 2002. Possible association of body dysmorphic disorder with an occupation or education in art and design. *American Journal of Psychiatry* 159: 1788-1790.

30. Aouizerate, B., H. Pujol, D. Grabot, M. Faytout, K. Suire, C. Braud, et al. 2003. Body dysmorphic disorder in a sample of cosmetic surgery applicants. *European Psychiatry* 18: 365-368.

31. Castle, D. J., M. Molton, K. Hoffman, N. J. Preston, and K. A. Phillips. 2004. Correlates of dysmorphic concern in people seeking cosmetic enhancement. *Australian and New Zealand Journal of Psychiatry* 38: 439-444.

32. McKay, D., J. Todaro, F. Neziroglu, and T. Campisi. 1997. Body dysmorphic disorder: A preliminary evaluation of treatment and maintenance using exposure with response prevention. *Behaviour Research and Therapy* 35: 67-70.

33. Veale, D., K. Gournay, W. Dryden, A. Boocock, F. Shah, R. Willson, et al. 1996. Body dysmorphic disorder: A cognitive behavioural model and pilot randomised controlled trial. *Behaviour Research and Therapy* 34: 717-729.

34. Rosen, J. C., J. Reiter, and P. Orosan. 1995. Cognitive behavioral body image therapy for body dysmorphic disorder. *Journal of Consulting and Clinical Psychology* 63: 263-269.

35. Wilhelm, S., M. W. Otto, B. Lohr, and T. Deckersbach. 1999. Cognitive behavior group therapy for body dysmorphic disorder: A case series. *Behaviour Research and Therapy* 37: 71-75.

36. Brown, K. W., T. McGoldrick, and R. Buchanan. 1997. Body dysmorphic disorder: Seven cases treated with eye movement desensitization and reprocessing. *Behavioural and Cognitive Psychotherapy* 25: 203-207.

37. Brady, K. T., L. Austin, and R. B. Lydiard. 1990. Body dysmorphic disorder: The relationship to obsessive-compulsive disorder. *Journal of Nervous and Mental Disease* 178: 538-540.

38. Phillips, K. A., R. S. Albertini, and S. A. Rasmussen. 2002. A randomized placebo controlled trial of fluoxetine in body dysmorphic disorder. *Archives of General Psychiatry* 59: 381-388.

39. Phillips, K. A., S. L. McElroy, M. M. Dwight, J. L. Eisen, and S. A. Rasmussen. 2001. Delusionality and response to open label fluvoxamine in body dysmorphic disorder. *Journal of Clinical Psychiatry* 62: 87-91.

40. Phillips, K. A., and S. A. Rasmussen. 2004. Change in psychosocial functioning and quality of life of patients with body dysmorphic disorder treated with fluoxetine: A placebo-controlled study. *Psychosomatics* 45: 438-444.

41. Phillips, K. A., M. M. Dwight, and S. L. McElroy. 1998. Efficacy and safety of fluvoxamine in body dysmorphic disorder. *Journal of Clinical Psychiatry* 59: 165-171.

Bulimia

1. American Psychiatric Association. 2000. *Diagnostic and Statistical Manual of Mental Disorders.* Text revision ed. Washington, DC: American Psychiatric Association.

2.   Keel, P. K., and J. E. Mitchell. 1997. Outcome in bulimia nervosa. *American Journal of Psychiatry* 154: 313-321.

3.   Zipfel, S., B. Lowe, D. L. Reas, H. C. Deter, and W. Herzog. 2000. Long-term prognosis in anorexia nervosa: Lessons from a 21-year follow-up study. *Lancet* 355: 721-722.

4.   Mehler, P. S. 2003. Bulimia nervosa. *New England Journal of Medicine* 349: 875-881.

5.   Mendell, D. A., and J. A. Logemann. 2001. Bulimia and swallowing: Cause for concern. *International Journal of Eating Disorders* 30: 252-258.

6.   Mehler, P. S. 1997. Constipation: Diagnosis and treatment in eating disorders. *Eating Disorders* 5: 41-46.

7.   Wolfe, B. E., E. D. Metzger, J. M. Levine, and DC Jimerson. 2001. Laboratory screening for electrolyte abnormalities and anemia in bulimia nervosa: A controlled study. *International Journal of Eating Disorders* 30: 288-293.

8.   Greenfeld, D., D. Mickley, D. M. Quinlan, and P. Roloff. 1995. Hypokalemia in outpatients with eating disorders. *American Journal of Psychiatry* 152: 60-63.

9.   Ho, P. C., R. Dweik, and M. C. Cohen. 1998. Rapidly reversible cardiomyopathy associated with chronic ipecac ingestion. *Clinical Cardiology* 21: 780-783.

10.   Brewerton, T. D., B. Lydiard, D. B. Herzog, A. W. Brotman, P. M. O'Neil, and J. C. Ballenger. 1995. Comorbidity of Axis I psychiatric disorders in bulimia nervosa. *Journal of Clinical Psychiatry* 56: 77-79.

11.   Dansky, B. S., T. D. Brewerton, D. G. Kilpatrick, P. M. O'Neil, H. S. Resnick, C. L. Best, et al. 1998. The nature and prevalence of binge eating disorder in a national sample of women. In *DSM-IV Sourcebook*, edited by T. A. Widiger, A. J. Frances, H. A. Pincus, R. Ross, M. B. First, W. F. Davis, et al. Washington, DC: APA Press.

12.   Rubenstein, C. S., T. A. Pigott, M. Altemus, F. L'Heureux, J. J. Gray, and D. L. Murphy. 1993. High rates of comorbid OCD in patients with bulimia nervosa. *Eating Disorders: The Journal of Treatment and Prevention* 1: 147-155.

13.   Lacey, J. H. 1993. Self-damaging and addictive behaviour in bulimia nervosa: A catchment area study. *British Journal of Psychiatry* 163: 190-194.

14.   Schmidt, N. B., and M. J. Telch. 1990. Prevalence of personality disorders among bulimics, nonbulimic binge eaters, and normal controls. *Journal of Psychopathology and Behavioral Assessment* 12: 169-185.

15.   Carroll, J. M., S. W. Touyz, and P. J. V. Beaumont. 1996. Specific comorbidity between bulimia nervosa and personality disorders. *International Journal of Eating Disorders* 19: 159-170.

16.   Lewinsohn, P. M., R. H. Striegel-Moore, and J. R. Seeley. 2000. Epidemiology and natural course of eating disorders in young women from adolescence to young adulthood. *Journal of the American Academy of Child and Adolescent Psychiatry* 39: 1284-1292.

17.   Kreipe, R. E., and S. A. Birndorf. 2000. Eating disorders in adolescents and young adults. *Medical Clinics of North America* 84: 1027-1049.

18.   Drewnowski, A., S. A. Hopkins, and R. C. Kessler. 1988. The prevalence of bulimia nervosa in the U.S. college student population. *American Journal of Public Health* 78: 1322-1325.

19.   Woodside, D. B., P. E. Garfinkel, E. Lin, P. Goering, A. S. Kaplan, D. S. Goldbloom, et al. 2001. Comparisons of men with full or partial eating disorders, men without eating disorders, and women with eating disorders in the community. *American Journal of Psychiatry* 158: 570-574.

20.   Ray, S. L. 2004. Eating disorders in adolescent males. *Professional School Counseling* 8: 98-101.

21.   Patel, D. R., H. D. Pratt, and D. E. Greydanus. 2003. Treatment of adolescents with anorexia nervosa. *Journal of Adolescent Research* 18: 244-260.

22.   Scheider, J. A. 1991. Gender identity issues in male bulimia nervosa. In *Psychodynamic Treatment of Anorexia Nervosa and Bulimia*, edited by C. Johnson. New York: The Guilford Press.

23.   Keel, P., K. L. Klump, G. Leon, and J. Fulkerson. 1998. Disordered eating in adolescent males from a school-based sample. *International Journal of Eating Disorders* 23: 125-132.

24.   Russell, C. J., and P. K. Keel. 2002. Homosexuality as a specific risk factor for eating disorders in men. *International Journal of Eating Disorders* 31: 300-306.

25. Bulik, C. M., B. Devlin, S. A. Bacanu, L. Thornton, K. L. Klump, M. M. Fichter, et al. 2003. Significant linkage on chromosome 10p in families with bulimia nervosa. *American Journal of Human Genetics* 72: 200-207.

26. Vaz, F. J. 1998. Outcome of bulimia nervosa: Prognostic indicators. *Journal of Psychosomatic Research* 45: 391-400.

27. Fairburn, C. G., S. L. Welch, H. A. Doll, B. A. Davies, and M. E. O'Connor. 1997. Risk factors for bulimia nervosa: A community-based case-control study. *Archives of General Psychiatry* 54: 509-517.

28. McCarthy, M. 1990. The thin ideal, depression and eating disorders in women. *Behaviour Research and Therapy* 28: 205-215.

29. Williams, M. S., S. R. Thomsen, and J. K. McCoy. 2003. Looking for an accurate mirror: A model for the relationship between media use and anorexia. *Eating Behaviors* 4: 127-134.

30. Harris, D. J., and S. A. Kuba. 1997. Ethnocultural identity and eating disorders in women of color. *Professional Psychology: Research and Practice* 28: 341-347.

31. Bacaltchuk, J., R. P. Trefiglio, I. R. Oliveira, P. Hay, M. S. Lima, and J. J. Mari. 2000. Combination of antidepressants and psychological treatments for bulimia nervosa: A systematic review. *Acta Psychiatrica Scandinavica* 101: 256-264.

32. Agras, W. S., T. Walsh, C. G. Fairburn, G. T. Wilson, and H. C. Kraemer. 2000. A multicenter comparison of cognitive-behavioral therapy and interpersonal psychotherapy for bulimia nervosa. *Archives of General Psychiatry* 57: 459-466.

33. Richards, P. S., B. M. Baldwin, H. A. Frost, J. B. Clark-Sly, M. E. Berrett, and R. K. Hardman. 2000. What works for treating eating disorders? Conclusions of 28 outcome reviews. *Eating Disorders: The Journal of Treatment and Prevention* 8: 189-206.

34. Chen, E., S. W. Touyz, P. J. V. Beumont, C. G. Fairburn, R. Griffiths, P. Butow, et al. 2003. Comparison of group and individual cognitive-behavioral therapy for patients with bulimia nervosa. *International Journal of Eating Disorders* 33: 241-254.

35. Openshaw, C., G. Waller, and D. Sperlinger. 2004. Group cognitive-behavior therapy for bulimia nervosa: Statistical versus clinical significance of changes in symptoms across treatment. *International Journal of Eating Disorders* 36: 363-375.

36. Fairburn, C. G., P. A. Norman, S. L. Welch, M. E. O'Connor, H. A. Doll, and R. C. Peveler. 1995. A prospective study of outcome in bulimia nervosa and the long-term effects of three psychological treatments. *Archives of General Psychiatry* 52: 304-312.

37. Bachar, E., Y. Latzer, S. Kreitler, and E. M. Berry. 1999. Empirical comparison of two psychological therapies. Self psychology and cognitive orientation in the treatment of anorexia and bulimia. *Journal of Psychotherapy Practice and Research* 8: 115-128.

38. Zhu, A. J., and B. T. Walsh. 2002. Pharmocologic treatment of eating disorders. *Canadian Journal of Psychiatry* 47: 227-234.

39. Latner, J. D., and G. T. Wilson. 2004. Binge eating and satiety in bulimia nervosa and binge eating disorder: Effects of macronutrient intake. *International Journal of Eating Disorders* 36: 402-415.

Dependent Personality

1. American Psychiatric Association. 2000. *Diagnostic and Statistical Manual of Mental Disorders.* Text revision ed. Washington, DC: American Psychiatric Association.

2. Overholser, J. C. 1996. The dependent personality and interpersonal problems. *Journal of Nervous and Mental Disease* 184: 8-16.

3. Grant, B. F., D. S. Hasin, F. S. Stinson, D. A. Dawson, S. P. Chou, W. J. Ruan, et al. 2005. Co-occurrence of 12-month mood and anxiety disorders and personality disorders in the US: Results from the national epidemiologic survey on alcohol and related conditions. *Journal of Psychiatric Research* 39: 1-9.

4. Oldham, J. M., A. E. Skodol, H. D. Kellman, S. E. Hyler, N. Doidge, L. Rosnick, et al. 1995. Comorbidity of axis I and axis II disorders. *American Journal of Psychiatry* 152: 571-578.

5. Skodol, A. E., R. L. Stout, T. H. McGlashan, C. M. Grilo, J. G. Gunderson, M. T. Shea, et al. 1999. Co-occurrence of mood and personality disorders: A report from the Collaborative Longitudinal Personality Disorders Study (CLPS). *Depression and Anxiety* 10: 175-182.

6. Skodol, A. E., P. E. Gallaher, and J. M. Oldham. 1996. Excessive dependency and depression: Is the relationship specific? *Journal of Nervous and Mental Disease* 184: 165-171.

7. Chioqueta, A. P., and T. C. Stiles. 2004. Assessing suicide risk in cluster C personality disorders. *Crisis* 25: 128-133.

8. Marchiori, E., S. Loschi, P. L. Marconi, D. Mioni, and L. Pavan. 1999. Dependence, locus of control, parental bonding, and personality disorders: A study in alcoholics and controls. *Alcohol and Alcoholism* 34: 396-401.

9. Grant, B. F., F. S. Stinson, D. A. Dawson, S. P. Chou, W. J. Ruan, and R. P. Pickering. 2004. Co-occurrence of 12-month alcohol and drug use disorders and personality disorders in the United States: Results from the National Epidemiologic Survey on Alcohol and Related Conditions. *Archives of General Psychiatry* 61: 361-368.

10. Grant, B. F., D. S. Hasin, F. S. Stinson, D. A. Dawson, S. P. Chou, W. J. Ruan, et al. 2004. Prevalence, correlates, and disability of personality disorders in the United States: Results from the National Epidemiologic Survey on Alcohol and Related Conditions. *Journal of Clinical Psychiatry* 65: 948-958.

11. Torgersen, S., E. Kringlen, and V. Cramer. 2001. The prevalence of personality disorders in a community sample. *Archives of General Psychiatry* 58: 590-596.

12. Ekselius, L., M. Tillfors, T. Furmark, and M. Fredrikson. 2001. Personality disorders in the general population: DSM-IV and ICD-10 defined prevalence as related to sociodemographic profile. *Personality and Individual Differences* 30: 311-320.

13. Torgersen, S., S. Lygren, P. A. Oien, I. Skre, S. Onstad, J. Edvardsen, et al. 2000. A twin study of personality disorders. *Comprehensive Psychiatry* 41: 416-425.

14. Kasen, S., P. Cohen, A. E. Skodol, J. G. Johnson, E. Smailes, and J. S. Brook. 2001. Childhood depression and adult personality disorder: Alternative pathways of continuity. *Archives of General Psychiatry* 58: 231-236.

15. Kasen, S., P. Cohen, A. E. Skodol, J. G. Johnson, E. Smailes, and J. S. Brook. 1999. The influence of child and adolescent psychiatric disorders on young adult personality disorder. *American Journal of Psychiatry* 156: 1529-1535.

16. Ojha, H., and R. R. Singh. 1988. Childrearing attitudes as related to insecurity and dependence proneness. *Psychological Studies* 33: 75-79.

17. Parker, G., and P. Lipscombe. 1980. The relevance of early parental experiences to adult dependency, hypochondriasis and utilization of primary physicians. *British Journal of Medical Psychology* 53: 355-363.

18. Vaillant, G. E. 1980. Natural history of male psychological health: VIII. Antecedents of alcoholism and orality. *American Journal of Psychiatry* 137: 181-186.

19. Baker, J. D., E. W. Capron, and J. Azorlosa. 1996. Family environment characteristics of persons with histrionic and dependent personality disorders. *Journal of Personality Disorders* 10: 82-87.

20. Bornstein, R. F. 1992. The dependent personality: Developmental, social, and clinical perspectives. *Psychological Bulletin* 112: 3-23.

21. Crits-Christoph, P., and J. P. Barber. 2002. Psychological treatments for personality disorders. In *A Guide to Treatments That Work*, edited by P. E. Nathan and J. M. Gorman. New York: Oxford University Press.

22. Winston, A., M. Laikin, J. Pollack, L. W. Samstag, L. McCullough, and J. C. Muran. 1994. Short-term psychotherapy of personality disorders. *American Journal of Psychiatry* 151: 190-194.

23. Winston, A., J. Pollack, L. McCullough, W. Flegenheimer, R. Kestenbaum, and M. Trujillo. 1991. Brief psychotherapy of personality disorders. *Journal of Nervous and Mental Disease* 179: 188-193.

24. Hardy, G. E., M. Barkham, D. A. Shapiro, W. B. Stiles, A. Rees, and S. Reynolds. 1995. Impact of Cluster C personality disorders on outcomes of contrasting brief psychotherapies for depression. *Journal of Consulting and Clinical Psychology* 63: 997-1004.

25. Beck, A. T., A. Freeman, J. Pretzer, D. D. Davis, B. Fleming, J. S. Beck, et al. 1990. *Cognitive Therapy of Personality Disorders*. New York: The Guilford Press.

26. Paterson, R. J. 2000. *The Assertiveness Workbook: How to Express Your Ideas and Stand Up for Yourself at Work and in Relationships*. Oakland, CA: New Harbinger Publications.

27. Bond, M., and J. C. Perry. 2004. Long-term changes in defense styles with psychodynamic psychotherapy for depressive, anxiety, and personality disorders. *American Journal of Psychiatry* 161: 1665-1671.

28. Perry, J. C. 1989. Dependent personality disorder. In *Treatments of Psychiatric Disorders: A Task Force Report of the American Psychiatric Association*, edited by American Psychiatric Association. Washington, DC: American Psychiatric Press.

29. Links, P. S., M. Stockwell, and M. M. MacFarlane. 2004. Is couple therapy indicated for patients with dependent personality disorder? *Journal of Family Psychotherapy* 15: 63-79.

30. Nichols, W. C. 2004. *Integrative Marital and Family Treatment of Dependent Personality Disorders*. Binghamton, NY: Haworth Clinical Practice Press.

31. Fava, M., A. H. Farabaugh, A. H. Sickinger, E. Wright, J. E. Alpert, S. Sonawalla, et al. 2002. Personality disorders and depression. *Psychological Medicine* 32: 1049-1057.

Depression

1. American Psychiatric Association. 2000. *Diagnostic and Statistical Manual of Mental Disorders*. Text revision ed. Washington, DC: American Psychiatric Association.

2. U.S. Department of Health and Human Services. 1999. *Mental Health: A Report of the Surgeon General*. Rockville, MD: U.S. Department of Health and Human Services, Substance Abuse and Mental Health Services Administration, Center for Mental Health Services, National Institutes of Health, National Institute of Mental Health.

3. Thase, M. E., and L. R. Sullivan. 1995. Relapse and recurrence of depression: A practical approach for prevention. *CNS Drugs* 4: 261-277.

4. Seligman, M. E. P. 1998. *Learned Optimism*. New York: Simon & Schuster, Inc.

5. Whisman, M. 2001. The association between depression and marital dissatisfaction. In *Marital and Family Processes in Depression: A Scientific Foundation for Clinical Practice*, edited by S. R. H. Beach. Washington, DC: American Psychological Association.

6. Uebelacker, L. A., and M. A. Whisman. 2005. Relationship beliefs, attributions, and partner behaviors among depressed married women. *Cognitive Therapy and Research* 29: 143-154.

7. Joiner, T. E., G. I. Metalsky, J. Katz, and S. R. H. Beach. 1999. Depression and excessive reassurance-seeking. *Psychological Inquiry* 10: 269-278.

8. Joiner, T. E. 1994. Contagious depression: Existence, specificity to depressed symptoms, and the role of reassurance seeking. *Journal of Personality and Social Psychology* 67: 287-296.

9. Angst, J., F. Angst, and H. H. Stassen. 1999. Suicide risk in patients with major depressive disorder. *Journal of Clinical Psychiatry* 60: 57-62.

10. Regier, D. A., D. S. Rae, W. E. Narrow, C. T. Kaelber, and A. F. Schatzberg. 1998. Prevalence of anxiety disorders and their comorbidity with mood and addictive disorders. *British Journal of Psychiatry* 173: 24-28.

11. Kessler, R. C., W. T. Chiu, O. Demler, and E. E. Walters. 2005. Prevalence, severity, and comorbidity of 12-month DSM-IV disorders in the National Comorbidity Survey Replication. *Archives of General Psychiatry* 62: 617-627.

12. Grant, B. F., D. S. Hasin, F. S. Stinson, D. A. Dawson, S. P. Chou, W. J. Ruan, et al. 2005. Co-occurrence of 12-month mood and anxiety disorders and personality disorders in the US: results from the national epidemiologic survey on alcohol and related conditions. *Journal of Psychiatric Research* 39: 1-9.

13. Skodol, A. E., R. L. Stout, T. H. McGlashan, C. M. Grilo, J. G. Gunderson, M. T. Shea, et al. 1999. Co-occurrence of mood and personality disorders: A report from the Collaborative Longitudinal Personality Disorders Study (CLPS). *Depression and Anxiety* 10: 175-182.

14. Merikangas, K. R., R. L. Mehta, B. E. Molnar, E. E. Walters, J. D. Swendsen, S. Auilar-Gaziola, et al. 1998. Comorbidity of substance use disorders with mood and anxiety disorders: Results of the international consortium in psychiatric epidemiology. *Addictive Behaviors* 23: 893-908.

15. Kessler, R. C., R. M. Crum, L. A. Warner, C. B. Nelson, J. Schulenber, and J. C. Anthony. 1997. Lifetime co-occurrence of DSM-III-R alcohol abuse and dependence with other psychiatric disorders in the National Comorbidity Survey. *Archives of General Psychiatry* 54: 313-321.

16. Grant, B. F., F. S. Stinson, D. A. Dawson, P. Chou, M. C. Dufour, W. Compton, et al. 2004. Prevalence and co-occurrence of substance use disorders and independent mood and anxiety disorders: Results from the National Epidemiologic Survey on Alcohol and Related Conditions. *Archives of General Psychiatry* 61: 807-816.

17. Wells, K. B., W. Rogers, M. A. Burnam, S. Greenfield, and J. E. Ware Jr. 1991. How the medical comorbidity of depressed patients differs across health care settings: Results from the Medical Outcomes Study. *American Journal of Psychiatry* 148: 1688-1696.

18. Taylor, W. D., D. R. McQuoid, and K. R. R. Krishnan. 2004. Medical comorbidity in late-life depression. *International Journal of Geriatric Psychiatry* 19: 935-943.

19. Oslin, D. W., C. J. Datto, M. J. Kallan, I. R. Katz, W. S. Edell, and T. TenHave. 2002. Association between medical comorbidity and treatment outcomes in late-life depression. *Journal of the American Geriatrics Society* 50: 823-828.

20. McCoy, D. M. 1996. Treatment considerations for depression in patients with significant medical comorbidity. *Journal of Family Practice* 43: S35-S44.

21. Lyness, J. M., and E. D. Caine. 2000. Vascular disease and depression: Models of the interplay between psychopathology and medical comorbidity. In *Physical Illness and Depression in Older Adults: A Handbook of Theory, Research, and Practice,* edited by G. M. Williamson, D. R. Shaffer, et al. Dordrecht, Netherlands: Kluwer Academic Publishers.

22. Katz, I. R. 1996. On the inseparability of mental and physical health in aged persons: Lessons from depression and medical comorbidity. *American Journal of Geriatric Psychiatry* 4: 1-16.

23. Appels, A. 2002. Depression and cardiac disease. *Current Opinion in Psychiatry* 15: 59-62.

24. Musselman, D. L., D. L. Evans, and C. B. Nemeroff. 1998. The relationship of depression to cardiovascular disease: Epidemiology, biology, and treatment. *Archives of General Psychiatry* 55: 580-592.

25. Lett, H. S., J. A. Blumenthal, M. A. Babyak, A. Sherwood, T. Strauman, C. Robins, et al. 2004. Depression as a risk factor for coronary artery disease: Evidence, mechanisms, and treatment. *Psychosomatic Medicine* 66: 305-315.

26. Murray, C. J. L., and A. D. Lopez, eds. 1996. *Summary: The Global Burden of Disease: A Comprehensive Assessment of Mortality and Disability from Diseases, Injuries, and Risk Factors in 1990 and Projected to 2020.* Cambridge, MA: Published by the Harvard School of Public Health on behalf of the World Health Organization and the World Bank, Harvard University Press.

27. Regier, D. A., W. E. Narrow, D. S. Rae, R. W. Manderscheid, B. Z. Locke, and F. K. Goodwin. 1993. The de facto US mental and addictive disorders service system: Epidemiologic catchment area prospective 1-year prevalence rates of disorders and services. *Archives of General Psychiatry* 50: 85-94.

28. Narrow, W. E. 1998. *One-Year Prevalence of Depressive Disorders Among Adults 18 and Over in the U.S.: NIMH ECA Prospective Data. Population Estimates Based on U.S. Census Estimated Residential Population Age 18 and Over on July 1, 1998.* Unpublished table.

29. Kessler, R. C., K. A. McGonagle, S. Zhao, C. B. Nelson, M. Hughes, S. Eshleman, et al. 1994. Lifetime and 12-month prevalence of DSM-III-R psychiatric disorders in the United States. *Archives of General Psychiatry* 51: 8-19.

30. Kessler, R. C., P. A. Berglund, O. Demler, R. Jin, and E. E. Walters. 2005. Lifetime prevalence and age-of-onset distributions of DSM-IV disorders in the National Comorbidity Survey Replication. *Archives of General Psychiatry* 62: 593-602.

31. Parker, G. B., and H. L. Brotchie. 2004. From diathesis to dimorphism: The biology of gender differences in depression. *Journal of Nervous and Mental Disease* 192: 210-216.

32. Simonds, V. M., and V. E. Whiffen. 2003. Are gender differences in depression explained by gender differences in co-morbid anxiety? *Journal of Affective Disorders* 77: 197-202.

33. Kuehner, C. 2003. Gender differences in unipolar depression: An update of epidemiological findings and possible explanations. *Acta Psychiatrica Scandinavica* 108: 163-174.

34. Brown, G. W., T. O. Harris, and C. Hepworth. 1994. Life events and endogenous depression. A puzzle reexamined. *Archives of General Psychiatry* 51: 525-534.

35. Galambos, N. L., B. J. Leadbeater, and E. T. Barker. 2004. Gender differences in and risk factors for depression in adolescence: A 4-year longitudinal study. *International Journal of Behavioral Development* 28: 16-25.

36.	Birmaher, B., N. D. Ryan, D. E. Williamson, D. Brent, J. Kauffman, R. E. Dahl, et al. 1996. Childhood and adolescent depression: A review of the past 10 years. Part 1. *Journal of the American Academy of Child and Adolescent Psychiatry* 35: 1427-1439.

37.	Weissman, M. M., R. Bland, P. R. Joyce, S. Newman, J. E. Wells, and H. U. Wittchen. 1993. Sex differences in rates of depression: Cross-national perspectives. *Journal of Affective Disorders* 29: 77-84.

38.	Robins, L. N., and D. A. Regier. 1991. *Psychiatric Disorders in America: The Epidemiologic Catchment Area Study.* New York: Free Press.

39.	Paterson, R. J. 2002. *Your Depression Map: Find the Source of Your Depression and Chart Your Own Recovery.* Oakland, CA: New Harbinger Publications.

40.	McGuffin, P., R. Katz, S. Watkins, and J. Rutherford. 1996. A hospital-based twin registry study of the heritability of DSM-IV unipolar depression. *Archives of General Psychiatry* 53: 129-136.

41.	National Institute of Mental Health. 2002. *Depression and Heart Disease.* In NIH Publication No. 02-5004. Bethesda, MD: National Institute of Mental Health, National Institutes of Health, U.S. Department of Health and Human Services.

42.	Delgado, P. L., and F. A. Moreno. 2000. Role of norepinephrine in depression. *Journal of Clinical Psychiatry* 61: 5-12.

43.	Rampello, L., F. Nicoletti, and F. Nicoletti. 2000. Dopamine and depression: Therapeutic implications. *CNS Drugs* 13: 35-45.

44.	Janowsky, D. S., and S. C. Risch. 1984. Adrenergic-cholinergic balance and affective disorders: A review of clinical evidence and therapeutic implications. *Psychiatric Hospital* 15: 163-171.

45.	Wetterberg, L. 1999. Melatonin and clinical application. *Reproduction, Nutrition, Development* 39: 367-382.

46.	Dilsaver, S. C., L. Wetterberg, M. C. Blehar, and N. E. Rosenthal. 1990. Onset of winter depression earlier than generally thought? *Journal of Clinical Psychiatry* 51: 258.

47.	Blehar, M. C., and N. E. Rosenthal. 1989. Seasonal affective disorders and phototherapy. Report of a National Institute of Mental Health-sponsored workshop. *Archives of General Psychiatry* 46: 469-474.

48.	Berkow, R., ed. 1987. *The Merck Manual.* 15th ed. New York: John Wiley and Sons, Inc.

49.	Lehne, R. A. 2004. *Pharmacology for Nursing Care.* 5th ed. St. Louis, MO: Saunders.

50.	Christensen, L., ed. 2005. *Springhouse Nurse's Drug Guide 2005.* 6th ed. Philadelphia: Lippincott Williams & Wilkins.

51.	Shea, A., C. Walsh, H. MacMillan, and M. Steiner. 2005. Child maltreatment and HPA axis dysregulation: Relationship to major depressive disorder and post traumatic stress disorder in females. *Psychoneuroendocrinology* 30: 162-178.

52.	Agid, O., B. Shapira, J. Zislin, M. Ritsner, B. Hanin, H. Murad, et al. 1999. Environment and vulnerability to major psychiatric illness: A case control study of early parental loss in major depression, bipolar disorder and schizophrenia. *Molecular Psychiatry* 4: 163-172.

53.	Hull, A. M. 2002. Neuroimaging findings in post-traumatic stress. *British Journal of Psychiatry* 181: 102-110.

54.	Beck, A. T., A. J. Rush, B. F. Shaw, and G. Emery. 1979. *Cognitive Therapy of Depression.* New York: The Guilford Press.

55.	Burns, D. 1999. *Feeling Good: The New Mood Therapy: The Clinically Proven Drug-Free Treatment for Depression.* New York: Avon Books.

56.	Young, J. 1990. *Cognitive Therapy for Personality Disorders: A Schema-Focused Approach.* Sarasota, FL: Professional Resource Exchange, Inc.

57.	Schmidt, N. B., T. E. Joiner, J. Young, and M. J. Telch. 1995. The Schema Questionnaire: Investigation of psychometric properties and the hierarchical structure of a measure of maladaptive schemas. *Cognitive Therapy and Research* 19: 295-321.

58.	Wang, P. S., M. Lane, M. Olfson, H. A. Pincus, K. B. Wells, and R. C. Kessler. 2005. Twelve-month use of mental health services in the United States. Results from the National Comorbidity Survey Replication. *Archives of General Psychiatry* 62: 629-640.

59. Wang, P. S., P. A. Berglund, M. Olfson, H. A. Pincus, K. B. Wells, and R. C. Kessler. 2005. Failure and delay in initial treatment contact after first onset of mental disorders in the National Comorbidity Survey Replication. *Archives of General Psychiatry* 62: 603-613.

60. Vos, T., M. M. Haby, J. J. Barendregt, M. Kruijshaar, J. Corry, and G. Andrews. 2004. The burden of major depression avoidable by longer-term treatment strategies. *Archives of General Psychiatry* 61: 1097-1103.

61. National Advisory Mental Health Council. 1999. Health care reform for Americans with severe mental illnesses. *American Journal of Psychiatry* 150: 1447-1465.

62. Olfson, M., S. C. Marcus, B. Druss, L. Elinson, T. Tanielian, and H. A. Pincus. 2002. National trends in the outpatient treatment of depression. *Journal of the American Medical Association* 287: 203-209.

63. Olfson, M., and G. L. Klerman. 1993. Trends in the prescription of antidepressants by office-based psychiatrists. *American Journal of Psychiatry* 150: 571-577.

64. Harris Interactive, Psychology Today, and PacifiCare Behavioral Health. 2004. Therapy in America 2004, May 5, 2004 [cited June 14, 2004]. Available from http://cms.psychologytoday.com/pto/press_release_050404.html.

65. Hollon, S. D., R. B. Jarrett, A. A. Nierenberg, M. E. Thase, M. Trivedi, and A. J. Rush. 2005. Psychotherapy and medication in the treatment of adult and geriatric depression: Which monotherapy or combined treatment? *Journal of Clinical Psychiatry* 66: 455-468.

66. National Institute of Mental Health. 2002. *Medications*. In NIH Publication No. 02-3929. Bethesda, MD: National Institute of Mental Health, National Institutes of Health, U. S. Department of Health and Human Services.

67. DeRubeis, R. J., S. D. Hollon, J. D. Amsterdam, R. C. Shelton, P. R. Young, R. M. Salomon, et al. 2005. Cognitive therapy vs medications in the treatment of moderate to severe depression. *Archives of General Psychiatry* 62: 409-416.

68. McPherson, S., P. Cairns, J. Carlyle, D. A. Shapiro, P. Richardson, and D. Taylor. 2005. The effectiveness of psychological treatments for treatment-resistant depression: A systematic review. *Acta Psychiatrica Scandinavica* 111: 331-340.

69. Craighead, W. E., A. B. Hart, L. W. Craighead, and S. S. Ilardi. 2002. Psychosocial treatments for major depressive disorder. In *A Guide to Treatments That Work*, edited by P. E. Nathan and J. M. Gorman. New York: Oxford University Press.

70. Depression Guideline Panel. 1993. Depression in primary care: Vol. 2. Treatment of major depression. In *Clinical Practice Guideline No. 5*. AHCPR Publication No. 93-0550. Rockville, MD: U.S. Department of Health and Human Services, Public Health Service, Agency for Health Care Policy and Research.

71. Skinner, B. F. 1953. *Science and Human Behavior*. New York: Macmillan.

72. Goldapple, K., Z. Segal, C. Garson, M. Lau, P. Bieling, S. Kennedy, et al. 2004. Modulation of cortical-limbic pathways in major depression. *Archives of General Psychiatry* 61: 34-41.

73. Hollon, S. D., M. E. Thase, and J. C. Markowitz. 2002. Treatment and prevention of depression. *Psychological Science in the Public Interest* 3: 39-77.

74. Gillies, L. A. 2001. Interpersonal psychotherapy for depression and other disorders. In *Clinical Handbook of Psychological Disorders: A Step-by-Step Treatment Manual*, edited by D. H. Barlow. New York: The Guilford Press.

75. Safran, J., and Z. Segal. 1996. *Interpersonal Process in Cognitive Therapy*. Northvale, NJ: Jason Aronson Inc.

76. Levenson, H. 2003. Time-limited dynamic psychotherapy: An integrationist perspective. *Journal of Psychotherapy Integration* 13: 300-333.

77. Blagys, M. D., and M. J. Hilsenroth. 2000. Distinctive features of short-term psychodynamic-interpersonal psychotherapy: A review of the comparative psychotherapy process literature. *Clinical Psychology: Science and Practice* 7: 167-188.

78. Jacobson, N. S., A. E. Fruzzetti, K. Dobson, M. Whisman, and H. Hops. 1993. Couple therapy as a treatment for depression. II. The effects of relationship quality and therapy on depressive relapse. *Journal of Consulting and Clinical Psychology* 61: 516-519.

79. Jacobson, N. S., A. Holtzworth-Munroe, and K. B. Schmaling. 1989. Marital therapy and spouse involvement in the treatment of depression, agoraphobia, and alcoholism. *Journal of Consulting and Clinical Psychology* 57: 5-10.

80.   O'Leary, K. D., and S. R. H. Beach. 1990. Marital therapy: A viable treatment for depression and marital discord. *American Journal of Psychiatry* 147: 183-186.

81.   Babyak, M., J. A. Blumenthal, S. Herman, P. Khatri, M. Doraiswamy, K. Moore, et al. 2000. Exercise treatment for major depression: Maintenance of therapeutic benefit at 10 months. *Psychosomatic Medicine* 62: 633-638.

82.   Schrader, E. 2000. Equivalence of St. John's wort extract (Ze 117) and fluoxetine: A randomized, controlled study in mild-moderate depression. *International Clinical Psychopharmacology* 15: 61-68.

83.   Volz, H.-P., and P. Laux. 2000. Potential treatment for subthreshold and mild depression: A comparison of St. John's wort extracts and fluoxetine. *Comprehensive Psychiatry* 41: 133-137.

84.   Hypericum Depression Trial Study Group. 2002. Effect of Hypericum perforatum (St. John's wort) in major depressive disorder: A randomized, controlled trial. *Journal of the American Medical Association* 287: 1807-1814.

85.   Mathew, S. J., J. M. Amiel, and H. A. Sackeim. 2005. Electroconvulsive therapy in treatment-resistant depression. *Primary Psychiatry* 12: 52-56.

86.   Bailine, S. H., A. Rifkin, E. Kayne, J. A. Selzer, J. Vital-Herne, M. Blieka, et al. 2000. Comparison of bifrontal and bitemporal ECT for major depression. *American Journal of Psychiatry* 157: 121-123.

87.   Rey, J. M., and G. Walter. 1997. Half a century of ECT use in young people. *American Journal of Psychiatry* 154: 595-602.

88.   Dilbaz, N., C. Sengal, T. Okay, G. Bayam, and A. Torkoglu. 2005. The combined treatment of venlafaxine and ECT in treatment-resistant depressive patients. *International Journal of Psychiatry in Clinical Practice* 9: 55-59.

89.   O'Leary, D., D. Gill, S. Gregory, and C. Shawcross. 1995. Which depressed patients respond to ECT? The Nottingham results. *Journal of Affective Disorders* 33: 245-250.

Dissociative Disorders

1.   American Psychiatric Association. 2000. *Diagnostic and Statistical Manual of Mental Disorders.* Text revision ed. Washington, DC: American Psychiatric Association.

2.   Kihlstrom, J. F., M. L. Glisky, and M. J. Angiulo. 1994. Dissociative tendencies and dissociative disorders. *Journal of Abnormal Psychology* 103: 117-124.

3.   Ross, C. A., S. Joshi, and R. Currie. 1990. Dissociative experiences in the general population. *American Journal of Psychiatry* 147: 1547-1552.

4.   Modestin, J., G. Ebner, M. Junghan, and T. Erni. 1996. Dissociative experiences and dissociative disorders in acute psychiatric inpatients. *Comprehensive Psychiatry* 37: 355-361.

5.   Lipsanen, T., J. Korkeila, P. Peltola, J. Järvinen, K. Langen, and H. Lauerma. 2004. Dissociative disorders among psychiatric patients: Comparison with a nonclinical sample. *European Psychiatry* 19: 53-55.

6.   Friedl, M. C., N. Draijer, and P. de Jonge. 2000. Prevalence of dissociative disorders in psychiatric inpatients: The impact of the study characteristics. *Acta Psychiatrica Scandinavica* 102: 423-428.

7.   Mulder, R. T., A. L. Beatrais, P. R. Joyce, and D. M. Fergusson. 1998. Relationship between dissociation, childhood sexual abuse, childhood physical abuse and mental illness in a general population sample. *American Journal of Psychiatry* 155: 806-811.

8.   Seedat, S., M. B. Stein, and D. R. Forde. 2003. Prevalence of dissociative experiences in a community sample. Relationship to gender, ethnicity, and substance use. *Journal of Nervous and Mental Disease* 191: 115-120.

9.   Saxe, G. N., B. A. van der Kolk, R. Berkowitz, G. Chinman, K. Hall, G. Lieberg, et al. 1993. Dissociative disorders in psychiatric inpatients. *American Journal of Psychiatry* 150: 1037-1042.

10.   Goff, DC, A. W. Brotman, D. Kindlon, M. Waites, and E. Amico. 1991. Self-reports of childhood abuse in chronically psychotic patients. *Psychiatric Research* 37: 73-80.

11.   Coons, P. M. 1994. Confirmation of childhood abuse in child and adolescent cases of multiple personality disorder and dissociative disorder not otherwise specified. *Journal of Nervous and Mental Disease* 182: 461-464.

12. Dancu, C. V., D. S. Riggs, D. Hearst-Ikeda, B. G. Shoyer, and E. B. Foa. 1996. Dissociative experiences and posttraumatic stress disorder among female victims of criminal assault and rape. *Journal of Traumatic Stress* 9: 253-267.

13. Witztum, E., H. Maragalit, and O. van der Hart. 2002. Combat-induced dissociative amnesia: Review and case example of generalized dissociative amnesia. *Journal of Trauma and Dissociation* 3: 35-55.

14. Cardena, E., and D. Spiegel. 1993. Dissociative reactions to the San Francisco Bay Area earthquake of 1989. *American Journal of Psychiatry* 150: 474-478.

15. Arrigo, J. M., and K. Pezdek. 1997. Lessons from the study of psychogenic amnesia. *Current Directions in Psychological Science* 6: 148-152.

16. Loewenstein, R. J. 1996. Dissociative amnesia and dissociative fugue. In *Handbook of Dissociation: Theoretical, Empirical, and Clinical Perspectives*, edited by L. K. Michelson and W. J. Ray. New York: Plenum Press.

17. Middleton, W. 2004. Dissociative disorders: A personal "work in progress." *Australasian Psychiatry* 12: 245-252.

18. Ishikura, R., and N. Tashiro. 2002. Frustration and fulfillment of needs in dissociative and conversion disorders. *Psychiatry and Clinical Neurosciences* 56: 381-390.

19. Maslow, A. H. 1943. A theory of human motivation. *Psychological Review* 50: 370-396.

20. Maslow, A. H. 1970. *Motivation and Personality.* 2nd ed. New York: Harper and Row.

21. Pope, H. G., Jr., P. S. Oliva, J. I. Hudson, J. A. Bodkin, and A. J. Gruber. 1999. Attitudes toward DSM-IV dissociative disorders diagnoses among board-certified American psychiatrists. *American Journal of Psychiatry* 156: 321-323.

22. Lalonde, J. K., J. I. Hudson, R. A. Gigante, and H. G. Pope Jr. 2001. Canadian and American psychiatrists' attitudes toward dissociative disorders diagnoses. *Canadian Journal of Psychiatry* 46: 407-412.

23. Middleton, W., and D. Higson. 2004. Establishing and running a trauma and dissociation unit: A contemporary experience. *Australasian Psychiatry* 12: 338-346.

24. Burton, N., and R. C. Lane. 2001. The relational treatment of dissociative identity disorder. *Clinical Psychology Review* 21: 301-320.

25. Degun-Mather, M. 2002. Hypnosis in the treatment of a case of dissociative amnesia for a 12-year period. *Contemporary Hypnosis* 19: 34-41.

26. Degun-Mather, M. 2001. The value of hypnosis in the treatment of chronic PTSD with dissociative fugues in a war veteran. *Contemporary Hypnosis* 18: 4-13.

27. Twombly, J. H. 2000. Incorporating EMDR and EMDR adaptations into the treatment of clients with dissociative identity disorder. *Journal of Trauma and Dissociation* 1: 61-81.

28. Fine, C. G. 1999. The tactical-integration model for the treatment of dissociative identity disorder and allied dissociative disorders. *American Journal of Psychotherapy* 53: 361-376.

29. Goldstein, L. H., A. C. Deale, S. J. Mitchell-O'Malley, B. K. Toone, and J. DC Mellers. 2004. An evaluation of cognitive behavioral therapy as a treatment for dissociative seizures: A pilot study. *Cognitive and Behavioral Neurology* 17: 41-49.

30. Sno, H. N., and H. F. A. Schalken. 1999. Dissociative identity disorder: Diagnosis and treatment in the Netherlands. *European Psychiatry* 14: 270-277.

31. Ballew, L., Y. Morgan, and S. Lippmann. 2003. Intravenous diazepam for dissociative disorder: Memory lost and found. *Psychosomatics: Journal of Consultation Liaison Psychiatry* 44: 346-347.

32. Eich, E., D. Macaulay, R. J. Loewenstein, and P. H. Dihle. 1997. Memory, amnesia, and dissociative identity disorder. *Psychological Science* 8: 417-422.

33. Elzinga, B. M., R. H. Phaf, A. M. Ardon, and R. van Dyck. 2003. Directed forgetting between, but not within, dissociative personality states. *Journal of Abnormal Psychology* 112: 237-243.

34. Huntjens, R. J. C., A. Postma, M. L. Peters, L. Woertman, and O. van der Hart. 2003. Interidentity amnesia for neutral, episodic information in Dissociative Identity Disorder. *Journal of Abnormal Psychology* 112: 290-297.

35. Kluft, R. P. 1996. Dissociative identity disorder. In *Handbook of Disassociation: Theoretical, Empirical, and Clinical Perspectives*, edited by L. K. Michelson and W. J. Ray. New York: Plenum Press.

36. Kihlstrom, J. F. 2001. Dissociative disorders. In *Comprehensive Handbook of Psychopathology*, edited by P. B. Sutker and H. E. Adams. New York: Plenum Press.

37. Coons, P. M., E. S. Bowman, and V. Milstein. 1988. Multiple personality disorder: A clinical investigation of 50 cases. *Journal of Nervous and Mental Disease* 176: 519-527.

38. Norton, G. R., C. A. Ross, and M. F. Novotny. 1990. Factors that predict scores on the Dissociative Experiences Scale. *Journal of Clinical Psychology* 46: 273-277.

39. Benner, D. G., and B. Joscelyne. 1984. Multiple personality as a borderline disorder. *Psychiatric Clinics of North America* 12: 98-104.

40. Ross, C. A., S. D. Miller, P. Reagor, L. Bjornson, and G. A. Fraser. 1990. Structured interview data on 102 cases of multiple personality disorder from four centers. *American Journal of Psychiatry* 147: 596-601.

41. Gast, U., F. Rodewald, V. Nickel, and H. M. Emrich. 2001. Prevalence of dissociative disorders among psychiatric inpatients in a German university clinic. *Journal of Nervous and Mental Disease* 189: 249-257.

42. Ellason, J. W., and C. A. Ross. 1997. Two-year follow-up of inpatients with dissociative disorder. *American Journal of Psychiatry* 154: 832-839.

43. Putnam, F. W., J. J. Guroff, E. K. Silberman, L. Barban, and R. M. Post. 1986. The clinical phenomenology of multiple personality disorder: Review of 100 recent cases. *Journal of Clinical Psychiatry* 47: 285-293.

44. Lewis, D. O., C. A. Yeager, Y. Swica, J. H. Pincus, and M. Lewis. 1997. Objective documentation of child abuse and dissociation in 12 murderers with dissociative identity disorder. *American Journal of Psychiatry* 154: 1703-1710.

45. Scroppo, J. C., S. L. Drob, J. L. Weinberger, and P. Eagle. 1998. Identifying dissociative identity disorder: A self-report and projective study. *Journal of Abnormal Psychology* 107: 272-284.

46. Guralnik, O., J. Schmeidler, and D. Simeon. 2000. Feeling unreal: Cognitive processes in depersonalization. *American Journal of Psychiatry* 157: 103-109.

47. Simeon, D., M. Knutelska, D. Nelson, and O. Guralnik. 2003. Feeling unreal: A depersonalization disorder update of 117 cases. *Journal of Clinical Psychiatry* 64: 990-997.

48. Steinberg, M. 1994. *Structured Clinical Interview for DSM-IV Dissociative Disorders, Revised* (SCID-D). Washington, DC: American Psychiatric Press.

49. Simeon, D., S. Gross, O. Guralnik, D. J. Stein, J. Schmeidler, and E. Hollander. 1997. Feeling unreal: 30 cases of DSM-III-R depersonalization disorder. *American Journal of Psychiatry* 154: 1107-1113.

50. Hunter, E. C. M., M. L. Phillips, T. Chalder, M. Sierra, and A. S. David. 2003. Depersonalisation disorder: A cognitive-behavioural conceptualisation. *Behaviour Research and Therapy* 41: 1451-1467.

51. Trueman, D. 1984. Depersonalization in a nonclinical population. *Journal of Psychology* 116: 107-112.

52. Sedman, G. 1966. Depersonalization in a group of normal subjects. *British Journal of Psychiatry* 112: 907-912.

53. Sedman, G. 1970. Theories of depersonalization: A re-appraisal. *British Journal of Psychiatry* 117: 1-14.

54. Dixon, J. C. 1963. Depersonalization phenomena in a sample of college students. *British Journal of Psychiatry* 109: 371-375.

55. Simeon, D., O. Guralnik, J. Schmeidler, B. Sirof, and M. Knutelska. 2001. The role of childhood interpersonal trauma in depersonalization disorder. *American Journal of Psychiatry* 158: 1027-1033.

56. Hunter, E. C. M., D. Baker, M. L. Phillips, M. Sierra, and A. S. David. 2002. Depersonalization disorder: A cognitive-behavioural conceptualization. Paper read at National Congress of the British Association of Behavioural and Cognitive Psychotherapies, at Warwick, England.

57. Holmes, E. A., R. J. Brown, W. Mansell, R. P. Fearon, E. C. M. Hunter, F. Frasquilho, et al. 2005. Are there two qualitatively distinct forms of dissociation? A review and some clinical implications. *Clinical Psychology Review* 25: 1-23.

58. Torch, E. M. 1987. The psychotherapeutic treatment of depersonalization disorder. *Hillside Journal of Clinical Psychiatry* 9: 133-143.

59. Cattell, J. P., and J. S. Cattell. 1974. Depersonalization: Psychological and social perspectives. In *American Handbook of Psychiatry*, edited by S. Arieti. New York: Basic Books.

Drug and Alcohol Addiction Problems

1. American Psychiatric Association. 2000. *Diagnostic and Statistical Manual of Mental Disorders.* Text revision ed. Washington, DC: American Psychiatric Association.

2. Denning, P. 2000. *Practicing Harm Reduction Psychotherapy: An Alternative Approach to Addictions.* New York: The Guilford Press.

3. Grant, B. F., F. S. Stinson, D. A. Dawson, P. Chou, M. C. Dufour, W. Compton, et al. 2004. Prevalence and co-occurrence of substance use disorders and independent mood and anxiety disorders: Results from the National Epidemiologic Survey on Alcohol and Related Conditions. *Archives of General Psychiatry* 61: 807-816.

4. Kessler, R. C., R. M. Crum, L. A. Warner, C. B. Nelson, J. Schulenber, and J. C. Anthony. 1997. Lifetime co-occurrence of DSM-III-R alcohol abuse and dependence with other psychiatric disorders in the National Comorbidity Survey. *Archives of General Psychiatry* 54: 313-321.

5. Kessler, R. C., W. T. Chiu, O. Demler, and E. E. Walters. 2005. Prevalence, severity, and comorbidity of 12-month DSM-IV disorders in the National Comorbidity Survey Replication. *Archives of General Psychiatry* 62: 617-627.

6. Grant, B. F., F. S. Stinson, D. A. Dawson, S. P. Chou, W. J. Ruan, and R. P. Pickering. 2004. Co-occurrence of 12-month alcohol and drug use disorders and personality disorders in the United States: Results from the National Epidemiologic Survey on Alcohol and Related Conditions. *Archives of General Psychiatry* 61: 361-368.

7. Oldham, J. M., A. E. Skodol, H. D. Kellman, S. E. Hyler, N. Doidge, L. Rosnick, et al. 1995. Comorbidity of Axis I and Axis II disorders. *American Journal of Psychiatry* 152: 571-578.

8. Regier, D. A., M. E. Farmer, D. S. Rae, B. Z. Locke, S. J. Keith, and L. L. Judd. 1990. Comorbidity of mental disorders with alcohol and other drug abuse: Results from the Epidemiologic Catchment Area (ECA) Study. *Journal of the American Medical Association* 264: 2511-2518.

9. Murray, C. J. L., and A. D. Lopez, eds. 1996. *Summary: The Global Burden of Disease: A Comprehensive Assessment of Mortality and Disability from Diseases, Injuries, and Risk Factors in 1990 and Projected to 2020.* Cambridge, MA: Published by the Harvard School of Public Health on behalf of the World Health Organization and the World Bank, Harvard University Press.

10. Kessler, R. C., K. A. McGonagle, S. Zhao, C. B. Nelson, M. Hughes, S. Eshleman, et al. 1994. Lifetime and 12-month prevalence of DSM-III-R psychiatric disorders in the United States. *Archives of General Psychiatry* 51: 8-19.

11. Kessler, R. C., P. A. Berglund, O. Demler, R. Jin, and E. E. Walters. 2005. Lifetime prevalence and age-of-onset distributions of DSM-IV disorders in the National Comorbidity Survey Replication. *Archives of General Psychiatry* 62: 593-602.

12. Oslin, D. W., W. Berrettini, H. R. Kranzler, H. Pettinati, J. Gelernter, J. R. Volpicelli, et al. 2003. A functional polymorphism of the mu-opioid receptor gene is associated with naltrexone response in alcohol-dependent patients. *Neuropsychopharmacology* 28: 1546-1552.

13. Nelson, E. C., A. C. Heath, K. K. Bucholz, P. A. Madden, Q. Fu, V. Knopik, et al. 2004. Genetic epidemiology of alcohol-induced blackouts. *Archives of General Psychiatry* 61: 257-263.

14. Conway, K. P., J. D. Swendsen, and K. R. Merikangas. 2003. Alcohol expectancies, alcohol consumption, and problem drinking: The moderating role of family history. *Addictive Behaviors* 28: 823-836.

15. Schuckit, M. A., G. P. Danko, and T. L. Smith. 2004. Patterns of drug-related disorders in a prospective study of men chosen for their family history of alcoholism. *Journal of Studies on Alcohol* 65: 613-620.

16. Boyd, S. J., B. W. Plemons, R. P. Schwartz, J. L. Johnson, and R. W. Pickens. 1999. The relationship between parental history and substance use severity in drug treatment patients. *American Journal on Addictions* 8: 15-23.

17. Self, D. 2004. Drug dependence and addiction. *American Journal of Psychiatry* 161: 223.

18. Yokel, R. A., and R. A. Wise. 1975. Increased lever pressing for amphetamine after pimozide in rats: Implications for a dopamine theory of reward. *Science* 187: 547-549.

19. Volkow, N. D., J. S. Fowler, G.-J. Wang, and J. M. Swanson. 2004. Dopamine in drug abuse and addiction: Results from imaging studies and treatment implications. *Molecular Psychiatry* 9: 557-569.

20. Koob, G. F., and M. Le Moal. 1997. Drug abuse: Hedonic homeostatic dysregulation. *Science* 278: 52-58.

21. Koob, G. F., S. B. Caine, L. Parsons, A. Markou, and F. Weiss. 1997. Opponent process model and psychostimulant addiction. *Pharmacology and Biochemistry of Behavior* 57: 513-521.

22. Robinson, T. E., and K. C. Berridge. 2003. Addiction. *Annual Review of Psychology* 54: 25-53.

23. Merikangas, K. R., R. L. Mehta, B. E. Molnar, E. E. Walters, J. D. Swendsen, S. Auilar-Gaziola, et al. 1998. Comorbidity of substance use disorders with mood and anxiety disorders: Results of the International Consortium in Psychiatric Epidemiology. *Addictive Behaviors* 23: 893-908.

24. Wang, P. S., M. Lane, M. Olfson, H. A. Pincus, K. B. Wells, and R. C. Kessler. 2005. Twelve-month use of mental health services in the United States. Results from the National Comorbidity Survey Replication. *Archives of General Psychiatry* 62: 629-640.

25. Wang, P. S., P. A. Berglund, M. Olfson, H. A. Pincus, K. B. Wells, and R. C. Kessler. 2005. Failure and delay in initial treatment contact after first onset of mental disorders in the National Comorbidity Survey Replication. *Archives of General Psychiatry* 62: 603-613.

26. Berglund, M., S. Thelander, M. Salaspuro, J. Franck, S. Andreasson, and A. Ojehagen. 2003. Treatment of alcohol abuse: An evidence-based review. *Alcoholism: Clinical and Experimental Research* 27: 1645-1656.

27. Mattson, M. E., J. P. Allen, R. Longabaugh, C. J. Nickless, G. J. Connors, and R. M. Kadden. 1994. A chronological review of empirical studies matching alcoholic clients to treatment. *Journal of Studies on Alcohol* 12:S16-S29.

28. Cornelius, J. R., I. M. Salloum, J. G. Ehler, P. J. Jarrett, M. D. Cornelius, J. M. Perel, et al. 1997. Fluoxetine in depressed alcoholics. *Archives of General Psychiatry* 54: 700-705.

29. Carroll, K. M., B. J. Rounsaville, L. T. Gordon, C. Nich, P. Jatlaw, R. M. Bisignini, et al. 1994. Psychotherapy and pharmacotherapy for ambulatory cocaine abusers. *Archives of General Psychiatry* 51: 177-187.

30. Nunes, E. V., P. J. McGrath, F. M. Quitkin, K. Ocepek-Wlikson, J. K. W. Stewart, T. Koenig, et al. 1995. Imipramine treatment of cocaine abuse: Possible boundaries of efficacy. *Drug and Alcohol Dependence* 39: 185-195.

31. Ling, W., C. Charuvastra, S. C. Kaim, and J. Klett. 1976. Methadyl acetate and methadone as maintenance treatments for heroin addicts. *Archives of General Psychiatry* 33: 709-720.

32. Washton, A. M., A. C. Pottash, and M. S. Gold. 1984. Naltrexone in addicted business executives and physicians. *Journal of Clinical Psychiatry* 34: 39-41.

Emotion Dysregulation

1. American Psychiatric Association. 2000. *Diagnostic and Statistical Manual of Mental Disorders*. Text revision ed. Washington, DC: American Psychiatric Association.

2. Koenigsberg, H. W., P. D. Harvey, V. Mitropoulou, J. Schmeidler, A. S. New, M. Goodman, et al. 2002. Characterizing affective instability in borderline personality disorder. *American Journal of Psychiatry* 159: 784-788.

3. Linehan, M. M. 1993. *Cognitive-Behavioral Treatment of Borderline Personality Disorder*. New York: The Guilford Press.

4. Lieb, K., M. C. Zanarini, C. Schmahl, M. M. Linehan, and M. Bohus. 2004. Borderline personality disorder. *Lancet* 364: 453-461.

5. Koenigsberg, H. W., P. D. Harvey, V. Mitropoulou, A. S. New, M. Goodman, J. Silverman, et al. 2001. Are the interpersonal and identity disturbances in the borderline personality disorder criteria linked to the traits of affective instability and impulsivity? *Journal of Personality Disorders* 15: 358-370.

6.   Butler, A. C., G. K. Brown, A. T. Beck, and J. R. Grisham. 2002. Assessment of dysfunctional beliefs in borderline personality disorder. *Behaviour Research and Therapy* 40: 1231-1240.

7.   Frankenburg, F. R., and M. C. Zanarini. 2004. The association between borderline personality disorder and chronic medical illnesses, poor health-related lifestyle choices, and costly forms of health care utilization. *Journal of Clinical Psychiatry* 65: 1660-1665.

8.   Zanarini, M. C., F. R. Frankenburg, C. J. DeLuca, J. Hennen, G. S. Khera, and J. G. Gunderson. 1998. The pain of being borderline: Dysphoric states specific to borderline personality disorder. *Harvard Review of Psychiatry* 6: 201-207.

9.   Zanarini, M. C., J. G. Gunderson, and F. R. Frankenburg. 1990. Cognitive features of borderline personality disorder. *American Journal of Psychiatry* 147: 57-63.

10. Black, D. W., N. Blum, B. Pfohl, and N. Hale. 2004. Suicidal behavior in borderline personality disorder: Prevalence, risk factors, prediction, and prevention. *Journal of Personality Disorders* 18: 226-239.

11. Paris, J. 1990. Completed suicide in borderline personality disorder. *Psychiatric Annals* 20: 19-21.

12. Paris, J., R. Brown, and D. Nowlis. 1987. Long-term follow-up of borderline patients in a general hospital. *Comprehensive Psychiatry* 28: 530-535.

13. Paris, J., and H. Zweig-Frank. 2001. The 27-year follow-up of patients with borderline personality disorder. *Comprehensive Psychiatry* 42: 482-487.

14. Paris, J. 2002. Chronic suicidality among patients with borderline personality disorder. *Psychiatric Services* 53: 738-742.

15. Yen, S., M. T. Shea, C. A. Sanislow, C. M. Grilo, A. E. Skodol, J. G. Gunderson, et al. 2004. Borderline personality disorder criteria associated with prospectively observed suicidal behavior. *American Journal of Psychiatry* 161: 1296-1298.

16. Skinstad, A. H., and A. Swain. 2001. Comorbidity in a clinical sample of substance abusers. *American Journal of Drug and Alcohol Abuse* 27: 45-64.

17. Oldham, J. M., A. E. Skodol, H. D. Kellman, S. E. Hyler, N. Doidge, L. Rosnick, et al. 1995. Comorbidity of Axis I and Axis II disorders. *American Journal of Psychiatry* 152: 571-578.

18. Zanarini, M. C., F. R. Frankenburg, J. Hennen, D. B. Reich, and K. R. Silk. 2004. Axis I comorbidity in patients with borderline personality disorder: 6-year follow-up and prediction of time to remission. *American Journal of Psychiatry* 161: 2108-2114.

19. Zanarini, M. C., F. R. Frankenburg, E. D. Dubo, A. E. Sickel, A. Trikha, A. Levin, et al. 1998. Axis I comorbidity of borderline personality disorder. *American Journal of Psychiatry* 155: 1733-1739.

20. Johnson, D. M., M. T. Shea, S. Yen, C. L. Battle, C. Zlotnick, C. A. Sanislow, et al. 2003. Gender differences in borderline personality disorder: Findings from the Collaborative Longitudinal Personality Disorders Study. *Comprehensive Psychiatry* 44: 284-292.

21. Zanarini, M. C., F. R. Frankenburg, E. D. Dubo, A. E. Sickel, A. Trikha, A. Levin, et al. 1998. Axis II comorbidity of borderline personality disorder. *Comprehensive Psychiatry* 39: 296-302.

22. Torgersen, S., E. Kringlen, and V. Cramer. 2001. The prevalence of personality disorders in a community sample. *Archives of General Psychiatry* 58: 590-596.

23. Ekselius, L., M. Tillfors, T. Furmark, and M. Fredrikson. 2001. Personality disorders in the general population: DSM-IV and ICD-10 defined prevalence as related to sociodemographic profile. *Personality and Individual Differences* 30: 311-320.

24. Jackson, H. J., and P. M. Burgess. 2000. Personality disorders in the community: A report from the Australian National Survey of Mental Health and Wellbeing. *Social Psychiatry and Psychiatric Epidemiology* 35: 531-538.

25. Swartz, M., D. Blazer, L. George, and I. Winfield. 1990. Estimating the prevalence of borderline personality disorder in the community. *Journal of Personality Disorders* 4: 257-272.

26. Widiger, T. A., and M. M. Weissman. 1991. Epidemiology of borderline personality disorder. *Hospital and Community Psychiatry* 42: 1015-1021.

27. Bernstein, D. P., P. Cohen, C. N. Velez, M. Schwab-Stone, L. J. Siever, and L. Shinsato. 1993. Prevalence and stability of the DSM-III-R personality disorders in a community-based survey of adolescents. *American Journal of Psychiatry* 150: 1237-1243.

28. Zanarini, M. C., F. R. Frankenburg, G. S. Khera, and J. Bleichmar. 2001. Treatment histories of borderline inpatients. *Comprehensive Psychiatry* 42: 144-150.

29. Becker, D., and S. Lamb. 1994. Sex bias in the diagnosis of borderline personality disorder and posttraumatic stress disorder. *Professional Psychology: Research and Practice* 25: 55-61.

30. Strain, B. A. 2003. Influence of gender bias on the diagnosis of borderline personality disorder. Dissertation Abstracts International: Section B: *The Sciences and Engineering* 64: 2941.

31. Bradley, R., J. Jenei, and D. Westen. 2005. Etiology of borderline personality disorder: Disentangling the contributions of intercorrelated antecedents. *Journal of Nervous and Mental Disease* 193: 24-31.

32. Torgersen, S., S. Lygren, P. A. Oien, I. Skre, S. Onstad, J. Edvardsen, et al. 2000. A twin study of personality disorders. *Comprehensive Psychiatry* 41: 416-425.

33. Livesley, W. J., K. L. Jang, and P. A. Vernon. 1998. Phenotypic and genetic structure of traits delineating personality disorder. *Archives of General Psychiatry* 55: 941-948.

34. Soloff, P. H., C. C. Meltzer, C. Becker, P. J. Greer, and D. Constantine. 2005. Gender differences in a fenfluramine-activated FDG PET study of borderline personality disorder. *Psychiatry Research: Neuroimaging* 138: 183-195.

35. Donegan, N. H., C. A. Sanislow, H. P. Blumberg, R. K. Fulbright, C. Lacadie, P. Skudlarski, et al. 2003. Amygdala hyperreactivity in borderline personality disorder: Implications for emotional dysregulation. *Biological Psychiatry* 54: 1284-1293.

36. Schmahl, C. G., E. Vermetten, B. M. Elzinga, and J. D. Bremner. 2003. Magnetic resonance imaging of hippocampal and amygdala volume in women with childhood abuse and borderline personality disorder. *Psychiatry Research: Neuroimaging* 122: 193-198.

37. Brambilla, P., P. H. Soloff, M. Sala, M. A. Nicoletti, M. S. Keshavan, and J. C. Soares. 2004. Anatomical MRI study of borderline personality disorder patients. *Psychiatry Research: Neuroimaging* 131: 125-133.

38. Zanarini, M. C., J. G. Gunderson, M. F. Marino, E. O. Schwartz, and F. R. Frankenburg. 1989. Childhood experiences of borderline patients. *Comprehensive Psychiatry* 30: 18-25.

39. Zanarini, M. C., A. A. Williams, R. E. Lewis, R. B. Reich, S. C. Vera, M. F. Marino, et al. 1997. Reported pathological childhood experiences associated with the development of borderline personality disorder. *American Journal of Psychiatry* 154: 1101-1106.

40. Shearer, S. L., C. P. Peters, M. S. Quaytman, and R. L. Ogden. 1990. Frequency and correlates of childhood sexual and physical abuse histories in adult female borderline inpatients. *American Journal of Psychiatry* 147: 214-216.

41. Paris, J., H. Zweig-Frank, and J. Guzder. 1994. Psychological risk factors for borderline personality disorder in female patients. *Comprehensive Psychiatry* 35: 301-305.

42. Paris, J., H. Zweig-Frank, and J. Guzder. 1994. Risk factors for borderline personality in male outpatients. *Journal of Nervous and Mental Disease* 182: 375-380.

43. Ogata, S. N., K. R. Silk, S. Goodrich, N. E. Lohr, D. Westen, and E. M. Hill. 1990. Childhood sexual and physical abuse in adult patients with borderline personality disorder. *American Journal of Psychiatry* 147: 1008-1013.

44. Westen, D., P. Ludolph, B. Misle, S. Ruffins, and J. Block. 1990. Physical and sexual abuse in adolescent girls with borderline personality disorder. *American Journal of Orthopsychiatry* 60: 55-66.

45. Zanarini, M. C., L. Yong, F. R. Frankenburg, J. Hennen, D. B. Reich, M. F. Marino, et al. 2002. Severity of reported childhood sexual abuse and its relationship to severity of borderline psychopathology and psychosocial impairment among borderline inpatients. *Journal of Nervous and Mental Disease* 190: 381-387.

46. Silk, K. R., S. Lee, E. M. Hill, and N. E. Lohr. 1995. Borderline personality disorder symptoms and severity of sexual abuse. *American Journal of Psychiatry* 152: 1059-1064.

47. Bandelow, B., J. Krause, D. Wedekind, A. Broocks, G. Hajak, and E. Ruther. 2005. Early traumatic life events, parental attitudes, family history, and birth risk factors in patients with borderline personality disorder and healthy controls. *Psychiatry Research* 134: 169-179.

48. Skodol, A. E., P. Buckley, and E. Charles. 1983. Is there a characteristic pattern to the treatment history of clinic outpatients with borderline personality? *Journal of Nervous and Mental Disease* 171: 405-410.

49. Perry, J. C., J. L. Herman, B. A. van der Kolk, and L. A. Hoke. 1990. Psychotherapy and psychological trauma in borderline personality disorder. *Psychiatric Annals* 20: 33-43.

50. Stevenson, J., and R. Meares. 1992. An outcome study of psychotherapy for patients with borderline personality disorder. *American Journal of Psychiatry* 149: 358-362.

51. Stevenson, J., R. Meares, and R. D'Angelo. 2005. Five-year outcome of outpatient psychotherapy with borderline patients. *Psychological Medicine* 35: 79-87.

52. Koons, C. R., C. J. Robins, J. L. Tweed, T. R. Lynch, A. M. Gonzalez, J. Q. Morse, et al. 2001. Efficacy of dialectical behavior therapy in women veterans with borderline personality disorder. *Behavior Therapy* 32: 371-390.

53. Verheul, R., L. M. C. van den Bosch, M. W. J. Koeter, M. A. J. de Ridder, T. Stijnen, and W. van den Brink. 2003. Dialectical behaviour therapy for women with borderline personality disorder: 12-month, randomised clinical trial in Netherlands. *British Journal of Psychiatry* 182: 135-140.

54. McQuillan, A., R. Nicastro, F. Guenot, M. Girard, C. Lissner, and F. Ferrero. 2005. Intensive dialectical behavior therapy for outpatients with borderline personality disorder who are in crisis. *Psychiatric Services* 56: 193-197.

55. Linehan, M. M., H. E. Armstrong, A. Suarez, D. Allmon, and H. Heard. 1991. Cognitive-behavioral treatment of chronically parasuicidal borderline patients. *Archives of General Psychiatry* 48: 1060-1064.

56. Linehan, M. M., H. Heard, and H. E. Armstrong. 1993. Naturalistic follow-up of a behavioral treatment for chronically parasuicidal borderline patients. *Archives of General Psychiatry* 50: 971-974.

57. Linehan, M. M., H. Schmidt III, L. A. Dimeff, J. C. Craft, J. Kanter, and K. A. Comtois. 1999. Dialectical behavior therapy for patients with borderline personality disorder and drug-dependence. *American Journal on Addictions* 8: 279-292.

58. van den Bosch, L. M. C., R. Verheul, G. M. Schippers, and W. van den Brink. 2002. Dialectical behavior therapy of borderline patients with and without substance use problems: Implementation and long-term effects. *Addictive Behaviors* 27: 911-923.

59. Zanarini, M. C., F. R. Frankenburg, J. Hennen, and K. R. Silk. 2004. Mental health service utilization by borderline personality disorder patients and Axis II comparison subjects followed prospectively for 6 years. *Journal of Clinical Psychiatry* 65: 28-36.

60. Rinne, T., W. van den Brink, L. Wouters, and R. van Dyck. 2002. SSRI treatment of borderline personality disorder: A randomized, placebo-controlled clinical trial for female patients with borderline personality disorder. *American Journal of Psychiatry* 159: 2048-2054.

61. Salzman, C., A. N. Wolfson, A. Schatzberg, J. Looper, R. Henke, M. Albanese, et al. 1995. Effect of fluoxetine on anger in symptomatic volunteers with borderline personality disorder. *Journal of Clinical Psychopharmacology* 15: 23-29.

62. Coccaro, E. F., and R. J. Kavoussi. 1997. Fluoxetine and impulsive aggressive behavior in personality-disordered subjects. *Archives of General Psychiatry* 54: 1081-1088.

63. Frankenburg, F. R., and M. C. Zanarini. 1993. Clozapine treatment of borderline patients: A preliminary study. *Comprehensive Psychiatry* 34: 402-405.

64. Chengappa, K. N. R., T. Ebeling, J. S. Kang, J. Levine, and H. Parepally. 1999. Clozapine reduces severe self-mutilation and aggression in psychotic patients with borderline personality disorder. *Journal of Clinical Psychiatry* 60: 477-484.

65. Rocca, P., L. Marchiaro, E. Cocuzza, and F. Bogetto. 2002. Treatment of borderline personality disorder with risperidone. *Journal of Clinical Psychiatry* 63: 241-244.

66. Schulz, S. C., K. L. Camlin, S. A. Berry, and J. A. Jesberger. 1999. Olanzapine safety and efficacy in patients with borderline personality disorder and comorbid dysthymia. *Biological Psychiatry* 46: 1429-1435.

67. Soler, J., J. C. Pascual, J. Campins, J. Barrachina, D. Puigdemont, E. Alvarez, et al. 2005. Double-blind, placebo-controlled study of dialectical behavior therapy plus olanzapine for borderline personality disorder. *American Journal of Psychiatry* 162: 1221-1224.

68. Frankenburg, F. R., and M. C. Zanarini. 2002. Divalproex sodium treatment of women with borderline personality disorder and bipolar II disorder: A double-blind placebo-controlled pilot study. *Journal of Clinical Psychiatry* 63: 442-446.

69. Nickel, M. K., C. Nickel, P. Kaplan, C. Lahmann, M. Muhlbacher, K. Tritt, et al. 2005. Treatment of aggression with topiramate in male borderline patients: A double-blind, placebo-controlled study. *Biological Psychiatry* 57: 495-499.

70. Tritt, K., C. Nickel, C. Lahmann, P. K. Leiberich, W. K. Rother, T. H. Loew, et al. 2005. Lamotrigine treatment of aggression in female borderline-patients: A randomized, double-blind, placebo-controlled study. *Journal of Psychopharmacology* 19: 287-291.

71. Zanarini, M. C., and F. R. Frankenburg. 2003. Omega-3 fatty acid treatment of women with borderline personality disorder: A double-blind, placebo-controlled pilot study. *American Journal of Psychiatry* 160: 167-169.

Extreme Suspicion of Others

1. American Psychiatric Association. 2000. *Diagnostic and Statistical Manual of Mental Disorders.* Text revision ed. Washington, DC: American Psychiatric Association.

2. Beck, A. T., A. Freeman, J. Pretzer, D. D. Davis, B. Fleming, J. S. Beck, et al. 1990. *Cognitive Therapy of Personality Disorders.* New York: The Guilford Press.

3. Seivewright, H., P. Tyrer, and T. Johnson. 2002. Change in personality status in neurotic disorders. *Lancet* 359: 2253-2254.

4. Grant, B. F., F. S. Stinson, D. A. Dawson, S. P. Chou, W. J. Ruan, and R. P. Pickering. 2004. Co-occurrence of 12-month alcohol and drug use disorders and personality disorders in the United States: Results from the National Epidemiologic Survey on Alcohol and Related Conditions. *Archives of General Psychiatry* 61: 361-368.

5. Grant, B. F., D. S. Hasin, F. S. Stinson, D. A. Dawson, S. P. Chou, W. J. Ruan, et al. 2005. Co-occurrence of 12-month mood and anxiety disorders and personality disorders in the US: Results from the National Epidemiologic Survey on Alcohol and Related Conditions. *Journal of Psychiatric Research* 39: 1-9.

6. Fava, M., A. H. Farabaugh, A. H. Sickinger, E. Wright, J. E. Alpert, S. Sonawalla, et al. 2002. Personality disorders and depression. *Psychological Medicine* 32: 1049-1057.

7. Ozkan, M., and A. Altindag. 2005. Comorbid personality disorders in subjects with panic disorder: Do personality disorders increase clinical severity? *Comprehensive Psychiatry* 46: 20-26.

8. Torgersen, S., E. Kringlen, and V. Cramer. 2001. The prevalence of personality disorders in a community sample. *Archives of General Psychiatry* 58: 590-596.

9. Ekselius, L., M. Tillfors, T. Furmark, and M. Fredrikson. 2001. Personality disorders in the general population: DSM-IV and ICD-10 defined prevalence as related to sociodemographic profile. *Personality and Individual Differences* 30: 311-320.

10. Grant, B. F., D. S. Hasin, F. S. Stinson, D. A. Dawson, S. P. Chou, W. J. Ruan, et al. 2004. Prevalence, correlates, and disability of personality disorders in the United States: Results from the National Epidemiologic Survey on Alcohol and Related Conditions. *Journal of Clinical Psychiatry* 65: 948-958.

11. Torgersen, S., S. Lygren, P. A. Oien, I. Skre, S. Onstad, J. Edvardsen, et al. 2000. A twin study of personality disorders. *Comprehensive Psychiatry* 41: 416-425.

12. Chang, C.-J., W. J. Chen, S. K. Liu, J. J. Cheng, W.-C. O. Yang, H.-J. Chang, et al. 2002. Morbidity risk of psychiatric disorders among the first degree relatives of schizophrenia patients in Taiwan. *Schizophrenia Bulletin* 28: 379-392.

13. Kasen, S., P. Cohen, A. E. Skodol, J. G. Johnson, E. Smailes, and J. S. Brook. 2001. Childhood depression and adult personality disorder: Alternative pathways of continuity. *Archives of General Psychiatry* 58: 231-236.

14. Johnson, J. G., P. Cohen, E. M. Smailes, A. E. Skodol, J. Brown, and J. M. Oldham. 2001. Childhood verbal abuse and risk for personality disorders during adolescence and early adulthood. *Comprehensive Psychiatry* 42: 16-23.

15. Coid, J. W. 1999. Aetiological risk factors for personality disorders. *British Journal of Psychiatry* 174: 530-538.

16. Bierer, L. M., R. Yehuda, J. Schmeidler, V. Mitropoulou, A. S. New, J. M. Silverman, et al. 2003. Abuse and neglect in childhood: Relationship to personality disorder diagnoses. *CNS Spectrums* 8: 737-740, 749-754.

17.   Griffith, E. E. H., and F. M. Baker. 1993. Psychiatric care of African Americans. In *Culture, Ethnicity, and Mental Illness*, edited by A. C. Gaw. Washington, DC: American Psychiatric Press.

18.   Cohen, C. I., C. Magai, R. Yaffee, and L. Walcott-Brown. 2004. Racial differences in paranoid ideation and psychoses in an older urban population. *American Journal of Psychiatry* 161: 864-871.

19.   Blazer, D. G., J. C. Hays, and M. E. Salive. 1996. Factors associated with paranoid symptoms in a community sample of older adults. *Gerontology* 36: 70-75.

20.   Tyrer, P., S. Mitchard, C. Methuen, and M. Ranger. 2003. Treatment rejecting and treatment seeking personality disorders: Type R and Type S. *Journal of Personality Disorders* 17: 263-267.

21.   Kuyken, W., N. Kurzer, R. J. DeRubeis, A. T. Beck, and G. K. Brown. 2001. Response to cognitive therapy in depression: The role of maladaptive beliefs and personality disorders. *Journal of Consulting and Clinical Psychology* 69: 560-566.

22.   Roth, A., and P. Fonagy. 1996. Personality disorders. In *What Works for Whom? A Critical Review of Psychotherapy Research*. New York: The Guilford Press.

23.   Stanley, B., E. Bundy, and R. Beberman. 2001. Skills training as an adjunctive treatment for personality disorders. *Journal of Psychiatric Practice* 7: 324-335.

24.   Linehan, M. M. 1993. *Cognitive-Behavioral Treatment of Borderline Personality Disorder*. New York: The Guilford Press.

25.   Leichsenring, F., and E. Leibing. 2003. The effectiveness of psychodynamic therapy and cognitive behavior therapy in the treatment of personality disorders: A meta-analysis. *American Journal of Psychiatry* 160: 1223-1232.

26.   Budman, S. H., A. Demby, S. Soldz, and J. Merry. 1996. Time-limited group psychotherapy for patients with personality disorders: Outcomes and dropouts. *International Journal of Group Psychotherapy* 46: 357-377.

27.   Karterud, S., G. Pedersen, E. Bjordal, J. Brabrand, S. Friis, O. Haaseth, et al. 2003. Day treatment of patients with personality disorders: Experiences from a Norwegian treatment research network. *Journal of Personality Disorders* 17: 243-262.

28.   Marziali, E., and H. Munroe-Blum. 1998. Interpersonal group psychotherapy for borderline personality disorder. *Psychotherapy in Practice* 4: 91-107.

Generalized Anxiety Disorder

1.   American Psychiatric Association. 2000. *Diagnostic and Statistical Manual of Mental Disorders*. Text revision ed. Washington, DC: American Psychiatric Association.

2.   Hunt, C., T. Slade, and G. Andrews. 2004. Generalized Anxiety Disorder and Major Depressive Disorder comorbidity in the National Survey of Mental Health and Well-Being. *Depression and Anxiety* 20: 23-31.

3.   Hoehn-Saric, R. 2005. Generalized anxiety disorder in medical practice. *Primary Psychiatry* 12: 30-34.

4.   Riskind, J. H., and N. L. Williams. 2005. The looming cognitive style and generalized anxiety disorder: Distinctive danger schemas and cognitive phenomenology. *Cognitive Therapy and Research* 29: 7-27.

5.   Beck, A. T., and G. Emery. 1985. *Anxiety Disorders and Phobias*. New York: Basic Books.

6.   Dugas, M. J., M. Hedayati, A. Karavidas, K. Buhr, K. Francis, and N. A. Phillips. 2005. Intolerance of uncertainty and information processing: Evidence of biased recall and interpretations. *Cognitive Therapy and Research* 29: 57-70.

7.   Dugas, M. J., A. Marchand, and R. Ladouceur. 2005. Further validation of a cognitive-behavioral model of generalized anxiety disorder: Diagnostic and symptom specificity. *Journal of Anxiety Disorders* 19: 329-343.

8.   Marten, P. A., T. A. Brown, D. H. Barlow, T. D. Borkovec, M. K. Shear, and R. B. Lydiard. 1993. Evaluation of the ratings comprising the associated symptom criterion of DSM-III-R generalized anxiety disorder. *Journal of Nervous and Mental Disease* 181: 676-682.

9. Wittchen, H. U., S. Zhao, R. C. Kessler, and W. W. Eaves. 1994. DSM-III-R generalized anxiety disorder in the National Comorbidity Survey. *Archives of General Psychiatry* 51: 355-364.

10. Kessler, R. C., R. L. DuPont, P. A. Berglund, and H. U. Wittchen. 1999. Impairment in pure and comorbid generalized anxiety disorder and major depression at 12 months in two national surveys. *American Journal of Psychiatry* 156: 1915-1923.

11. Merikangas, K. R., R. L. Mehta, B. E. Molnar, E. E. Walters, J. D. Swendsen, S. Auilar-Gaziola, et al. 1998. Comorbidity of substance use disorders with mood and anxiety disorders: Results of the International Consortium in Psychiatric Epidemiology. *Addictive Behaviors* 23: 893-908.

12. Grant, B. F., F. S. Stinson, D. A. Dawson, P. Chou, M. C. Dufour, W. Compton, et al. 2004. Prevalence and co-occurrence of substance use disorders and independent mood and anxiety disorders: Results from the National Epidemiologic Survey on Alcohol and Related Conditions. *Archives of General Psychiatry* 61: 807-816.

13. Kessler, R. C., W. T. Chiu, O. Demler, and E. E. Walters. 2005. Prevalence, severity, and comorbidity of 12-month DSM-IV disorders in the National Comorbidity Survey Replication. *Archives of General Psychiatry* 62: 617-627.

14. Grant, B. F., D. S. Hasin, F. S. Stinson, D. A. Dawson, S. P. Chou, W. J. Ruan, et al. 2005. Co-occurrence of 12-month mood and anxiety disorders and personality disorders in the US: Results from the National Epidemiologic Survey on Alcohol and Related Conditions. *Journal of Psychiatric Research* 39: 1-9.

15. Pini, S., G. B. Cassano, E. Simonini, M. Savino, A. Russo, and S. A. Montgomery. 1997. Prevalence of anxiety disorders comorbidity in bipolar depression, unipolar depression and dysthymia. *Journal of Affective Disorders* 42: 145-153.

16. Logue, M. B., A. M. Thomas, J. G. Barbee, R. Hoehn-Saric, R. J. Maddock, J. J. Schwab, et al. 1993. Generalized anxiety disorder patients seek evaluation for cardiological symptoms at the same frequency as patients with panic disorder. *Journal of Psychiatric Research* 27: 55-59.

17. Blanchard, E. B., L. Scharff, S. P. Schwarz, J. M. Suls, and D. H. Barlow. 1990. The role of anxiety and depression in the irritable bowel syndrome. *Behaviour Research and Therapy* 28: 401-405.

18. Kennedy, B. L., and J. J. Schwab. 1997. Utilization of medical specialists by anxiety disorder patients. *Psychosomatics* 38: 109-112.

19. Maier, W., and P. Falkai. 1999. The epidemiology of comorbidity between depression, anxiety disorders and somatic diseases. *International Clinical Psychopharmacology* 14: S1-S6.

20. Sherbourne, C. D., C. A. Jackson, L. S. Meredith, P. Camp, and K. B. Wells. 1996. Prevalence of comorbid anxiety disorders in primary care outpatients. *Archives of Family Medicine* 5: 27-34.

21. Kessler, R. C., P. A. Berglund, O. Demler, R. Jin, and E. E. Walters. 2005. Lifetime prevalence and age-of-onset distributions of DSM-IV disorders in the National Comorbidity Survey Replication. *Archives of General Psychiatry* 62: 593-602.

22. Kessler, R. C., K. A. McGonagle, S. Zhao, C. B. Nelson, M. Hughes, S. Eshleman, et al. 1994. Lifetime and 12-month prevalence of DSM-III-R psychiatric disorders in the United States. *Archives of General Psychiatry* 51: 8-19.

23. Sanderson, W. C., and D. H. Barlow. 1990. A description of patients diagnosed with DSM-III-R generalized anxiety disorder. *Journal of Nervous and Mental Disease* 178: 588-591.

24. Blazer, D. G., D. Hughes, and L. K. George. 1987. Stressful life events and the onset of the generalized anxiety disorder syndrome. *American Journal of Psychiatry* 144: 1178-1183.

25. Kendler, K. S., M. C. Neale, R. C. Kessler, A. C. Heath, and L. J. Eaves. 1992. Generalized anxiety disorder in women: A population-based twin study. *Archives of General Psychiatry* 49: 267-272.

26. Hettema, J. M., M. C. Neale, and K. S. Kendler. 2001. A review and meta-analysis of the genetic epidemiology of anxiety disorders. *American Journal of Psychiatry* 158: 1568-1578.

27. Kagan, J., N. Snidman, D. Arcus, and J. S. Reznick. 1997. *Galen's Prophesy*. New York: Basic Books.

28. Hoehn-Saric, R., D. R. McLeod, F. Funderburk, and P. Kowalski. 2004. Somatic symptoms and physiologic responses in generalized anxiety disorder and panic disorder. *Archives of General Psychiatry* 61: 913-921.

29. Borkovec, T. D., and J. Inz. 1990. The nature of worry in generalized anxiety disorder: A predominance of thought activity. *Behaviour Research and Therapy* 28: 153-158.

30. Borkovec, T. D. 1994. The nature, functions, and origins of worry. In *Worrying: Perspectives on Theory, Assessment, and Treatment*, edited by G. Davey and F. Tallis. New York: Wiley.

31. Roemer, L., K. Salters, S. D. Raffa, and S. M. Orsillo. 2005. Fear and avoidance of internal experiences in GAD: Preliminary tests of a conceptual model. *Cognitive Therapy and Research* 29: 71-88.

32. Mogg, K., and B. P. Bradley. 2005. Attentional bias in generalized anxiety disorder versus depressive disorder. *Cognitive Therapy and Research* 29: 29-45.

33. Barlow, D. H. 1988. *Anxiety and Its Disorders: The Nature and Treatment of Anxiety and Panic.* New York: The Guilford Press.

34. Blazer, D. G., L. K. George, and D. Hughes. 1991. The epidemiology of anxiety disorders: An age comparison. In *Anxiety in the Elderly*, edited by C. Salzman and B. D. Lebowitz. New York: Springer.

35. Blazer, D. G. 1991. Generalized anxiety disorder. In *Psychiatric Disorders in America*, edited by L. N. Robins and D. A. Regier. New York: Free Press.

36. Wang, P. S., P. A. Berglund, M. Olfson, H. A. Pincus, K. B. Wells, and R. C. Kessler. 2005. Failure and delay in initial treatment contact after first onset of mental disorders in the National Comorbidity Survey Replication. *Archives of General Psychiatry* 62: 603-613.

37. Durham, R. C., T. Murphy, T. Allan, K. Richard, L. R. Treliving, and G. W. Fenton. 1994. Cognitive therapy, analytic psychotherapy and anxiety management training for generalised anxiety disorder. *British Journal of Psychiatry* 165: 315-323.

38. Fisher, P. L., and R. C. Durham. 1999. Recovery rates in generalized anxiety disorder following psychological therapy: An analysis of clinically significant change in the STAI-T across outcome studies since 1990. *Psychological Medicine* 29: 1425-1434.

39. White, J. 1999. *Overcoming Generalized Anxiety Disorder: A Relaxation, Cognitive Restructuring, and Exposure-Based Protocol for the Treatment of GAD.* Oakland, CA: New Harbinger Publications.

40. Brown, T. A., T. A. O'Leary, and D. H. Barlow. 2001. Generalized anxiety disorder. In *Clinical Handbook of Psychological Disorders*, edited by D. H. Barlow. New York: The Guilford Press.

41. Ost, L. G., and E. Breitholtz. 2000. Applied relaxation vs. cognitive therapy in the treatment of generalized anxiety disorder. *Behaviour Research and Therapy* 38: 777-790.

42. Mitte, K., P. Noack, R. Steil, and M. Hautzinger. 2001. A meta-analytic review of the efficacy of drug treatment in generalized anxiety disorder. *Journal of Clinical Psychopharmacology* 25: 141-150.

43. Baldwin, D. S., and C. Polkinghorn. 2005. Evidence-based pharmacotherapy of generalized anxiety disorder. *International Journal of Neuropsychopharmacology* 8: 293-302.

Impulse Control Disorders

1. American Psychiatric Association. 2000. *Diagnostic and Statistical Manual of Mental Disorders.* Text revision ed. Washington, DC: American Psychiatric Association.

2. Treuer, T., Z. Fabian, and J. Furedi. 2001. Internet addiction associated with features of impulse control disorder: Is it a real psychiatric disorder? *Journal of Affective Disorders* 66: 283.

3. Johansson, A., and K. G. Gotestam. 2004. Problems with computer games without monetary reward: Similarity to pathological gambling. *Psychological Reports* 95: 641-650.

4. Grant, J. E., and S. W. Kim. 2005. Quality of life in kleptomania and pathological gambling. *Comprehensive Psychiatry* 46: 34-37.

5. Mavromatis, M., and J. R. Lion. 1977. A primer on pyromania. *Diseases of the Nervous System* 38: 954-955.

6. Galovski, T., and E. B. Blanchard. 2002. Psychological characteristics of aggressive drivers with and without intermittent explosive disorder. *Behaviour Research and Therapy* 40: 1157-1168.

7.   Diefenbach, G. J., D. F. Tolin, S. Hannan, J. Crocetto, and P. Worhunsky. 2005. Trichotillomania: Impact on psychosocial functioning and quality of life. *Behaviour Research and Therapy* 43: 869-884.

8.   Gerstein, D. R., R. A. Volberg, M. T. Toce, H. Harwood, R. A. Johnson, T. Bule, et al. 1999. *Gambling Impact and Behavior Study: Report to the National Gambling Impact Study Commission*. Chicago, IL: National Opinion Research Center at the University of Chicago.

9.   Murray, J. B. 1992. Kleptomania: A review of the research. *Journal of Psychology: Interdisciplinary and Applied* 126: 131-137.

10.   Wiedemann, G. 1998. Kleptomania: Characteristics of 12 cases. *European Psychiatry* 13: 67-77.

11.   Grant, J. E., and S. W. Kim. 2002. Clinical characteristics and associated psychopathology of 22 patients with kleptomania. *Comprehensive Psychiatry* 43: 378-384.

12.   U. S. Fire Administration. 2004. *Fire in the United States: 1992–2001: Executive Summary*. In FA-286. Emmitsburg, MD: Federal Emergency Management Association.

13.   Diefenbach, G. J., S. Mouton-Odum, and M. A. Stanley. 2002. Affective correlates of trichotillomania. *Behaviour Research and Therapy* 40: 1305-1315.

14.   Kress, V. E. W., B. L. Kelly, and L. J. McCormick. 2004. Trichotillomania: Assessment, diagnosis, and treatment. *Journal of Counseling and Development* 82: 185-190.

15.   McElroy, S. L., C. A. Soutullo, D. A. Beckman, P. Taylor Jr., and P. E. Keck Jr. 1998. DSM-IV intermittent explosive disorder: A report of 27 cases. *Journal of Clinical Psychiatry* 59: 203-210.

16.   Kausch, O. 2003. Suicide attempts among veterans seeking treatment for pathological gambling. *Journal of Clinical Psychiatry* 64: 1031-1038.

17.   Ledgerwood, D. M., and N. M. Petry. 2004. Gambling and suicidality in treatment-seeking pathological gamblers. *Journal of Nervous and Mental Disease* 192: 711-714.

18.   Petry, N. M., F. S. Stinson, and B. F. Grant. 2005. Comorbidity of DSM-IV pathological gambling and other psychiatric disorders: Results from the National Epidemiologic Survey on Alcohol and Related Conditions. *Journal of Clinical Psychiatry* 66: 564-574.

19.   Dannon, P. N., K. Lowengrub, M. Sasson, B. Shalgi, L. Tuson, Y. Saphir, et al. 2004. Comorbid psychiatric diagnoses in kleptomania and pathological gambling: A preliminary comparison study. *European Psychiatry* 19: 299-302.

20.   Durst, R., G. Katz, A. Teitelbaum, J. Zislin, and P. N. Dannon. 2001. Kleptomania: Diagnosis and treatment options. *CNS Drugs* 15: 185-195.

21.   Bayle, F. J., H. Caci, B. Millet, S. Richa, and J.-P. Olio. 2003. Psychopathology and comorbidity of psychiatric disorders in patients with kleptomania. *American Journal of Psychiatry* 160: 1509-1513.

22.   McElroy, S., H. G. J. Pope, P. E. Keck, and K. L. White. 1991. Kleptomania: A report of 20 cases. *American Journal of Psychiatry* 148: 652-657.

23.   Galovski, T., E. B. Blanchard, and C. Veazey. 2002. Intermittent explosive disorder and other psychiatric comorbidity among court-referred and self-referred aggressive drivers. *Behaviour Research and Therapy* 40: 641-651.

24.   Christenson, G. A., T. B. Mackenzie, and J. E. Mitchell. 1991. Characteristics of 60 adult chronic hair pullers. *American Journal of Psychiatry* 148: 365-370.

25.   Swedo, S. E., and H. L. Leonard. 1992. Trichotillomania: An obsessive compulsive spectrum disorder? *Psychiatric Clinics of North America* 15: 777-790.

26.   Murry, J. B. 1993. Review on research on pathological gambling. *Psychological Reports* 72: 791-810.

27.   Shaffer, H. J., M. N. Hall, and J. Vander Bilt. 1999. Estimating the prevalence of disordered gambling behavior in the United States and Canada: A research synthesis. *American Journal of Public Health* 89: 1369-1376.

28.   Lepkifker, E., P. N. Dannon, R. Ziv, I. Iancu, N. Horesh, and M. Kotler. 1999. The treatment of kleptomania with serotonin reuptake inhibitors. *Clinical Neuropharmacology* 22: 40-43.

29.   Goldman, M. J. 1992. Kleptomania: An overview. Psychiatric Annals 22: 68-71.

30.   Bouwer, C., and D. J. Stein. 1998. Trichobezoars in trichotillomania: Case report and literature overview. *Psychosomatic Medicine* 60: 658-660.

31. Diefenbach, G. J., D. Reitman, and D. A. Williamson. 2000. Trichotillomania: A challenge to research and practice. *Clinical Psychology Review* 20: 289-309.

32. Coccaro, E. F., C. A. Schmidt, J. F. Samuels, and G. Nestadt. 2004. Lifetime and 1-month prevalence rates of intermittent explosive disorder in a community sample. *Journal of Clinical Psychiatry* 65: 820-824.

33. Kessler, R. C., P. A. Berglund, O. Demler, R. Jin, and E. E. Walters. 2005. Lifetime prevalence and age-of-onset distributions of DSM-IV disorders in the National Comorbidity Survey Replication. *Archives of General Psychiatry* 62: 593-602.

34. Goudriaan, A. E., J. Oosterlaan, E. de Beurs, and W. Van den Brink. 2004. Pathological gambling: A comprehensive review of biobehavioral findings. *Neuroscience and Biobehavioral Reviews* 28: 123-141.

35. Olvera, R. L. 2002. Intermittent explosive disorder: Epidemiology, diagnosis and management. *CNS Drugs* 16: 517-526.

36. Pérez, de Castro, I., A. Ibáñez, J. Saiz-Ruiz, and J. Fernández-Piqueras. 2002. Concurrent positive association between pathological gambling and functional DNA polymorphisms at the MAO-A and the 5-HT transporter genes. *Molecular Psychiatry* 7: 927-928.

37. Kavoussi, R. J., P. Armstead, and E. F. Coccaro. 1997. The neurobiology of impulsive aggression. *Psychiatric Clinics of North America* 20: 395-403.

38. Shah, K. R., S. A. Eisen, H. Xian, and M. N. Potenza. 2005. Genetic studies of pathological gambling: A review of methodology and analyses of data from the Vietnam Era Twin Registry. *Journal of Gambling Studies* 21: 179-203.

39. Scherrer, J. F., H. Xian, K. R. Shah, R. Volberg, W. Slutske, and S. A. Eisen. 2005. Effect of genes, environment, and lifetime co-occurring disorders on health-related quality of life in problem and pathological gamblers. *Archives of General Psychiatry* 62: 677-683.

40. Vythilingum, B., J. Warwick, J. van Kradenburg, C. Hugo, B. van Heerden, and D. J. Stein. 2002. SPECT scans in identical twins with trichotillomania. *Journal of Neuropsychiatry and Clinical Neurosciences* 14: 340-342.

41. Lochner, C., P. L. du Toit, N. Zungu-Dirwayi, A. Marais, J. van Kradenburg, S. Seedat, et al. 2002. Childhood trauma in obsessive-compulsive disorder, trichotillomania, and controls. *Depression and Anxiety* 15: 66-68.

42. Boughn, S., and J. J. Holdom. 2003. The relationship of violence and trichotillomania. *Journal of Nursing Scholarship* 35: 165-170.

43. Petry, N. M., and K. L. Steinberg. 2005. Childhood maltreatment in male and female treatment-seeking pathological gamblers. *Psychology of Addictive Behaviors* 19: 226-229.

44. Kolko, D., and A. E. Kazdin. 1990. Matchplay and firesetting in children: Relationship to parent, marital, and family dysfunction. *Journal of Clinical Child Psychology* 19: 229-238.

45. Grant, J. E., and S. W. Kim. 2002. Temperament and early environmental influences in kleptomania. *Comprehensive Psychiatry* 43: 223-228.

46. Kohn, C. S., and D. O. Antonuccio. 2002. Treatment of kleptomania using cognitive and behavioral strategies. *Clinical Case Studies* 1: 25-38.

47. McConaghy, N., and A. Blaszczynski. 1988. Imaginal desensitization: A cost-effectiveness treatment in two shop-lifters and a binge-eater resistant to previous therapy. *Australian and New Zealand Journal of Psychiatry* 22: 78-82.

48. Toneatto, T., and R. Ladoceur. 2003. Treatment of pathological gambling: A critical review of the literature. *Psychology of Addictive Behaviors* 17: 284-292.

49. van Minnen, A., K. A. L. Hoogduin, G. P. J. Keijsers, I. Hellenbrand, and G.-J. Hendriks. 2003. Treatment of trichotillomania with behavioral therapy or fluoxetine: A randomized, waiting-list controlled study. *Archives of General Psychiatry* 60: 517-522.

50. Pélissier, M.-C., and K. O'Connor. 2004. Cognitive-behavioral treatment of trichotillomania, targeting perfectionism. *Clinical Case Studies* 3: 57-69.

51. Edmondson, C. B., and J. C. Conger. 1996. A review of treatment efficacy for individuals with anger problems: Conceptual, assessment and methodological issues. *Clinical Psychology Review* 16: 251-275.

52. Bumpass, E. R., F. D. Fagelman, and R. J. Brix. 1983. Intervention with children who set fires. *American Journal of Psychotherapy* 37: 328-345.

53. Petry, N. M. 2005. Gamblers Anonymous and cognitive-behavioral therapies for pathological gamblers. *Journal of Gambling Studies* 21: 27-33.

54. Christenson, G. A., and S. Crow. 1996. The characterization and treatment of trichotillomania. *Journal of Clinical Psychiatry* 57: 42-47.

55. Chong, S. A., and B. L. Low. 1996. Treatment of kleptomania with fluvoxamine. *Acta Psychiatrica Scandinavica* 93: 314-315.

56. Dannon, P. N. 2002. Kleptomania: An impulse control disorder? *International Journal of Psychiatry in Clinical Practice* 6: 3-7.

57. McElroy, S. L. 1999. Recognition and treatment of DSM-IV intermittent explosive disorder. *Journal of Clinical Psychiatry* 60: 12-16.

58. Hollander, E., E. Sood, S. Pallanti, N. Baldini-Rossi, and B. Baker. 2005. Pharmacological treatments of pathological gambling. Journal of Gambling Studies 21: 101-110.

59. Stewart, R. S., and V. A. Nejtek. 2003. An open-label, flexible-dose study of olanzapine in the treatment of trichotillomania. *Journal of Clinical Psychiatry* 64: 49-52.

60. Srivastava, R. K., S. Sharma, N. Tiwari, and B. Saluja. 2005. Olanzapine augmentation of fluoxetine in trichotillomania: Two cases. *Australian and New Zealand Journal of Psychiatry* 39: 112-113.

Obsessive-Compulsive Disorder

1. American Psychiatric Association. 2000. *Diagnostic and Statistical Manual of Mental Disorders.* Text revision ed. Washington, DC: American Psychiatric Association.

2. Roberts, A. R., K. Yeager, and A. Seigel. 2003. Obsessive-compulsive disorder, comorbid depression, substance abuse, and suicide attempts: Clinical presentations, assessments, and treatment. *Brief Treatment and Crisis Intervention* 3: 145-167.

3. Foa, E. B., M. J. Kozak, W. K. Goodman, E. Hollander, M. A. Jenike, and P. R. Rasmussen. 1995. DSM-IV field trial: Obsessive-compulsive disorder. *American Journal of Psychiatry* 152: 90-96.

4. Karno, M. G., M. Golding, S. B. Sorensin, and A. Burnam. 1988. The epidemiology of OCD in five U.S. communities. *Archives of General Psychiatry* 45: 1094-1099.

5. Gunstad, J., and K. A. Phillips. 2003. Axis I comorbidity in body dysmorphic disorder. *Comprehensive Psychiatry* 44: 270-276.

6. Brady, K. T., L. Austin, and R. B. Lydiard. 1990. Body dysmorphic disorder: The relationship to obsessive-compulsive disorder. *Journal of Nervous and Mental Disease* 178: 538-540.

7. Pini, S., G. B. Cassano, E. Simonini, M. Savino, A. Russo, and S. A. Montgomery. 1997. Prevalence of anxiety disorders comorbidity in bipolar depression, unipolar depression and dysthymia. *Journal of Affective Disorders* 42: 145-153.

8. McElroy, S. L., L. L. Altschuler, T. Suppes, P. E. Keck Jr., M. A. Frye, K. D. Denicoff, et al. 2001. Axis I psychiatric comorbidity and its relationship to historical illness variables in 288 patients with bipolar disorder. *American Journal of Psychiatry* 158: 420-426.

9. Rasmussen, S. A., and M. T. Tsuang. 1986. Clinical characteristics and family history in DSM-III obsessive-compulsive disorder. *American Journal of Psychiatry* 143: 317-322.

10. Kessler, R. C., W. T. Chiu, O. Demler, and E. E. Walters. 2005. Prevalence, severity, and comorbidity of 12-month DSM-IV disorders in the National Comorbidity Survey Replication. *Archives of General Psychiatry* 62: 617-627.

11. Zanarini, M. C., F. R. Frankenburg, J. Hennen, D. B. Reich, and K. R. Silk. 2004. Axis I comorbidity in patients with borderline personality disorder: 6-year follow-up and prediction of time to remission. *American Journal of Psychiatry* 161: 2108-2114.

12. Zanarini, M. C., F. R. Frankenburg, E. D. Dubo, A. E. Sickel, A. Trikha, A. Levin, et al. 1998. Axis I comorbidity of borderline personality disorder. *American Journal of Psychiatry* 155: 1733-1739.

13. O'Brien, K. M., and N. K. Vincent. 2003. Psychiatric comorbidity in anorexia and bulimia nervosa: Nature, prevalence and causal relationships. *Clinical Psychology Review* 23: 57-74.

14. Baker, D., E. Hunter, E. Lawrence, N. Medford, M. Patel, C. Senior, et al. 2003. Depersonalisation disorder: Clinical features of 204 cases. *British Journal of Psychiatry* 182: 428-433.

15. Christenson, G. A., T. B. Mackenzie, and J. E. Mitchell. 1991. Characteristics of 60 adult chronic hair pullers. *American Journal of Psychiatry* 148: 365-370.

16. Swedo, S. E., and H. L. Leonard. 1992. Trichotillomania: An obsessive compulsive spectrum disorder? *Psychiatric Clinics of North America* 15: 777-790.

17. Murray, C. J. L., and A. D. Lopez, eds. 1996. *Summary: The Global Burden of Disease: A Comprehensive Assessment of Mortality and Disability from Diseases, Injuries, and Risk Factors in 1990 and Projected to 2020.* Cambridge, MA: Published by the Harvard School of Public Health on behalf of the World Health Organization and the World Bank, Harvard University Press.

18. Kessler, R. C., P. A. Berglund, O. Demler, R. Jin, and E. E. Walters. 2005. Lifetime prevalence and age-of-onset distributions of DSM-IV disorders in the National Comorbidity Survey Replication. *Archives of General Psychiatry* 62: 593-602.

19. National Institute of Mental Health. 2004. The numbers count: Mental disorders in America. National Institute of Mental Health 2001 [cited June 19, 2004]. Available from www.nimh.nih.gov/publicat/numbers.cfm.

20. Rachman, S., and P. de Silva. 1978. Abnormal and normal obsessions. *Behaviour Research and Therapy* 16: 233-248.

21. Bilgic, B., I. Baral-Kulaksizoglu, H. Hanagasi, M. Saylan, E. Aykutlu, H. Gurvit, et al. 2004. Obsessive-compulsive disorder secondary to bilateral frontal damage due to a closed head injury. *Cognitive Behavioral Neurology* 17: 118-120.

22. Isaacs, K. L., J. W. Philbeck, W. B. Barr, O. Devinsky, and K. Alper. 2004. Obsessive-compulsive symptoms in patients with temporal lobe epilepsy. *Epilepsy and Behavior* 5: 569-574.

23. Abramowitz, J., K. Moore, C. Carmin, P. S. Wiegartz, and C. Purdon. 2001. Acute onset of obsessive-compulsive disorder in males following childbirth. *Psychosomatics* 42: 429-431.

24. Pujol, J., C. Soriano-Mas, P. Alonso, N. Cardoner, J. M. Menchon, J. Deus, et al. 2004. Mapping structural brain alterations in obsessive-compulsive disorder. *Archives of General Psychiatry* 61: 720-730.

25. Saxena, S., A. L. Brody, J. M. Schwartz, and L. R. Baxter. 1998. Neuroimaging and frontal-subcortical circuitry in obsessive-compulsive disorder. *British Journal of Psychiatry* 173: 26-37.

26. Delgado, M. R., V. A. Stenger, and J. A. O. Fiez. 2004. Motivation-dependent responses in the human caudate nucleus. *Cerebral Cortex* 14: 1022-1030.

27. Carbon, M., Y. Ma, A. Barnes, V. Dhawan, T. Chaly, M. F. Ghilardi, et al. 2004. Caudate nucleus: Influence of dopaminergic input on sequence learning and brain activation in Parkinsonism. *Neuroimage* 21: 1497-1507.

28. Haruno, M., T. Kuroda, K. Doya, K. Toyama, M. Kimura, K. Samejima, et al. 2004. A neural correlate of reward-based learning in caudate nucleus: A functional magnetic resonance imaging study of a schastic decision task. *Journal of Neuroscience* 24: 1660-1665.

29. Obsessive Compulsive Cognitions Working Group. 1997. Cognitive assessment of obsessive-compulsive disorder. *Behaviour Research and Therapy* 35: 667-681.

30. Steketee, G. S. 1999. *Overcoming Obsessive-Compulsive Disorder: A Behavioral and Cognitive Protocol for the Treatment of OCD.* Best Practices for Therapy. Oakland, CA: New Harbinger Publications.

31. Wegner, D. 1994. *White Bears and Other Unwanted Thoughts.* New York: The Guilford Press.

32. Narrow, W. E., D. A. Regier, D. S. Rae, R. W. Manderscheid, and B. Z. Locke. 1993. Use of services by persons with mental and addictive disorders: Findings from the National Institute of Mental Health Epidemiologic Catchment Area Program. *Archives of General Psychiatry* 50: 95-107.

33. Mathew, S. J., H. B. Simpson, and B. A. Fallon. 2000. Treatment strategies for obsessive-compulsive disorder. *Psychiatric Annals* 30: 699-708.

34. Foa, E. B., and M. J. Kozak. 1996. Obsessive-compulsive disorder: Long term outcome of psychological treatment. In *Long-Term Treatments of Anxiety Disorders,* edited by M. R. Mavissakalian and R. F. Prien. Washington, DC: American Psychiatric Press.

35. Kozak, M. J., M. L. Liebowitz, and E. B. Foa. 2001. Cognitive behavior therapy and pharmacotherapy for OCD. In *Treatment Challenges in Obsessive Compulsive Disorder,* edited by W. K. Goodman, J. D. Maser, and M. Rudorfer. Mahwah, NJ: Lawrence Erlbaum.

36.	Hansen, E. S., S. Hasselbalch, I. Law, and T. G. Bolwig. 2002. The caudate nucleus in obsessive-compulsive disorder. Reduced metabolism following treatment with paroxetine: A PET study. *International Journal of Neuropsychopharmacology* 5: 1-10.

37.	Schwartz, J. M., P. W. Stoessel, L. R. Baxter, K. M. Martin, and M. E. Phelps. 1996. Systematic changes in cerebral glucose metabolic rate after successful behavior modification treatment of obsessive-compulsive disorder. *Archives of General Psychiatry* 53: 109-113.

38.	Baxter, L. R., J. M. Schwartz, K. S. Bergman, M. P. Szuba, B. H. Guze, J. C. Mazziotta, et al. 1992. Caudate glucose metabolic rate changes with both drug and behavior therapy for obsessive-compulsive disorder. *Archives of General Psychiatry* 49: 681-689.

39.	Van Noppen, B., and G. S. Steketee. 2003. Family responses and multifamily behavioral treatment for obsessive-compulsive disorder. *Brief Treatment and Crisis Intervention* 3: 231-247.

40.	Biondi, M., and A. Picardi. 2005. Increased maintenance of obsessive-compulsive disorder remission after integrated serotonergic treatment and cognitive psychotherapy compared with medication alone. *Psychotherapy and Psychosomatics* 74: 123-128.

41.	Franklin, M. E., J. Abramowitz, D. A. Bux, L. A. Zoellner, and N. C. Feeny. 2002. Cognitive-behavioral therapy with and without medication in the treatment of obsessive-compulsive disorder. *Professional Psychology: Research and Practice* 33: 162-168.

42.	Foa, E. B., M. L. Liebowitz, M. J. Kozak, S. Davies, R. Campeas, M. E. Franklin, et al. 2005. Randomized, placebo-controlled trial of exposure and ritual prevention, clomipramine, and their combination in the treatment of obsessive-compulsive disorder. *American Journal of Psychiatry* 162: 151-161.

43.	Pato, M. T., and K. A. Phillips. 2003. Biological, pharmacological, and somatic treatments for obsessive-compulsive disorder. *Brief Treatment and Crisis Intervention* 3: 275-290.

44.	Jenike, M. A. 1998. Neurosurgical treatment of obsessive-compulsive disorder. *British Journal of Psychiatry* 173: 79-90.

45.	Mindus, P., and M. A. Jenike. 1992. Neurosurgical treatment of malignant obsessive compulsive disorder. *Psychiatric Clinics of North America* 15: 921-938.

46.	Dougherty, D. D., L. Baer, G. R. Cosgrove, E. H. Cassem, B. H. Price, A. A. Nierenberg, et al. 2002. Prospective long-term follow-up of 44 patients who received cingulotomy for treatment-refractory obsessive-compulsive disorder. *American Journal of Psychiatry* 159: 269-275.

Panic Disorder

1.	American Psychiatric Association. 2000. *Diagnostic and Statistical Manual of Mental Disorders.* Text revision ed. Washington, DC: American Psychiatric Association.

2.	U.S. Department of Health and Human Services. 1999. *Mental Health: A Report of the Surgeon General.* Rockville, MD: U.S. Department of Health and Human Services, Substance Abuse and Mental Health Services Administration, Center for Mental Health Services, National Institutes of Health, National Institute of Mental Health.

3.	Katerndahl, D. A., and J. P. Realini. 1995. Where do panic attack sufferers seek care? *Journal of Family Practice* 40: 237-243.

4.	Wang, P. S., M. Lane, M. Olfson, H. A. Pincus, K. B. Wells, and R. C. Kessler. 2005. Twelve-month use of mental health services in the United States. Results from the National Comorbidity Survey Replication. *Archives of General Psychiatry* 62: 629-640.

5.	Ballenger, J. C. 1997. Panic disorder in the medical setting. *Journal of Clinical Psychiatry* 38: 13-17.

6.	Stahl, S. M., and S. Soefje. 1995. Panic attacks and panic disorder: The great neurologic imposters. *Seminars in Neurology* 15: 126-132.

7.	Carter, C. S., D. Servan-Schreiber, and W. M. Perlstein. 1997. Anxiety disorders and the syndrome of chest pain with normal coronary arteries: Prevalence and pathophysiology. *Journal of Clinical Psychiatry* 58: 70-73.

8.	Pollock, M. H., R. Kradin, M. W. Otto, J. Worthington, R. Gould, S. A. Sabatino, et al. 1996. Prevalence of panic in patients referred for pulmonary function testing at a major medical center. *American Journal of Psychiatry* 153: 110-113.

9.	Cox, B. J., N. S. Endler, and R. P. Swinson. 1995. An examination of levels of agoraphobic severity in panic disorder. *Behaviour Research and Therapy* 33: 57-62.

10. Grant, B. F., F. S. Stinson, D. A. Dawson, P. Chou, M. C. Dufour, W. Compton, et al. 2004. Prevalence and co-occurrence of substance use disorders and independent mood and anxiety disorders: Results from the National Epidemiologic Survey on Alcohol and Related Conditions. *Archives of General Psychiatry* 61: 807-816.

11. Kessler, R. C., W. T. Chiu, O. Demler, and E. E. Walters. 2005. Prevalence, severity, and comorbidity of 12-month DSM-IV disorders in the National Comorbidity Survey Replication. *Archives of General Psychiatry* 62: 617-627.

12. Grant, B. F., D. S. Hasin, F. S. Stinson, D. A. Dawson, S. P. Chou, W. J. Ruan, et al. 2005. Co-occurrence of 12-month mood and anxiety disorders and personality disorders in the US: Results from the National Epidemiologic Survey on Alcohol and Related Conditions. *Journal of Psychiatric Research* 39: 1-9.

13. Murray, C. J. L., and A. D. Lopez, eds. 1996. *Summary: The Global Burden of Disease: A Comprehensive Assessment of Mortality and Disability from Diseases, Injuries, and Risk Factors in 1990 and Projected to 2020.* Cambridge, MA: Published by the Harvard School of Public Health on behalf of the World Health Organization and the World Bank, Harvard University Press.

14. Kessler, R. C., K. A. McGonagle, S. Zhao, C. B. Nelson, M. Hughes, S. Eshleman, et al. 1994. Lifetime and 12-month prevalence of DSM-III-R psychiatric disorders in the United States. *Archives of General Psychiatry* 51: 8-19.

15. Kessler, R. C., P. A. Berglund, O. Demler, R. Jin, and E. E. Walters. 2005. Lifetime prevalence and age-of-onset distributions of DSM-*IV d*isorders in the National Comorbidity Survey Replication. *Archives of General Psychiatry* 62: 593-602.

16. National Institute of Mental Health. 2004. The numbers count: Mental disorders in America. National Institute of Mental Health 2001 [cited June 19, 2004]. Available from www.nimh.nih.gov/publicat/numbers.cfm.

17. Norton, G. R., B. J. Cox, and J. Malan. 1992. Non-clinical panickers: A critical review. *Clinical Psychology Review* 12: 121-139.

18. McKay, M., M. Davis, and P. Fanning. 1997. *Thoughts and Feelings: Taking Control of Your Moods and Your Life.* Oakland, CA: New Harbinger Publications.

19. Craske, M. G., P. P. Miller, R. Rotunda, and D. H. Barlow. 1990. A descriptive report of features of initial unexpected panic attacks in minimal and extensive avoiders. *Behaviour Research and Therapy* 28: 395-400.

20. Ehlers, A., and P. Breuer. 1996. How good are patients with panic disorder at perceiving their heartbeats? *Biological Psychology* 42: 165-182.

21. Ehlers, A., P. Breuer, D. Dohn, and W. Geigenbaum. 1995. Heartbeat perception and panic disorder: Possible explanations for discrepant findings. *Behaviour Research and Therapy* 33: 69-76.

22. Craske, M. G., and D. H. Barlow. 2001. Panic disorder and agoraphobia. In *Clinical Handbook of Psychological Disorders: A Step-by-Step Treatment Manual*, edited by D. H. Barlow. New York: The Guilford Press.

23. Williams, S. L., P. J. Kinney, S. T. Harap, and M. Liebmann. 1997. Thoughts of agoraphobic people during scary tasks. *Journal of Abnormal Psychology* 106: 511-520.

24. Narrow, W. E., D. A. Regier, D. S. Rae, R. W. Manderscheid, and B. Z. Locke. 1993. Use of services by persons with mental and addictive disorders: Findings from the National Institute of Mental Health Epidemiologic Catchment Area Program. *Archives of General Psychiatry* 50: 95-107.

25. Wang, P. S., P. A. Berglund, M. Olfson, H. A. Pincus, K. B. Wells, and R. C. Kessler. 2005. Failure and delay in initial treatment contact after first onset of mental disorders in the National Comorbidity Survey Replication. *Archives of General Psychiatry* 62: 603-613.

26. Barlow, D. H. 1990. Long-term outcome for patients with panic disorder treated with cognitive-behavioral therapy. *Journal of Clinical Psychiatry* 51: 17-23.

27. Barlow, D. H., M. G. Craske, J. A. Cerny, and J. S. Klosko. 1989. Behavioral treatment of panic disorder. *Behavior Therapy* 20: 261-282.

28. Craske, M. G., T. A. Brown, and D. H. Barlow. 1991. Behavioral treatment of panic disorder: A two-year follow-up. *Behavior Therapy* 22: 289-304.

29. Zuercher-White, E. 1999. *Overcoming Panic Disorder and Agoraphobia: A Cognitive Restructuring and Exposure-Based Protocol for the Treatment of Panic and Agoraphobia.* Oakland, CA: New Harbinger Publications.

30. American Psychiatric Association. 1998. Practice guideline for the treatment of patients with panic disorder. *American Journal of Psychiatry* 155: 1-34.

31. Marks, I. M., R. P. Swinson, M. Basoglu, K. Kuch, H. Noshirvani, G. O'Sullivan, et al. 1993. Alprazolam and exposure alone and combined in panic disorder with agoraphobia: A controlled study in London and Toronto. *British Journal of Psychiatry* 162: 776-787.

32. Barlow, D. H., J. M. Gorman, M. K. Shear, and S. W. Woods. 2000. Cognitive-behavioral therapy, imipramine, or their combination for panic disorder: A randomized controlled trial. *Journal of the American Medical Association* 283: 2529-2536.

Phobia

1. American Psychiatric Association. 2000. *Diagnostic and Statistical Manual of Mental Disorders.* Text revision ed. Washington, DC: American Psychiatric Association.

2. U.S. Department of Health and Human Services. 1999. *Mental Health: A Report of the Surgeon General.* Rockville, MD: U.S. Department of Health and Human Services, Substance Abuse and Mental Health Services Administration, Center for Mental Health Services, National Institutes of Health, National Institute of Mental Health.

3. Grant, B. F., F. S. Stinson, D. A. Dawson, P. Chou, M. C. Dufour, W. Compton, et al. 2004. Prevalence and co-occurrence of substance use disorders and independent mood and anxiety disorders: Results from the National Epidemiologic Survey on Alcohol and Related Conditions. *Archives of General Psychiatry* 61: 807-816.

4. Kessler, R. C., W. T. Chiu, O. Demler, and E. E. Walters. 2005. Prevalence, severity, and comorbidity of 12-month DSM-IV disorders in the National Comorbidity Survey Replication. *Archives of General Psychiatry* 62: 617-627.

5. Schneier, F. R., J. R. Johnson, C. D. Hornig, M. R. Liebowitz, and M. M. Weissman. 1992. Social phobia: Comorbidity and morbidity in an epidemiologic sample. *Archives of General Psychiatry* 49: 282-288.

6. Grant, B. F., D. S. Hasin, F. S. Stinson, D. A. Dawson, S. P. Chou, W. J. Ruan, et al. 2005. Co-occurrence of 12-month mood and anxiety disorders and personality disorders in the US: Results from the National Epidemiologic Survey on Alcohol and Related Conditions. *Journal of Psychiatric Research* 39: 1-9.

7. Norquist, G. S., and D. A. Regier. 1996. The epidemiology of psychiatric disorders and the de facto mental health care system. *Annual Review of Medicine* 47: 473-479.

8. Regier, D. A., W. E. Narrow, D. S. Rae, R. W. Manderscheid, B. Z. Locke, and F. K. Goodwin. 1993. The de facto US mental and addictive disorders service system: Epidemiologic Catchment Area prospective 1-year prevalence rates of disorders and services. *Archives of General Psychiatry* 50: 85-94.

9. Kessler, R. C., K. A. McGonagle, S. Zhao, C. B. Nelson, M. Hughes, S. Eshleman, et al. 1994. Lifetime and 12-month prevalence of DSM-III-R psychiatric disorders in the United States. *Archives of General Psychiatry* 51: 8-19.

10. Kessler, R. C., P. A. Berglund, O. Demler, R. Jin, and E. E. Walters. 2005. Lifetime prevalence and age-of-onset distributions of DSM-IV disorders in the National Comorbidity Survey Replication. *Archives of General Psychiatry* 62: 593-602.

11. Bourne, E. J. 1998. *Overcoming Specific Phobia: A Hierarchy and Exposure-Based Protocol for the Treatment of All Specific Phobias.* Oakland, CA: New Harbinger Publications.

12. Kagan, J., J. S. Reznick, and N. Snidman. 1988. Biological bases of childhood shyness. *Science* 240: 167-171.

13. Wang, P. S., P. A. Berglund, M. Olfson, H. A. Pincus, K. B. Wells, and R. C. Kessler. 2005. Failure and delay in initial treatment contact after first onset of mental disorders in the National Comorbidity Survey Replication. *Archives of General Psychiatry* 62: 603-613.

14. Barlow, D. H., S. D. Raffa, and E. M. Cohen. 2002. Psychosocial treatments for panic disorders, phobias, and generalized anxiety disorder. In *A Guide to Treatments That Work*, edited by P. E. Nathan and B. S. Gorman. New York: Oxford University Press.

15. Agras, S. 1985. *Panic: Facing Fears, Phobias and Anxiety.* New York: W. H. Freeman.

16. Turk, C. L., R. G. Heimberg, and D. A. Hope. 2001. Social anxiety disorder. In *Clinical Handbook of Psychological Disorders: A Step-by-Step Treatment Manual*, edited by D. H. Barlow. New York: The Guilford Press.

17. Wang, P. S., M. Lane, M. Olfson, H. A. Pincus, K. B. Wells, and R. C. Kessler. 2005. Twelve-month use of mental health services in the United States. Results from the National Comorbidity Survey Replication. *Archives of General Psychiatry* 62: 629-640.

18. Roy-Byrne, P., and D. S. Cowley. 2002. Pharmacological treatments for panic disorder, generalized anxiety disorder, specific phobia, and social anxiety disorder. In *A Guide to Treatments That Work*, edited by P. E. Nathan and J. M. Gorman. New York: Oxford University Press.

Post-traumatic Stress Disorder

1. American Psychiatric Association. 2000. *Diagnostic and Statistical Manual of Mental Disorders.* Text revision ed. Washington, DC: American Psychiatric Association.

2. Kessler, R. C., W. T. Chiu, O. Demler, and E. E. Walters. 2005. Prevalence, severity, and comorbidity of 12-month DSM-IV disorders in the National Comorbidity Survey Replication. *Archives of General Psychiatry* 62: 617-627.

3. Boudewyns, P. A., J. Albrecht, F. Talbert, and L. Hyer. 1991. Co-morbidity and treatment outcome of inpatients with chronic combat-related PTSD. *Hospital and Community Psychiatry* 42: 847-849.

4. Boudewyns, P. A., L. Hyer, M. G. Woods, W. R. Harrison, and E. McCranie. 1990. PTSD among Vietnam veterans: An early look at treatment outcome using direct therapeutic exposure. *Journal of Traumatic Stress* 3: 359-368.

5. Davidson, J. R. T., H. S. Kudler, W. B. Saunders, and R. D. Smith. 1990. Symptoms and comorbidity patterns in World War II and Vietnam veterans with posttraumatic stress disorder. *Comprehensive Psychiatry* 31: 162-170.

6. Grant, B. F. 1996. DSM-IV, DSM-III-R, and ICD-10 alcohol and drug abuse/harmful use and dependence, United States, 1992. *Alcoholism: Clinical and Experimental Research* 10: 1481-1488.

7. Regier, D. A., M. E. Farmer, D. S. Rae, B. Z. Locke, S. J. Keith, and L. L. Judd. 1990. Comorbidity of mental disorders with alcohol and other drug abuse: Results from the Epidemiologic Catchment Area (ECA) Study. *Journal of the American Medical Association* 264: 2511-2518.

8. Ouimette, P., R. Cronkite, A. Prins, and R. Moos. 2004. Posttraumatic stress disorder, anger and hostility, and physical health status. *Journal of Nervous and Mental Disease* 192: 563-566.

9. Schnurr, P. P., and M. K. Jankowski. 1999. Physical health and post-traumatic stress disorder: Review and synthesis. *Seminars in Clinical Neuropsychiatry* 68: 258-268.

10. Murray, C. J. L., and A. D. Lopez, eds. 1996. *Summary: The Global Burden of Disease: A Comprehensive Assessment of Mortality and Disability from Diseases, Injuries, and Risk Factors in 1990 and Projected to 2020.* Cambridge, MA: Published by the Harvard School of Public Health on behalf of the World Health Organization and the World Bank, Harvard University Press.

11. National Institute of Mental Health. 2004. The numbers count: Mental disorders in America. National Institute of Mental Health 2001 [cited June 19 2004]. Available from www.nimh.nih.gov/publicat/numbers.cfm.

12. Kessler, R. C., A. Sonnega, E. Bromet, M. Hughes, and C. B. Nelson. 1995. Posttraumatic stress disorder in the National Co-morbidity Survey. *Archives of General Psychiatry* 52: 1048-1060.

13. Kramer, T. L., J. D. Lindy, B. L. Green, M. C. Grace, and A. C. Leonard. 1994. The comorbidity of post-traumatic stress disorder and suicidality in Vietnam veterans. *Suicide and Life Threatening Behaviors* 24: 58-67.

14. Kessler, R. C., P. A. Berglund, O. Demler, R. Jin, and E. E. Walters. 2005. Lifetime prevalence and age-of-onset distributions of DSM-IV disorders in the National Comorbidity Survey Replication. *Archives of General Psychiatry* 62: 593-602.

15.   U.S. Department of Justice. National crime victimization survey: Violence against women: Estimates from the redesigned survey 1995 [cited August 16, 2005. Available from www.ojp.usdoj.gov/bjs/pub/pdf/femvied.pdf.

16.   Baker, R. 1992. Psychological consequences for tortured refugees seeking asylum and refugee status in Europe. In *Torture and Its Consequences: Current Treatment Approaches*, edited by M. Basolgu. New York: Cambridge University Press.

17.   Van Ommeren, M., J. T. V. M. de Jong, B. Sharma, I. Komproe, S. B. Thapa, and E. Cardena. 2001. Psychiatric disorders among tortured Bhutanese refugees in Nepal. *Archives of General Psychiatry* 58: 475-482.

18.   Davidson, J. R. T., D. J. Stein, A. Y. Shalev, and R. Yehuda. 2004. Posttraumatic stress disorder: Acquisition, recognition, course, and treatment. *Journal of Neuropsychiatry and Clinical Neurosciences* 16: 135-147.

19.   Yehuda, R., L. M. Bierer, J. Schmeidler, D. H. Aferiat, I. Breslau, and S. Dolan. 2000. Low cortisol and risk for PTSD in adult offspring of Holocaust survivors. *American Journal of Psychiatry* 157: 1252-1259.

20.   Yehuda, R., S. L. Halligan, and L. M. Bierer. 2002. Cortisol levels in adult offspring of Holocaust survivors: Relation to PTSD symptom severity in the parent and child. *Psychoneuroendocrinology* 27: 171-180.

21.   Hull, A. M. 2002. Neuroimaging findings in post-traumatic stress. *British Journal of Psychiatry* 181: 102-110.

22.   Larkin, M. 1999. Can post-traumatic stress disorder be put on hold? *Lancet* 354: 1008.

23.   Foa, E. B., G. S. Steketee, and B. O. Rothbaum. 1989. Behavior/cognitive conceptualizations of post-traumatic stress disorder. *Behavior Therapy* 20: 155-176.

24.   Horowitz, M. 1986. *Stress Response Syndromes*. 2nd ed. New York: Aronson.

25.   Wang, P. S., P. A. Berglund, M. Olfson, H. A. Pincus, K. B. Wells, and R. C. Kessler. 2005. Failure and delay in initial treatment contact after first onset of mental disorders in the National Comorbidity Survey Replication. *Archives of General Psychiatry* 62: 603-613.

26.   Resick, P. A., and K. S. Calhoun. 2001. Posttraumatic stress disorder. In *Clinical Handbook of Psychological Disorders: A Step-by-Step Treatment Manual*, edited by D. H. Barlow. New York: The Guilford Press.

27.   Foa, E. B., J. R. T. Davidson, and A. J. Frances. 1999. The Expert Consensus Guideline Series: Treatment of posttraumatic stress disorder. *Journal of Clinical Psychiatry* 60: 4-79.

28.   Bradley, B. P., J. Greene, E. Russ, L. Dutra, and D. Westen. 2005. A multidimensional meta-analysis of psychotherapy for PTSD. *American Journal of Psychiatry* 162: 214-227.

29.   Foa, E. B., B. O. Rothbaum, D. S. Riggs, and T. B. Murdock. 1991. Treatment of posttraumatic stress disorder in rape victims: A comparison between cognitive-behavioral procedures and counseling. *Journal of Consulting and Clinical Psychology* 59: 155-176.

30.   Lee, C., H. Gavriel, P. Drummond, J. Richards, and R. Greenwald. 2002. Treatment of PTSD: Stress inoculation training with prolonged exposure compared to EMDR. *Journal of Clinical Psychology* 58: 1071-1089.

31.   Rothbaum, B. O., and E. B. Foa. 1992. Exposure therapy for rape victims with post-traumatic stress disorder. *Behavior Therapist* 15: 219-222.

32.   Foa, E. B., C. V. Dancu, E. A. Hembree, L. H. Jaycox, E. A. Meadows, and G. P. Street. 1999. A comparison of exposure therapy, stress inoculation training, and their combination for reducing posttraumatic stress disorder in female assault victims. *Journal of Consulting and Clinical Psychology* 67: 194-200.

33.   Fecteau, G., and R. Nicki. 1999. Cognitive behavioural treatment of posttraumatic stress disorder after motor vehicle accidents. *Behavioural and Cognitive Psychotherapy* 27: 201-214.

34.   Resick, P. A., P. Nishith, T. L. Weaver, M. C. Astin, and C. A. Feuer. 2002. A comparison of cognitive-processing therapy with prolonged exposure and a waiting condition for the treatment of chronic posttraumatic stress disorder in female rape victims. *Journal of Consulting and Clinical Psychology* 70: 867-879.

35.   Resick, P. A., and M. K. Schnicke. 1993. *Cognitive Processing Therapy for Rape Victims: A Treatment Manual*. Newbury Park, CA: Sage.

36. Ironson, G., B. Freund, J. L. Strauss, and J. I. Williams. 2002. Comparison of two treatments for traumatic stress: A community-based study of EMDR and prolonged exposure. *Journal of Clinical Psychology* 58: 113-128.

37. Krupnick, J. L. 2002. Brief psychodynamic treatment of PTSD. *Journal of Clinical Psychology* 58: 919-932.

38. Brom, D., R. J. Kleber, and P. B. Defares. 1989. Brief psychotherapy for posttraumatic stress disorders. *Journal of Consulting and Clinical Psychology* 57: 607-612.

39. Orsillo, S. M., and S. V. Batten. 2005. Acceptance and commitment therapy in the treatment of posttraumatic stress disorder. *Behavior Modification* 29: 95-129.

40. Batten, S. V., and S. C. Hayes. 2005. Acceptance and commitment therapy in the treatment of comorbid substance abuse and post-traumatic stress disorder: A case study. *Clinical Case Studies* 4: 246-262.

41. Wang, P. S., M. Lane, M. Olfson, H. A. Pincus, K. B. Wells, and R. C. Kessler. 2005. Twelve-month use of mental health services in the United States. Results from the National Comorbidity Survey Replication. *Archives of General Psychiatry* 62: 629-640.

42. Ahearn, E. P., A. Krohn, K. M. Connor, and J. R. T. Davidson. 2003. Pharmacologic treatment of posttraumatic stress disorder: A focus on antipsychotic use. *Annals of Clinical Psychiatry* 15: 193-201.

Schema-Focused Relationship Problems

1. Young, J. 1999. *Cognitive Therapy for Personality Disorders: A Schema-Focused Approach.* 3rd ed. Sarasota, FL: Professional Resources Press.

2. Baldwin, M. W. 1992. Relational schemas and the processing of social information. *Psychological Bulletin* 112: 461-484.

3. Waldinger, R. J., L. Diguer, F. Guastella, R. Lefebvre, J. P. Allen, L. Luborsky, et al.. 2002. The same old song?—Stability and change in relationship schemas from adolescence to young adulthood. *Journal of Youth and Adolescence* 31: 17-29.

4. Dattilio, F. M. 2005. The restructuring of family schemas: A cognitive-behavior perspective. *Journal of Marital and Family Therapy* 31: 15-30.

5. Young, J. 1998. *Early Maladaptive Schemas.* New York: Cognitive Therapy Center of New York.

6. Beck, A. T., A. J. Rush, B. F. Shaw, and G. Emery. 1979. *Cognitive Therapy of Depression.* New York: The Guilford Press.

7. Evans, J., J. Heron, G. Lewis, R. Araya, and D. Wolke. 2005. Negative self-schemas and the onset of depression in women: Longitudinal study. *British Journal of Psychiatry* 186: 302-307.

8. Young, J., A. D. Weinberger, and A. T. Beck. 2001. Cognitive therapy for depression. In *Clinical Handbook of Psychological Disorders: A Step-by-Step Treatment Manual*, edited by D. H. Barlow. New York: The Guilford Press.

9. Ball, S. A., and J. J. Cecero. 2002. Addicted patients with personality disorders: Traits, schemas and presenting problems. *Journal of Personality Disorders* 15: 72-83.

10. Ball, S. A., and J. Young. 2000. Dual focus schema therapy for personality disorders and substance dependence: Case study results. *Cognitive and Behavioral Practice* 7: 270-281.

11. Beck, A. T., F. D. Wright, C. F. Newman, and B. S. Liese. 1993. *Cognitive Therapy of Substance Abuse.* New York: The Guilford Press.

12. Hedley, L. M., A. Hoffart, and H. Sexton. 2001. Early maladaptive schemas in patients with panic disorder with agoraphobia. *Journal of Cognitive Psychotherapy* 15: 131-142.

13. Beck, A. T., and G. Emery. 1985. *Anxiety Disorders and Phobias.* New York: Basic Books.

14. Waller, G., C. Meyer, and V. Ohanian. 2001. Psychometric properties of the long and short versions of the Young Schema Questionnaire: Core beliefs among bulimic and comparison women. *Cognitive Therapy and Research* 25: 137-147.

15. Leung, N., G. Waller, and G. Thomas. 2000. Outcome of cognitive-behavior therapy for bulimia nervosa: The role of core beliefs. *Behaviour Research and Therapy* 38: 145-156.

16. Beck, A. T., A. Freeman, J. Pretzer, D. D. Davis, B. Fleming, J. S. Beck, et al. 1990. *Cognitive Therapy of Personality Disorders.* New York: The Guilford Press.

17.   Petrocelli, J. V., B. A. Glaser, G. B. Calhoun, and L. F. Campbell. 2001. Early maladaptive schemas of personality disorder subtypes. *Journal of Personality Disorders* 15: 546-559.

18.   Nordahl, H. M., H. Holthe, and J. A. Haugum. 2005. Early maladaptive schemas in patients with or without personality disorders: Does schema modification predict symptomatic relief? *Clinical Psychology and Psychotherapy* 12: 142-149.

19.   Beck, A. T. 1976. *Cognitive Therapy and the Emotional Disorders*. New York: International Universities Press.

20.   Schmidt, N. B., and T. E. Joiner. 2004. Global maladaptive schemas, negative life events, and psychological distress. *Journal of Psychopathology and Behavioral Assessment* 26: 65-72.

21.   Tilden, T., and F. M. Dattilio. 2005. Vulnerability schemas of individuals in couples relationships: A cognitive perspective. *Contemporary Family Therapy* 27: 139-162.

22.   McKay, M., and P. Fanning. 1991. *Prisoners of Belief: Exposing and Changing Beliefs That Control Your Life*. Oakland, CA: New Harbinger Publications.

23.   Baucom, D. H., S. L. Sayers, and T. G. Sher. 1990. Supplementing behavioral marital therapy with cognitive restructuring and emotional expressiveness training: An outcome investigation. *Journal of Consulting and Clinical Psychology* 58: 636-645.

Schizoid Personality

1.   American Psychiatric Association. 2000. *Diagnostic and Statistical Manual of Mental Disorders*. Text revision ed. Washington, DC: American Psychiatric Association.

2.   Rasmussen, P. R. 2005. The schizoid prototype. In *Personality-Guided Cognitive-Behavioral Therapy*. Washington, DC: American Psychological Association.

3.   Birtchnell, J. 1996. Detachment. In *Personality Characteristics of the Personality Disordered*, edited by C. G. Costello. New York: Wiley.

4.   Beck, A. T., A. Freeman, J. Pretzer, D. D. Davis, B. Fleming, J. S. Beck, et al. 1990. *Cognitive Therapy of Personality Disorders*. New York: The Guilford Press.

5.   Comer, R. J. 2001. Personality disorders. In *Abnormal Psychology*. New York: Worth Publishers.

6.   Chen, H., P. Cohen, J. G. Johnson, S. Kasen, J. R. Sneed, and T. N. Crawford. 2004. Adolescent personality disorders and conflict with romantic partners during the transition to adulthood. *Journal of Personality Disorders* 18: 507-525.

7.   Grant, B. F., D. S. Hasin, F. S. Stinson, D. A. Dawson, S. P. Chou, W. J. Ruan, et al. 2005. Co-occurrence of 12-month mood and anxiety disorders and personality disorders in the US: Results from the National Epidemiologic Survey on Alcohol and Related Conditions. *Journal of Psychiatric Research* 39: 1-9.

8.   Skodol, A. E., R. L. Stout, T. H. McGlashan, C. M. Grilo, J. G. Gunderson, M. T. Shea, et al. 1999. Co-occurrence of mood and personality disorders: A report from the Collaborative Longitudinal Personality Disorders Study (CLPS). *Depression and Anxiety* 10: 175-182.

9.   Grant, B. F., F. S. Stinson, D. A. Dawson, S. P. Chou, W. J. Ruan, and R. P. Pickering. 2004. Co-occurrence of 12-month alcohol and drug use disorders and personality disorders in the United States: Results from the National Epidemiologic Survey on Alcohol and Related Conditions. *Archives of General Psychiatry* 61: 361-368.

10.   Marchiori, E., S. Loschi, P. L. Marconi, D. Mioni, and L. Pavan. 1999. Dependence, locus of control, parental bonding, and personality disorders: A study in alcoholics and controls. *Alcohol and Alcoholism* 34: 396-401.

11.   Skinstad, A. H., and A. Swain. 2001. Comorbidity in a clinical sample of substance abusers. *American Journal of Drug and Alcohol Abuse* 27: 45-64.

12.   Rodriguez Solano, J. J., and M. Gonzalez De Chavez. 2000. Premorbid personality disorders in schizophrenia. *Schizophrenia Research* 44: 137-144.

13.   Camisa, K. M., M. A. Bockbrader, P. Lysaker, L. L. Rae, C. A. Brenner, and B. F. O'Donnell. 2005. Personality traits in schizophrenia and related personality disorders. *Psychiatry Research* 133: 23-33.

14.   Rouff, L. 2000. Schizoid personality traits among the homeless mentally ill: A quantitative and qualitative report. *Journal of Social Distress and the Homeless* 9: 127-141.

15. Grant, B. F., D. S. Hasin, F. S. Stinson, D. A. Dawson, S. P. Chou, W. J. Ruan, et al. 2004. Prevalence, correlates, and disability of personality disorders in the United States: Results from the National Epidemiologic Survey on Alcohol and Related Conditions. *Journal of Clinical Psychiatry* 65: 948-958.

16. Ekselius, L., M. Tillfors, T. Furmark, and M. Fredrikson. 2001. Personality disorders in the general population: DSM-IV and ICD-10 defined prevalence as related to sociodemographic profile. *Personality and Individual Differences* 30: 311-320.

17. Jackson, H. J., and P. M. Burgess. 2000. Personality disorders in the community: A report from the Australian National Survey of Mental Health and Wellbeing. *Social Psychiatry and Psychiatric Epidemiology* 35: 531-538.

18. Torgersen, S., E. Kringlen, and V. Cramer. 2001. The prevalence of personality disorders in a community sample. *Archives of General Psychiatry* 58: 590-596.

19. Torgersen, S., S. Lygren, P. A. Oien, I. Skre, S. Onstad, J. Edvardsen, et al. 2000. A twin study of personality disorders. *Comprehensive Psychiatry* 41: 416-425.

20. Wolff, S., and R. J. McGuire. 1995. Schizoid personality in girls: A follow-up study: What are the links with Asperger's syndrome? *Journal of Child Psychology and Psychiatry* 36: 793-817.

21. Wolff, S. 1998. Schizoid personality in childhood: The links with Asperger syndrome, schizophrenia spectrum disorders, and elective mutism. In *Asperger Syndrome or High-Functioning Autism? Current Issues in Autism*, edited by E. Schopler and G. B. Mesibov. New York: Plenum Press.

22. Wolff, S. 1991. "Schizoid" personality in childhood and adult life. I. The vagaries of diagnostic labelling. *British Journal of Psychiatry* 159: 615-620.

23. Ramklint, M., A.-L. von Knorring, L. von Knorring, and L. Ekselius. 2003. Child and adolescent psychiatric disorders predicting adult personality disorder: A follow-up study. *Nordic Journal of Psychiatry* 57: 23-28.

24. Kasen, S., P. Cohen, A. E. Skodol, J. G. Johnson, E. Smailes, and J. S. Brook. 2001. Childhood depression and adult personality disorder: Alternative pathways of continuity. *Archives of General Psychiatry* 58: 231-236.

25. Hebebrand, J., K. Hennighausen, S. Nau, G. W. Himmelmann, E. Schulz, H. Schafer, et al. 1997. Low body weight in male children and adolescents with schizoid personality disorder or Asperger's disorder. *Acta Psychiatrica Scandinavica* 96: 64-67.

26. Hoek, H. W., E. Susser, K. A. Buck, and L. H. Lumey. 1996. Schizoid personality disorder after prenatal exposure to famine. *American Journal of Psychiatry* 153: 1637-1639.

27. Johnson, J. G., P. Cohen, E. M. Smailes, A. E. Skodol, J. Brown, and J. M. Oldham. 2001. Childhood verbal abuse and risk for personality disorders during adolescence and early adulthood. *Comprehensive Psychiatry* 42: 16-23.

28. Bernstein, D. P., J. A. Stein, and L. Handelsman. 1998. Predicting personality pathology among adult patients with substance use disorders: Effects of childhood maltreatment. *Addictive Behaviors* 23: 855-868.

29. Crits-Christoph, P., and J. P. Barber. 2002. Psychological treatments for personality disorders. In *A Guide to Treatments That Work*, edited by P. E. Nathan and J. M. Gorman. New York: Oxford University Press.

30. Millon, T. 1999. *Personality-Guided Therapy*. New York: John Wiley and Sons, Inc.

31. Quality Assurance Project. 1990. Treatment outlines for paranoid, schizotypal and schizoid personality disorders. *Australian and New Zealand Journal of Psychiatry* 24: 339-350.

32. Bateman, A. W., and P. Fonagy. 2000. Effectiveness of psychotherapeutic treatment of personality disorder. *British Journal of Psychiatry* 177: 138-143.

33. Leichsenring, F., and E. Leibing. 2003. The effectiveness of psychodynamic therapy and cognitive behavior therapy in the treatment of personality disorders: A meta-analysis. *American Journal of Psychiatry* 160: 1223-1232.

34. Roth, A., and P. Fonagy. 1996. Personality disorders. In *What Works for Whom? A Critical Review of Psychotherapy Research*. New York: The Guilford Press.

Schizophrenia

1. American Psychiatric Association. 2000. *Diagnostic and Statistical Manual of Mental Disorders*. Text revision ed. Washington, DC: American Psychiatric Association.
2. RANZCP Guidelines Team. 2005. Royal Australian and New Zealand College of Psychiatrists clinical practice guidelines for the treatment of schizophrenia and related disorders. *Australian and New Zealand Journal of Psychiatry* 39: 1-30.
3. Cutting, J. 1985. *The Psychology of Schizophrenia*. Edinburgh, UK: Churchill-Livingstone.
4. Flashman, L. A., and M. F. Green. 2004. Review of cognition and brain structure in schizophrenia: Profiles, longitudinal course, and effects of treatment. *Psychiatric Clinics of North America* 27: 1-18.
5. Heinrichs, R. W. 2005. The primacy of cognition in schizophrenia. *American Psychologist* 60: 229-242.
6. Heinrichs, R. W., and W. T. Carpenter. 1985. Prospective study of prodromal symptoms in schizophrenic relapse. *American Journal of Psychiatry* 3: 371-373.
7. Bustillo, J. R., R. W. Buchanan, and W. T. Carpenter. 1995. Prodromal symptoms vs. early warning signs and clinical action in schizophrenia. *Schizophrenia Bulletin* 4: 553-559.
8. Herz, M. I., and J. S. Lamberti. 1995. Prodromal symptoms and relapse prevention in schizophrenia. *Schizophrenia Bulletin* 4: 541-551.
9. Norman, R. M. G., and A. K. Malla. 1995. Prodromal symptoms of relapse in schizophrenia: A review. *Schizophrenia Bulletin* 4: 527-539.
10. Cassano, G. B., S. Pini, M. Saettoni, P. Rucci, and L. Dell'Osso. 1998. Occurrence and clinical correlates of psychiatric comorbidity in patients with psychotic disorders. *Journal of Clinical Psychiatry* 59: 60-68.
11. Peet, M. 2004. Diet, diabetes and schizophrenia: Review and hypothesis. *British Journal of Psychiatry* 184: s102-s105.
12. Green, A. I., C. M. Canuso, M. J. Brenner, and J. D. Wojcik. 2003. Detection and management of comorbidity in patients with schizophrenia. *Psychiatric Clinics of North America* 26: 115-139.
13. Goodwin, R. D., X. F. Amador, D. Malaspina, S. A. Yale, R. R. Goetz, and J. M. Gorman. 2003. Anxiety and substance use comorbidity among inpatients with schizophrenia. *Schizophrenia Research* 61: 89-95.
14. Pallanti, S., L. Quercioli, and E. Hollander. 2004. Social anxiety in outpatients with schizophrenia: A relevant cause of disability. *American Journal of Psychiatry* 161: 53-58.
15. Black, D. W., G. Warrack, and G. Winokur. 1985. The Iowa record-linkage study. I. Suicides and accidental deaths among psychiatric patients. *Archives of General Psychiatry* 42: 71-75.
16. Tsuang, M. T., J. A. Fleming, and J. C. Simpson. 1999. Suicide and schizophrenia. In *The Harvard Medical School Guide to Suicide Assessment and Intervention*, edited by D. G. Jacobs. San Francisco: Jossey-Bass.
17. Susnick, L. C., and J. R. Belcher. 1995. Why are they homeless? The chronically mentally ill in Washington, DC. *International Journal of Mental Health* 24: 70-84.
18. Torrey, E. F. 1997. *Out of the Shadows: Confronting America's Mental Illness Crisis*. New York: Wiley.
19. Manderscheid, R. W., and M. Rosenstein. 1992. Homeless persons with mental illness and alcohol or other drug abuse: Current research, policy, and prospects. *Current Opinion in Psychiatry* 5: 273-278.
20. Murray, C. J. L., and A. D. Lopez, eds. 1996. *Summary: The Global Burden of Disease: A Comprehensive Assessment of Mortality and Disability from Diseases, Injuries, and Risk Factors in 1990 and Projected to 2020*. Cambridge, MA: Published by the Harvard School of Public Health on behalf of the World Health Organization and the World Bank, Harvard University Press.
21. Berry, N., V. Jobanputra, and H. Pal. 2003. Molecular genetics of schizophrenia: A critical review. *Journal of Psychiatry and Neuroscience* 28: 415-429.
22. Norquist, G. S., and D. A. Regier. 1996. The epidemiology of psychiatric disorders and the de facto mental health care system. *Annual Review of Medicine* 47: 473-479.

23. Wyatt, R. J., R. C. Alexander, M. F. Egan, and D. G. Kirch. 1988. Schizophrenia, just the facts: What do we know, how well do we know it? *Schizophrenia Research* 1: 3-18.

24. Bradshaw, W., and D. Roseborough. 2004. Evaluating the effectiveness of cognitive-behavioral treatment of residual symptoms and impairment in schizophrenia. *Research on Social Work Practice* 14: 112-120.

25. Aleman, A., R. S. Kahn, and J. P. Selten. 2003. Sex differences in the risk of schizophrenia: Evidence from meta-analysis. *Archives of General Psychiatry* 60: 565-571.

26. van Meijel, B., M. van der Gaag, R. K. Sylvain, and M. H. F. Grypdonck. 2004. Recognition of early warning signs in patients with schizophrenia: A review of the literature. *International Journal of Mental Health Nursing* 13: 107-116.

27. Gottesman, I. I. 2001. Psychopathology through a life span-genetic prism. *American Psychologist* 56: 867-878.

28. Ananth, J., S. Parameswaran, and B. Hara. 2004. Drug therapy in schizophrenia. *Current Pharmaceutical Design* 10: 2205-2217.

29. Glatt, S. J., S. V. Faraone, and M. T. Tsuang. 2003. Meta-analysis identifies an association between the dopamine D2 receptor gene and schizophrenia. *Molecular Psychiatry* 8: 911-915.

30. Nelson, M. D., A. J. Saykin, L. A. Flashman, and H. J. Riordan. 1998. Hippocampal volume reduction in schizophrenia as assessed by magnetic resonance imaging: A meta-analytic study. *Archives of General Psychiatry* 55: 433-440.

31. Shenton, M. E., C. C. Dickey, M. Frumin, and R. W. McCarley. 2001. A review of MRI findings in schizophrenia. *Schizophrenia Research* 49: 1-52.

32. Tamminga, C. A., and H. H. Holcomb. 2005. Phenotype of schizophrenia: A review and formulation. *Molecular Psychiatry* 10: 27-39.

33. Harrison, P. J., N. Freemantle, and J. R. Geddes. 2003. Meta-analysis of brain weight in schizophrenia. *Schizophrenia Research* 64: 25-34.

34. Antonova, E., T. Sharma, R. Morris, and V. Kumari. 2004. The relationship between brain structure and neurocognition in schizophrenia: A selective review. *Schizophrenia Research* 70: 117-145.

35. Christensen, L., ed. 2005. *Springhouse Nurse's Drug Guide 2005*. 6th ed. Philadelphia: Lippincott Williams & Wilkins.

36. Lenroot, R., J. R. Bustillo, J. Lauriello, and S. J. Keith. 2003. Integrated treatment of schizophrenia. *Psychiatric Services* 54: 1499-1507.

37. Hale, A. S. 1995. Atypical antipsychotics and compliance in schizophrenia. *Nordic Journal of Psychiatry* 49: 31-39.

38. Pitschel-Walz, G., S. Leucht, J. Baeuml, W. Kissling, and R. R. Engel. 2001. The effect of family interventions on relapse and rehospitalization in schizophrenia—A meta-analysis. *Schizophrenia Bulletin* 27: 73-92.

39. Pilling, S., P. Bebbington, E. Kuipers, P. Garety, J. Geddes, G. Orbach, et al. 2002. Psychological treatments in schizophrenia. I. Meta-analysis of family intervention and cognitive behaviour therapy. *Psychological Medicine* 32: 763-782.

40. Bechdolf, A., B. Knost, C. Kuntermann, S. Schiller, J. Klosterkotter, M. Hambrecht, et al. 2004. A randomized comparison of group cognitive-behavioural therapy and group psychoeducation in patients with schizophrenia. *Acta Psychiatrica Scandinavica* 110: 21-28.

41. Marcinko, L., and M. Read. 2004. Cognitive therapy for schizophrenia: Treatment and dissemination. *Current Pharmaceutical Design* 10: 2269-2275.

42. Rector, N. A., and A. T. Beck. 2001. Cognitive behavioral therapy for schizophrenia: An empirical review. *Journal of Nervous and Mental Disease* 189: 278-287.

43. Tarrier, N., A. Wittkowski, C. Kinney, E. McCarthy, J. Morris, and L. Humphreys. 1999. Durability of the effects of cognitive-behavioral therapy in the treatment of chronic schizophrenia: 12-month follow-up. *British Journal of Psychiatry* 174: 500-504.

44. Pinto, A., S. La Pia, R. Mannella, G. Domenico, and L. DeSimone. 1999. Cognitive-behavioral therapy and clozapine for clients with treatment-refractory schizophrenia. *Psychiatric Services* 50: 901-904.

45. Sensky, T., D. Turkington, D. Kingdon, J. L. Scott, J. Scott, R. Siddle, et al. 2000. A randomized controlled trial of cognitive-behavioral therapy for persistent symptoms in schizophrenia resistant to medication. *Archives of General Psychiatry* 57: 165-172.

46.   Tarrier, N., R. Beckett, S. Harwood, A. Baker, L. Yusupoff, and I. Ugarteburu. 1993. A trial of two cognitive-behavioural methods of treating drug-resistant residual psychotic symptoms in schizophrenic patients. I. Outcome. *British Journal of Psychiatry* 162: 524-532.

47.   Tarrier, N., L. Yusupoff, C. Kinney, E. McCarthy, A. Gledhill, G. Haddock, et al. 1998. Randomized controlled trial of intensive cognitive behavior therapy for patients with chronic schizophrenia. *British Journal of Psychiatry* 317: 303-307.

48.   Bach, P., and S. C. Hayes. 2002. The use of acceptance and commitment therapy to prevent the rehospitalization of psychotic patients: A randomized controlled trial. *Journal of Consulting and Clinical Psychology* 70: 1129-1139.

49.   Gaudiano, B. A., and J. D. Herbert. 2006. Acute treatment of inpatients with psychotic symptoms using Acceptance and Commitment Therapy: Pilot results. *Behaviour Research and Therapy* 44: 415-437.

50.   Bellack, A. S., and K. T. Mueser. 1993. Psychosocial treatment for schizophrenia. *Schizophrenia Bulletin* 19: 317-336.

51.   Bond, G. R., R. E. Drake, K. T. Mueser, and D. R. Becker. 1997. An update on supported employment for people with severe mental illness. *Psychiatric Services* 48: 335-346.

52.   Mueser, K. T., G. R. Bond, R. E. Drake, and S. G. Resnick. 1998. Models of community care for severe mental illness: A review of research on case management. *Schizophrenia Bulletin* 42: 37-74.

53.   Scott, J., and L. Dixon. 1995. Assertive community treatment and case management. *Schizophrenia Bulletin* 21: 657-668.

Self-Focused Personality

1.   American Psychiatric Association. 2000. *Diagnostic and Statistical Manual of Mental Disorders.* Text revision ed. Washington, DC: American Psychiatric Association.

2.   Campbell, W. K., A. S. Goodie, and J. D. Foster. 2004. Narcissism, confidence, and risk attitude. *Journal of Behavioral Decision Making* 17: 297-311.

3.   McKay, M., and P. Fanning. 1992. *Self-Esteem: A Proven Program of Cognitive Techniques for Assessing, Improving, and Maintaining Your Self-Esteem.* 2nd ed. Oakland, CA: New Harbinger Publications.

4.   Sedikides, C., E. A. Rudich, A. P. Gregg, M. Kumashiro, and C. Rusbult. 2004. Are normal narcissists psychologically healthy?: Self-esteem matters. *Journal of Personality and Social Psychology* 87: 400-416.

5.   Emmons, R. A. 1984. Factor analysis and construct validity of the Narcissistic Personality Inventory. *Journal of Personality Assessment* 48: 291-300.

6.   Raskin, R., and H. Terry. 1988. A principal-components analysis of the Narcissistic Personality Inventory and further evidence of its construct validity. *Journal of Personality and Social Psychology* 54: 890-902.

7.   Wallace, H. M., and R. F. Baumeister. 2002. The performance of narcissists rises and falls with perceived opportunity for glory. *Journal of Personality and Social Psychology* 82: 819-834.

8.   Exline, J. J., R. F. Baumeister, B. J. Bushman, W. K. Campbell, and E. J. Finkel. 2004. Too proud to let go: Narcissistic entitlement as a barrier to forgiveness. *Journal of Personality and Social Psychology* 87: 894-912.

9.   Brown, R. P. 2004. Vengeance is mine: Narcissism, vengeance, and the tendency to forgive. *Journal of Research in Personality* 38: 576-584.

10.   Wink, P. 1991. Two faces of narcissism. *Journal of Personality and Social Psychology* 61: 590-597.

11.   Bushman, B. J., and R. F. Baumeister. 1998. Threatened egotism, narcissism, self-esteem, and direct and displaced aggression: Does self-love or self-hate lead to violence? *Journal of Personality and Social Psychology* 75: 219-229.

12.   Campbell, W. K., and C. A. Foster. 2002. Narcissism and commitment in romantic relationships: An investment model analysis. *Personality and Social Psychology Bulletin* 28: 484-495.

13.   Campbell, W. K., C. A. Foster, and E. J. Finkel. 2002. Does self-love lead to love for others? A story of narcissistic game playing. *Journal of Personality and Social Psychology* 83: 340-354.

14. Schiavone, P., S. Dorz, D. Conforti, C. Scarso, and G. Borgherini. 2004. Co-morbidity of DSM-IV personality disorders in unipolar and bipolar affective disorders: A comparative study. *Psychological Reports* 95: 121-128.

15. Brieger, P., U. Ehrt, and A. Marneros. 2003. Frequency of comorbid personality disorders in bipolar and unipolar affective disorders. *Comprehensive Psychiatry* 44: 28-34.

16. Oldham, J. M., A. E. Skodol, H. D. Kellman, S. E. Hyler, N. Doidge, L. Rosnick, et al. 1995. Comorbidity of Axis I and Axis II disorders. *American Journal of Psychiatry* 152: 571-578.

17. Tschanz, B. T., C. C. Morf, and C. W. Turner. 1998. Gender differences in the structure of narcissism: A multi-sample analysis of the Narcissistic Personality Inventory. *Sex Roles* 38: 863-870.

18. Casillas, A., and L. A. Clark. 2002. Dependency, impulsivity, and self-harm: Traits hypothesized to underlie the association between Cluster B personality and substance use disorders. *Journal of Personality Disorders* 16: 424-436.

19. Blaszczynski, A., and Z. Steel. 1998. Personality disorders among pathological gamblers. *Journal of Gambling Studies* 14: 51-71.

20. Davis, C., G. Claridge, and D. Cerullo. 1997. Personality factors and weight preoccupation: A continuum approach to the association between eating disorders and personality disorders. *Journal of Psychiatric Research* 31: 467-480.

21. Brunton, J. N., J. H. Lacey, and G. Waller. 2005. Narcissism and eating characteristics in young nonclinical women. *Journal of Nervous and Mental Disease* 193: 140-143.

22. Links, P. S., B. Gould, and R. Ratnayake. 2003. Assessing suicidal youth with antisocial, borderline, or narcissistic personality disorder. *Canadian Journal of Psychiatry* 48: 301-310.

23. Apter, A., A. Bleich, R. A. King, S. Kron, A. Fluch, M. Kotler, et al. 1993. Death without warning? A clinical postmortem study of suicide in 43 Israeli adolescent males. *Archives of General Psychiatry* 50: 138-142.

24. Stone, M. H. 1989. Long-term follow-up of narcissistic personality disorder. *Psychiatric Clinics of North America* 12: 621-641.

25. Ronningstam, E. F., and J. T. Maltsberger. 1998. Pathological narcissism and sudden suicide-related collapse. *Suicide and Life Threatening Behaviors* 28: 262-271.

26. Perry, J. C. 1989. Personality disorders, suicide, and self-destructive behavior. In *Suicide: Understanding and Responding: Harvard Medical School Perspectives*, edited by D. Jacobs and H. N. Brown. Madison, CT: International Universities Press, Inc.

27. Torgersen, S., E. Kringlen, and V. Cramer. 2001. The prevalence of personality disorders in a community sample. *Archives of General Psychiatry* 58: 590-596.

28. Samuels, J. F., W. Eaton, J. Bienvenu III, C. H. Brown, P. T. Costa, and G. Nestadt. 2002. Prevalence and correlates of personality disorders in a community sample. *British Journal of Psychiatry* 180: 536-542.

29. Ekselius, L., M. Tillfors, T. Furmark, and M. Fredrikson. 2001. Personality disorders in the general population: DSM-IV and ICD-10 defined prevalence as related to sociodemographic profile. *Personality and Individual Differences* 30: 311-320.

30. Golomb, M., M. Fava, M. Abraham, and J. F. Rosenbaum. 1995. Gender differences in personality disorders. *American Journal of Psychiatry* 152: 579-582.

31. Grant, B. F., D. S. Hasin, F. S. Stinson, D. A. Dawson, S. P. Chou, W. J. Ruan, et al. 2004. Prevalence, correlates, and disability of personality disorders in the United States: Results from the National Epidemiologic Survey on Alcohol and Related Conditions. *Journal of Clinical Psychiatry* 65: 948-958.

32. Torgersen, S., S. Lygren, P. A. Oien, I. Skre, S. Onstad, J. Edvardsen, et al. 2000. A twin study of personality disorders. *Comprehensive Psychiatry* 41: 416-425.

33. Kasen, S., P. Cohen, A. E. Skodol, J. G. Johnson, E. Smailes, and J. S. Brook. 2001. Childhood depression and adult personality disorder: Alternative pathways of continuity. *Archives of General Psychiatry* 58: 231-236.

34. Kasen, S., P. Cohen, A. E. Skodol, J. G. Johnson, E. Smailes, and J. S. Brook. 1999. The influence of child and adolescent psychiatric disorders on young adult personality disorder. *American Journal of Psychiatry* 156: 1529-1535.

35. Capron, E. W. 2004. Types of pampering and the narcissistic personality trait. *Journal of Individual Psychology* 60: 77-93.

36.   Gramzow, R., and J. P. Tangney. 1992. Proneness to shame and the narcissistic personality. *Personality and Social Psychology Bulletin* 18: 369-376.

37.   Rhodewalt, F., and C. C. Morf. 1998. On self-aggrandizement and anger: A temporal analysis of narcissism and affective reactions to success and failure. *Journal of Personality and Social Psychology* 74: 672-685.

38.   Rhodewalt, F., J. C. Madrian, and S. Cheney. 1998. Narcissism, self-knowledge organization, and emotional reactivity: The effect of daily experiences on self-esteem and affect. *Personality and Social Psychology Bulletin* 24: 75-87.

39.   Bogart, L. M., E. G. Benotsch, and J. D. Pavlovic. 2004. Feeling superior but threatened: The relation of narcissism to social comparison. *Basic and Applied Social Psychology* 26: 35-44.

40.   Lawrence, C. 1987. An integrated spiritual and psychological growth model in the treatment of narcissism. *Journal of Psychological Theology* 15: 205-213.

41.   Beck, A. T., A. Freeman, J. Pretzer, D. D. Davis, B. Fleming, J. S. Beck, et al. 1990. *Cognitive Therapy of Personality Disorders*. New York: The Guilford Press.

42.   Crits-Christoph, P., and J. P. Barber. 2002. Psychological treatments for personality disorders. In *A Guide to Treatments That Work*, edited by P. E. Nathan and J. M. Gorman. New York: Oxford University Press.

43.   Bateman, A. W., and P. Fonagy. 2000. Effectiveness of psychotherapeutic treatment of personality disorder. *British Journal of Psychiatry* 177: 138-143.

44.   Leichsenring, F., and E. Leibing. 2003. The effectiveness of psychodynamic therapy and cognitive behavior therapy in the treatment of personality disorders: A meta-analysis. *American Journal of Psychiatry* 160: 1223-1232.

45.   Callaghan, G. M., C. J. Summers, and M. Weidman. 2003. The treatment of histrionic and narcissistic personality disorder behaviors: A single-subject demonstration of clinical improvement using functional analytic psychotherapy. *Journal of Contemporary Psychotherapy* 33: 321-339.

46.   McWilliams, N. 1994. *Psychoanalytic Diagnosis: Understanding Personality Structure in the Clinical Process*. New York: The Guilford Press.

47.   Fava, M., A. H. Farabaugh, A. H. Sickinger, E. Wright, J. E. Alpert, S. Sonawalla, et al. 2002. Personality disorders and depression. *Psychological Medicine* 32: 1049-1057.

Somatoform Disorders

1.   American Psychiatric Association. 2000. *Diagnostic and Statistical Manual of Mental Disorders*. Text revision ed. Washington, DC: American Psychiatric Association.

2.   de Waal, M. W. M., I. A. Arnold, J. A. H. Eekhof, and A. M. van Hemert. 2004. Somatoform disorders in general practice: Prevalence, functional impairment and comorbidity with anxiety and depressive disorders. *British Journal of Psychiatry* 184: 470-476.

3.   Fink, P., M. S. Hansen, and M.-L. Oxhoj. 2004. The prevalence of somatoform disorders among internal medical inpatients. *Journal of Psychosomatic Research* 56: 413-418.

4.   Skapinakis, P., G. Lewis, and V. Mavreas. 2003. Cross-cultural differences in the epidemiology of unexplained fatigue syndromes in primary care. *British Journal of Psychiatry* 184: 205-209.

5.   Looper, K. J., and L. J. Kirmayer. 2002. Behavioral medicine approaches to somatoform disorders. *Journal of Consulting and Clinical Psychology* 70: 810-827.

6.   Hiller, W., M. M. Fichter, and W. Rief. 2003. A controlled treatment study of somatoform disorders including analysis of healthcare utilization and cost-effectiveness. *Journal of Psychosomatic Research* 54: 369-380.

7.   Grabe, H. J., C. Meyer, U. Hapke, H.-J. Rumpf, H. J. Freyberger, H. Dilling, et al. 2003. Specific somatoform disorder in the general population. *Psychosomatics: Journal of Consultation Liaison Psychiatry* 44: 304-311.

8.   Kashner, T. M., K. Rost, B. Cohen, M. Anderson, and G. R. Smith. 1995. Enhancing the health of somatization disorder patients: Effectiveness of short-term group therapy. *Psychosomatics* 36: 462-470.

9.   Lidbeck, J. 1997. Group therapy for somatization disorders in general practice: Effectiveness of a short cognitive-behavioral treatment model. *Acta Psychiatrica Scandinavica* 96: 14-24.

10. Speckens, A. E. M., A. M. van Hemert, P. Spinhoven, K. E. Hawton, J. H. Bolk, and H. G. M. Rooijmnas. 1995. Cognitive behavioural therapy for medically unexplained physical symptoms: A randomised controlled trial. *British Medical Journal* 311: 1328-1332.

11. Volz, H. P., H. Murck, S. Kasper, and H. J. Moller. 2002. St. John's wort extract (LI 160) in somatoform disorders: Results of a placebo-controlled trial. *Psychopharmacology* 164: 294-300.

12. Speed, J. 1996. Behavioral management of conversion disorder: Retrospective study. *Archives of Physical Medicine and Rehabilitation* 77: 147-154.

13. Moene, F. C., K. E. L. Hoogduin, and R. Van Dyck. 1998. The inpatient treatment of patients suffering from (motor) conversion symptoms: A description of eight cases. *International Journal of Clinical and Experimental Hypnosis* 46: 171-190.

14. Griffith, J. L., A. Polles, and M. E. Griffith. 1989. Pseudoseizures, families, and unspeakable dilemmas. *Psychosomatics* 39: 144-153.

15. Fishbain, D. A., M. Goldbery, T. M. Khalil, S. S. Asfour, E. Abdel-Moty, R. Meagher, et al. 1988. The utility of electromyographic biofeedback in the treatment of conversion paralysis. *American Journal of Psychiatry* 145: 1572-1575.

16. Elliott, A. M., B. H. Smith, K. I. Penny, W. C. Smith, and W. A. Chambers. 1999. The epidemiology of chronic pain in the community. *Lancet* 354: 1248-1252.

17. Smith, B. H., A. M. Elliott, W. A. Chambers, W. C. Smith, P. C. Hannaford, and K. Penny. 2001. The impact of chronic pain in the community. *Family Practice* 18: 292-299.

18. Mantyselka, P., E. Kumpusalo, R. Ahonen, A. Kumpusalo, J. Kauhanen, H. Viinamaki, et al. 2001. Pain as a reason to visit the doctor: A study in Finnish primary health care. *Pain* 89: 175-180.

19. Waxman, R., A. Tennant, and P. Helliwell. 2000. A prospective follow-up study of low back pain in the community. *Spine* 25: 2085-2090.

20. Stewart, W. F., R. B. Lipton, D. D. Celentano, and M. L. Reed. 1992. Prevalence of migraine headache in the United States. Relation to age, income, race, and other sociodemographic factors. *Journal of the American Medical Association* 267: 64-69.

21. Becker, N., A. Bondegaard Thomsen, A. K. Olsen, P. Sjogren, P. Bech, and J. Eriksen. 1997. Pain epidemiology and health related quality of life in chronic non-malignant pain patients referred to a Danish multidisciplinary pain center. *Pain* 73: 393-400.

22. Arnow, B. A., E. M. Hunkeler, C. M. Blasey, J. Lee, M. J. Constantino, B. Fireman, et al. 2006. Comorbid depression, chronic pain, and disability in primary care. *Psychosomatic Medicine* 68: 262-268.

23. Scharff, L. 1997. Recurrent abdominal pain in children: A review of psychological factors and treatment. *Clinical Psychology Review* 17: 145-166.

24. Sharpe, M., and A. C. DC Williams. 2002. Treating patients with somatoform pain disorder and hypochondriasis. In *Psychological Approaches to Pain Management: A Practitioner's Handbook*, edited by DC Turk and R. J. Gatchel. New York: The Guilford Press.

25. Masheb, R. M., and R. D. Kerns. 2000. Pain disorder. In *Effective Brief Therapies: A Clinician's Guide*, edited by M. Hersen and M. Biaggio. San Diego, CA: Academic Press, Inc.

26. Turk, D. C. 1994. Perspectives on chronic pain: The role of psychological factors. *Current Directions in Psychological Science* 3: 45-48.

27. Dahl, J., K. G. Wilson, and A. Nilsson. 2004. Acceptance and commitment therapy and the treatment of persons at risk for long-term disability resulting from stress and pain symptoms: A preliminary randomized trial. *Behavior Therapy* 35: 785-801.

28. Gutierrez, O., C. Luciano, M. Rodriguez, and B. C. Fink. 2004. Comparison between an acceptance-based and a cognitive-control-based protocol for coping with pain. *Behavior Therapy* 35: 767-783.

29. McCracken, L. M., K. E. Vowles, and C. Eccleston. 2005. Acceptance-based treatment for persons with complex, long standing chronic pain: A preliminary analysis of treatment outcome in comparison to a waiting phase. *Behaviour Research and Therapy* 43: 1335-1346.

30. Middaugh, S. J., and K. Pawlick. 2002. Biofeedback and behavioral treatment of persistent pain in the older adult: A review and a study. *Applied Psychophysiology and Biofeedback* 27: 185-202.

31.   Sarafino, E. P., and P. Goehring. 2000. Age comparisons in acquiring biofeedback control and success in reducing headache pain. *Annals of Behavioral Medicine* 22: 10-16.

32.   Newton-John, T. R., S. H. Spence, and D. Schotte. 1995. Cognitive-behavioural therapy versus EMG biofeedback in the treatment of chronic low back pain. *Behaviour Research and Therapy* 33: 691-697.

33.   Brinkhaus, B., C. M. Witt, S. Jena, K. Linde, A. Streng, S. Wagenpfeil, et al. 2006. Acupuncture in patients with chronic low back pain: A randomized controlled trial. *Archives of Internal Medicine* 166: 450-457.

34.   Manheimer, E., A. White, B. Berman, K. Forys, and E. Ernst. 2005. Meta-analysis: Acupuncture for low back pain. *Annals of Internal Medicine* 142: 651-663.

35.   Thomas, K. J., H. MacPherson, J. Ratcliffe, L. Thorpe, J. Brazier, M. Campbell, et al. 2005. Longer term clinical and economic benefits of offering acupuncture care to patients with chronic low back pain. *Health Technology Assessment* 9: iii-iv, ix-x, 1-109.

36.   Langenfeld, M. C., E. Cipani, and J. J. Borckardt. 2002. Hypnosis for the control of HIV/AIDS-related pain. *International Journal of Clinical and Experimental Hypnosis* 50: 170-188.

37.   Lu, D. P., G. P. Lu, and L. Kleinman. 2001. Acupuncture and clinical hypnosis for facial and head and neck pain: a single crossover comparison. *American Journal of Clinical Hypnosis* 44: 141-148.

38.   Holroyd, J. 1996. Hypnosis treatment of clinical pain: Understanding why hypnosis is useful. *International Journal of Clinical and Experimental Hypnosis* 44: 33-51.

39.   Liddle, S. D., G. D. Baxter, and J. H. Gracey. 2004. Exercise and chronic back pain: What works? *Pain* 107: 176-190.

40.   Kabat-Zinn, J., L. Lipworth, and R. Burney. 1985. The clinical use of mindfulness meditation for the self-regulation of chronic pain. *Journal of Behavioral Medicine* 8: 163-190.

41.   Kabat-Zinn, J., L. Lipworth, R. Burney, and W. Sellers. 1987. Four-year follow-up of a meditation-based program for the self-regulation of chronic pain: Treatment outcomes and compliance. *Clinical Journal of Pain* 2: 159-173.

42.   Wallis, C. 2005. The right (and wrong) way to treat pain. *Time*, Feb. 28, 47-57.

43.   Marcus, D. A. 2002. Pharmacoeconomics of opioid therapy for chronic non-malignant pain. *Expert Opinion on Pharmacotherapy* 3: 229-235.

44.   Nicholas, M. K., A. R. Molloy, and C. Brooker. 2006. Using opioids with persisting noncancer pain: A biopsychosocial perspective. *Clinical Journal of Pain* 22: 137-146.

45.   Warwick, H. M., D. M. Clark, M. Cobb, and P. M. Salkovskis. 1996. A controlled trial of cognitive-behavioural treatment of hypochondriasis. *British Journal of Psychiatry* 169: 189-195.

46.   Clark, D. M., P. M. Salkovskis, A. Hackmann, A. Wells, M. Fennell, J. Ludgate, et al. 1998. Two psychological treatments for hypochondriasis. *British Journal of Psychiatry* 173: 218-225.

47.   Fallon, B. A. 2004. Pharmacotherapy of somatoform disorders. *Journal of Psychosomatic Research* 56: 455-460.

Chapter 3
Acceptance and Commitment Therapy

1.   Hayes, S. C., K. D. Strosahl, and K. G. Wilson. 1999. *Acceptance and Commitment Therapy: An Experiential Approach to Behavior Change*. New York: The Guilford Press.

2.   Hayes, S. C., and S. Smith. 2005. *Get Out of Your Mind and into Your Life: The New Acceptance and Commitment Therapy*. Oakland, CA: New Harbinger Publications.

Analytical/Jungian Psychotherapy

1.   Jung, C. G. 1957. *The Practice of Psychotherapy. The Collected Works of C. G. Jung*, Vol. 16. Princeton, NJ: Princeton University.

2.   Jung, C. G. 1935/1956. *Two Essays on Analytical Psychology. The Collected Works of C. G. Jung*, Vol. 17. Princeton, NJ: Princeton University.

3.   Jung, C. G. 1934/1966. *The Practical Use of Dream Analysis. The Practice of Psychotherapy, Collected Works*, Vol. 16. Princeton, NJ: Princeton University.

Behavior Therapy

1. Bandura, A., D. Ross, and S. A. Ross. 1963. Vicarious reinforcement and imitative learning. *Journal of Abnormal and Social Psychology* 67: 601-607.
2. Skinner, B. F. 1953. *Science and Human Behavior*. New York: Macmillan.
3. Wolpe, J. 1958. *Psychotherapy by Reciprocal Inhibition*. Stanford, CA: Stanford University Press.
4. Foa, E. B., and M. E. Franklin. 2001. Obsessive-compulsive disorder. In *Clinical Handbook of Psychological Disorders: A Step-by-Step Treatment Manual*, edited by D. H. Barlow. New York: The Guilford Press.

Brief Psychodynamic Therapy

1. Budman, S. H., and A. S. Gurman. 1988. *Theory and Practice of Brief Therapy*. New York: The Guilford Press.
2. Malan, D. H. 1976. *The Frontier of Brief Psychotherapy*. New York: Plenum Press.
3. Mann, J. J. 1973. *Time-Limited Psychotherapy*. Cambridge, MA: Harvard University Press.
4. Strupp, H. H., and J. L. Binder. 1984. *Psychotherapy in a New Key*. New York: Basic Books.
5. Levenson, H. 2003. Time-limited dynamic psychotherapy: An integrationist perspective. *Journal of Psychotherapy Integration* 13: 300-333.
6. Levenson, H. 1995. *Time-Limited Dynamic Psychotherapy: A Guide to Clinical Practice*. New York: Basic Books.

Cognitive Behavioral Therapy

1. Butler, A. C., J. E. Chapman, E. M. Forman, and A. T. Beck. 2006. The empirical status of cognitive-behavioral therapy: A review of meta-analyses. *Clinical Psychology Review* 26: 17-31.
2. Beck, A. T., A. J. Rush, B. F. Shaw, and G. Emery. 1979. *Cognitive Therapy of Depression*. New York: The Guilford Press.
3. Beck, J. S. 1995. *Cognitive Therapy: Basics and Beyond*. New York: The Guilford Press.

Couples Therapy

1. Weiss, R. L., and R. E. Heyman. 1990. Observation of marital interaction. In *The Psychology of Marriage: Basic Issues and Applications*, edited by F. D. Fincham and T. N. Bradbury. New York: The Guilford Press.
2. Gottman, J. M. 1994. *What Predicts Divorce? The Relationship Between Marital Processes and Marital Outcomes*. Hillsdale, NJ: Lawrence Erlbaum.
3. Christensen, A., and J. L. Shenk. 1991. Communication, conflict, and psychological distance in nondistressed, clinic, and divorcing couples. *Journal of Consulting and Clinical Psychology* 59: 458-463.
4. Stuart, R. B. 1980. *Helping Couples Change: A Social Learning Approach to Marital Therapy*. New York: The Guilford Press.
5. Christensen, A., N. S. Jacobson, and J. C. Babcock. 1995. Integrative behavioral couple therapy. In *Clinical Handbook of Couple Therapy*, edited by N. S. Jacobson and A. S. Gurman. New York: The Guilford Press.
6. Gottman, J. M., and R. W. Levenson. 1988. The social psychophysiology of marriage. In *Perspectives on Marital Interaction. Monographs in Social Psychology of Language*, No. 1., edited by P. Noller and M. A. Fitzpatrick. Clevedon, England: Multilingual Matters, Ltd.
7. Noller, P., S. Beach, and S. Osgarby. 1997. Cognitive and affective processes in marriage. In *Clinical Handbook of Marriage and Couples Interventions*, edited by W. K. Halford and H. J. Markman. Chichester, England: Wiley.
8. Pretzer, J., N. Epstein, and B. Fleming. 1991. Marital Attitude Survey: A measure of dysfunctional attributions and expectancies. *Journal of Cognitive Psychotherapy* 5: 131-148.

9. Weiss, R. L., H. Hops, and G. R. Patterson. 1973. A framework for conceptualizing marital conflict, a technology for altering it, some data for evaluating it. In *Behavior Change: Methodology, Concepts, and Practice*, edited by L. A. Hamerlynck, L. C. Handy, and E. J. Mash. Champaign, IL: Research Press.

10. Kobak, R., K. Ruckdeschel, and C. Hazan. 1994. From symptom to signal: An attachment view of emotion in marital therapy. In *The Heart of the Matter: Perspectives on Emotion in Marital Therapy*, edited by S. M. Johnson and L. S. Greenberg. New York: Brunner/Mazel.

11. Johnson, S. M., and L. S. Greenberg. 1995. The emotionally focused approach to problems in adult attachment. In *Clinical Handbook of Couple Therapy*, edited by N. S. Jacobson and A. S. Gurman. New York: The Guilford Press.

12. Minuchin, S. 1974. *Families and Family Therapy*. Cambridge, MA: Harvard University Press.

Dialectical Behavior Therapy

1. Linehan, M. M. 1993. *Cognitive-Behavioral Treatment of Borderline Personality Disorder*. New York: The Guilford Press.

2. Linehan, M. M. 1993. *Skills Training Manual for Treating Borderline Personality Disorder*. New York: The Guilford Press.

3. Marra, T. 2005. *Dialectical Behavior Therapy in Private Practice: A Practical and Comprehensive Guide*. Oakland, CA: New Harbinger Publications.

Existential Psychotherapy

1. Frankl, V. E. 1984. *Man's Search for Meaning: An Introduction to Logotherapy*. New York: Simon and Schuster, Inc.

2. Yalom, I. 1981. *Existential Psychotherapy*. New York: Basic Books.

Eye-Movement Desensitization and Reprocessing (EMDR)

1. Shapiro, F. 2001. *Eye Movement Desensitization and Reprocessing: Basic Principles, Protocols and Procedures*. 2nd ed. New York: The Guilford Press.

2. Shapiro, F. 2002. EMDR 12 years after its introduction: Past and future research. *Journal of Clinical Psychology* 58: 1-22.

3. Shapiro, F., and L. Maxfield. 2002. Eye movement desensitization and reprocessing (EMDR): Information processing in the treatment of trauma. *Journal of Clinical Psychology* 58: 933-946.

4. Barrowcliff, A. L., N. S. Gray, S. MacCulloch, T. C. A. Freeman, and M. J. MacCulloch. 2003. Horizontal rhythmical eye movements consistently diminish the arousal provoked by auditory stimuli. *British Journal of Clinical Psychology* 42: 289-302.

5. Barrowcliff, A. L., N. S. Gray, T. C. A. Freeman, and M. J. MacCulloch. 2004. Eye-movements reduce the vividness, emotional valence and electrodermal arousal associated with negative autobiographical memories. *Journal of Forensic Psychiatry and Psychology* 15: 325-345.

6. Stickgold, R. 2002. EMDR: A putative neurobiological mechanism of action. *Journal of Clinical Psychology* 58: 61-75.

7. Friedberg, F. 2001. *Do-It-Yourself Eye Movement Technique for Emotional Healing*. Oakland, CA: New Harbinger Publications.

8. Smyth, L. 1999. *Overcoming Post-Traumatic Stress Disorder: A Cognitive-Behavioral Exposure-Based Protocol for the Treatment of PTSD and the Other Anxiety Disorders*. Oakland, CA: New Harbinger Publications.

Family Therapy

1. Kerr, M. E., and M. Bowen. 1988. *Family Evaluation: An Approach Based on Bowen Theory*. New York: W. W. Norton.

2. Kliman, J. 1994. The interweaving of gender, class, and race in family therapy. In *Women in Context: Toward a Feminist Reconstruction of Psychotherapy*, edited by M. P. Mirkin. New York: The Guilford Press.

3. Minuchin, S. 1974. *Families and Family Therapy.* Cambridge, MA: Harvard University Press.

4. Watzlawick, P., J. H. Weakland, and R. Fisch. 1974. *Change: Principles of Problem Formation and Problem Resolution.* New York: W. W. Norton.

5. White, M., and D. Epston. 1990. *Narrative Means to Therapeutic Ends.* New York: W. W. Norton.

Gestalt Psychotherapy

1. Perls, F., R. Hefferline, and P. Goodman. 1951/1994. *Gestalt Therapy: Excitement and Growth in the Human Personality.* New York: The Gestalt Journal Press.

2. Perls, F. 1969/1992. *Gestalt Therapy Verbatim.* Highland, NY: The Gestalt Journal Press.

3. Kepner, J. 1987. *Body Process: A Gestalt Approach to Working with the Body in Psychotherapy.* New York: Gestalt Institute of Cleveland Press.

Humanistic/Client-Centered Therapy/ Person-Centered Therapy

1. Rogers, C. R. 1951. *Client-Centered Therapy.* Boston: Houghton Mifflin.

2. Rogers, C. R. 1957. The necessary and sufficient conditions of therapeutic personality change. *Journal of Consulting Psychology* 21: 95-103.

3. Rogers, C. R. 1986. Client-centered therapy. In *Psychotherapist's Casebook: Therapy and Technique in Practice*, edited by I. L. Kutash and A. Wolf. San Francisco: Jossey-Bass.

Hypnotherapy

1. Breuer, J., and S. Freud. 1895. Studies on hysteria. In *Standard Edition of the Complete Psychological Works of Sigmund Freud,* edited by J. Strachey. London: Hogarth Press.

2. Patterson, D. R. 2004. Treating pain with hypnosis. *Current Directions in Psychological Science* 13: 252-255.

3. Patterson, D. R., and M. P. Jensen. 2003. Hypnosis and clinical pain. *Psychological Bulletin* 129: 495-521.

4. Jensen, M. P., M. A. Hanley, J. M. Engel, J. M. Romano, J. Barber, D. D. Cardenas, et al. 2005. Hypnotic analgesia for chronic pain in persons with disabilities: A case series. *International Journal of Clinical and Experimental Hypnosis* 53: 198-228.

5. Hill, R., and G. Bannon-Ryder. 2005. The use of hypnosis in the treatment of driving phobia. *Contemporary Hypnosis* 22: 99-103.

6. Pates, J., I. Maynard, and T. Westbury. 2001. An investigation into the effects of hypnosis on basketball performance. *Journal of Applied Sport Psychology* 13: 84-102.

7. Pates, J., R. Oliver, and I. Maynard. 2001. The effects of hypnosis on flow states and golf-putting performance. *Journal of Applied Sport Psychology* 13: 341-354.

8. Martin, A. A., P. G. Schauble, S. H. Rai, and R. W. Curry Jr. 2001. The effects of hypnosis on the labor processes and birth outcomes of pregnant adolescents. *Journal of Family Practice* 50: 441-443.

9. Elkins, G. R., and M. H. Rajab. 2004. Clinical hypnosis for smoking cessation: Preliminary results of a three-session intervention. *International Journal of Clinical and Experimental Hypnosis* 52: 73-81.

10. Ahijevych, K., R. Yerardi, and N. Nedilsky. 2000. Descriptive outcomes of the American Lung Association of Ohio hypnotherapy smoking cessation program. *International Journal of Clinical and Experimental Hypnosis* 48: 374-387.

11. Green, J. P., and S. J. Lynn. 2000. Hypnosis and suggestion-based approaches to smoking cessation: An examination of the evidence. *International Journal of Clinical and Experimental Hypnosis* 48: 195-224.

12. Lynn, S. J., I. Kirsch, A. Barabasz, E. Cardena, and D. Patterson. 2000. Hypnosis as an empirically supported clinical intervention: The state of the evidence and a look to the future. *International Journal of Clinical and Experimental Hypnosis* 48: 239-259.

13. Kosslyn, S. M., W. L. Thompson, M. F. Costantini-Ferrando, N. M. Alpert, and D. Spiegel. 2000. Hypnotic visual illusion alters color processing in the brain. *American Journal of Psychiatry* 157: 1279-1284.

14. Szechtman, H., E. Woody, K. S. Bowers, and C. Nahmias. 1998. Where the imaginal appears real: A positron emission tomography study of auditory hallucinations. *Proceedings of the National Academy of Sciences of the United States of America* 95: 1956-1960.

15. Hilgard, E. R. 1965. *Hypnotic Susceptibility*. New York: Harcourt, Brace & World.

16. Bertrand, L. D. 1989. The assessment and modification of hypnotic susceptibility. In *Hypnosis: The Cognitive-Behavioral Perspective*, edited by N. P. Spanos and J. F. Chaves. Buffalo, NY: Prometheus.

Interpersonal Therapy

1. Sullivan, H. S. 1953. *The Interpersonal Theory of Psychiatry*. New York: W. W. Norton.

2. Klerman, G. L., M. M. Weissman, B. J. Rounsaville, and E. S. Chevron. 1984. *Interpersonal Psychotherapy of Depression*. New York: Basic Books.

Medications

1. Preston, J. D., J. H. O'Neal, and M. C. Talaga. 2004. *Handbook of Clinical Psychopharmacology for Therapists*. 4th ed. Oakland, CA: New Harbinger Publications.

2. Wang, P. S., M. Lane, M. Olfson, H. A. Pincus, K. B. Wells, and R. C. Kessler. 2005. Twelve-month use of mental health services in the United States. Results from the National Comorbidity Survey Replication. *Archives of General Psychiatry* 62: 629-640.

3. Narrow, W. E., D. A. Regier, D. S. Rae, R. W. Manderscheid, and B. Z. Locke. 1993. Use of services by persons with mental and addictive disorders: Findings from the National Institute of Mental Health Epidemiologic Catchment Area Program. *Archives of General Psychiatry* 50: 95-107.

4. Llewellyn-Jones, S., G. Jones, and P. Donnelly. 2001. Questions patients ask psychiatrists. *Psychiatric Bulletin* 25: 21-24.

5. Harris Interactive, Psychology Today, and PacifiCare Behavioral Health. 2004. Therapy in America 2004, May 5, 2004 [cited June 14, 2004]. Available from http://cms.psychologytoday.com/pto/press_release_050404.html.

6. U.S. Food and Drug Administration. FDA public health advisory: Suicidality in children and adolescents being treated with antidepressant medications, October 15, 2004 [cited January 2, 2006]. Available from http://www.fda.gov/cder/drug/antidepressants/SSRIPHA200410.htm.

7. U.K. Medicines and Health Care Products Regulatory Agency. 2006. Safety review of antidepressants used by children completed, December 10, 2003 [cited January 6, 2006]. Available from http://www.mhra.gov.uk/home/idcplg?IdcService=SS_GET_PAGEanduseSecondary=trueandssDocName=CON002045andssTargetNodeId=389.

8. Simon, G., J. Savarino, B. Operskalski, and P. S. Wang. 2006. Suicide risk during antidepressant treatment. *American Journal of Psychiatry* 163: 41-47.

9. Keltner, N. L., and D. G. Folks. 2001. *Psychotropic Drugs*. 3rd ed. St. Louis, MO: Mosby.

10. Lieberman, J. A., and A. Tasman. 2000. *Psychiatric Drugs*. St. Louis, MO: W.B. Saunders.

11. Neppe, V. M. 1989. Buspirone: An anxioselective neuromodulator. In *Innovative Psychopharmacotherapy*, edited by V. M. Neppe. New York: Raven.

12. Rosenbaum, J. F., M. Fava, S. L. Hoog, R. C. Ascroft, and W. B. Krebs. 1998. Selective serotonin reuptake inhibitor discontinuation syndrome: A randomized clinical trial. *Biological Psychiatry* 44: 77-87.

13. Guelfi, J. D., C. White, D. Hackett, J. Y. Guichoux, and G. Magni. 1995. Effectiveness of venlafaxine in patients hospitalized for major depression and melancholia. *Journal of Clinical Psychiatry* 56: 450-458.

14. Mendels, J., R. Johnston, J. A. Mattes, and R. Riesenberg. 1993. Efficacy and safety of b.i.d. doses of venlafaxine in a dose-response study. *Psychopharmacology Bulletin* 29: 169-174.

15. Ascher, J. A., J. O. Cole, J.-N. Colin, J. P. Feighner, R. M. Ferris, H. C. Fibiger, et al. 1995. Bupropion: A review of its mechanism of antidepressant activity. *Journal of Clinical Psychiatry* 56: 395-401

16. Potter, W. Z., and L. E. Hollister. 2004. Antipsychotic agents and lithium. In *Basic and Clinical Pharmacology*, edited by B. G. Katzung. New York: Lange Medical Books/McGraw-Hill.

17. National Institute of Mental Health. 2002. *Medications*. In NIH Publication No. 02-3929. Bethesda, MD: National Institute of Mental Health, National Institutes of Health, U.S. Department of Health and Human Services.

18. Bowden, C. L., and V. Singh. 2005. Valproate in bipolar disorder: 2000 onwards. *Acta Psychiatrica Scandinavica* 111: 13-20.

19. Bowden, C. L., J. R. Calabrese, S. L. McElroy, L. Gyulai, A. Wassef, F. Petty, et al., for the Divalproex Maintenance Study Group. 2000. A randomized, placebo-controlled 12-month trial of divalproex and lithium in treatment of outpatients with bipolar I disorder. *Archives of General Psychiatry* 57: 481-489.

20. Porter, R. J., and B. S. Meldrum. 2004. Antiseizure drugs. In *Basic and Clinical Pharmacology*, edited by B. G. Katzung. New York: Lange Medical Books/McGraw-Hill.

21. McIntyre, R. S., D. A. Mancini, S. McCann, J. Srinivasan, and S. H. Kennedy. 2003. Valproate, bipolar disorder and polycystic ovarian syndrome. *Bipolar Disorder* 5: 28-35.

22. Weisler, R. H., T. A. Ketter, and A. H. Kalali. 2004. A 6-month, multicenter, open-label evaluation of beaded, extended-release carbamazepine capsule monotherapy in bipolar disorder patients with manic or mixed episodes. *Journal of Clinical Psychiatry* 65: 668-673.

23. Weisler, R. H., P. E. Keck Jr., A. C. Swann, A. J. Cutler, T. A. Ketter, and A. H. Kalali. 2005. Extended-release carbamazepine capsules as monotherapy for acute mania in bipolar disorder: A multicenter, randomized, double-blind, placebo-controlled trial. *Journal of Clinical Psychiatry* 66: 323-330.

24. Lieberman, J. A., T. S. Stroup, J. P. McEvoy, M. S. Swartz, R. Rosenheck, D. O. Perkins, et al. 2006. Effectiveness of antipsychotic drugs in patients with chronic schizophrenia. *New England Journal of Medicine* 353: 1209-1223.

25. RANZCP Guidelines Team. 2005. Royal Australian and New Zealand College of Psychiatrists clinical practice guidelines for the treatment of schizophrenia and related disorders. *Australian and New Zealand Journal of Psychiatry* 39: 1-30.

26. Schooler, N., J. Rabinowitz, M. Davidson, R. Emsley, P. D. Harvey, L. Kopala, et al. 2005. Risperidone and haloperidol in first-episode psychosis: A long-term randomized trial. *American Journal of Psychiatry* 162: 947-953.

Mindfulness Therapy

1. Bishop, S. R., M. Lau, S. Shapiro, L. Carlson, N. D. Anderson, J. Carmody, et al. 2004. Mindfulness: A proposed operational definition. *Clinical Psychology: Science and Practice* 11: 230-241.

2. Rahula, W. 1974. *What the Buddha Taught*. 2nd ed. New York: Grove Press.

3. Chodron, P. 2003. How we get hooked, how we get unhooked. *Shambala Sun*, March, 30-35.

4. Kabat-Zinn, J. 1982. An out-patient program in behavioral medicine for chronic pain patients based on the practice of mindfulness meditation: Theoretical considerations and preliminary results. *General Hospital Psychiatry* 4: 33-47.

5. Kabat-Zinn, J. 1990. *Full Catastrophe Living: Using the Wisdom of Your Body and Mind to Face Stress, Pain and Illness*. New York: Delacorte.

6. Segal, Z. V., J. M. G. Williams, and J. D. Teasdale. 2002. *Mindfulness-Based Cognitive Therapy for Depression: A New Approach to Preventing Relapse*. New York: The Guilford Press.

7. Baer, R. A. 2003. Mindfulness training as a clinical intervention: A conceptual and empirical review. *Clinical Psychology: Science and Practice* 10: 125-143.

8. Davidson, R. J., J. Kabat-Zinn, J. Schumacher, M. Rosenkranz, D. Muller, S. F. Santorelli, et al. 2003. Alterations in brain and immune function produced by mindfulness meditation. *Psychosomatic Medicine* 65: 564-570.

9. Kabat-Zinn, J., L. Lipworth, and R. Burney. 1985. The clinical use of mindfulness meditation for the self-regulation of chronic pain. *Journal of Behavioral Medicine* 8: 163-190.

10. Kabat-Zinn, J., L. Lipworth, R. Burney, and W. Sellers. 1987. Four-year follow-up of a meditation-based program for the self-regulation of chronic pain: Treatment outcomes and compliance. *Clinical Journal of Pain* 2: 159-173.

11. Kristeller, J. L., and C. B. Hallett. 1999. An exploratory study of a meditation-based intervention for binge eating disorder. *Journal of Health Psychology* 4: 357-363.

12. Speca, M., L. E. Carlson, E. Goodey, and M. Angen. 2000. A randomized, wait-list controlled clinical trial: The effect of a mindfulness meditation-based stress reduction program on mood and symptoms of stress in cancer outpatients. *Psychosomatic Medicine* 62: 613-622.

13. Tacon, A. M., Y. M. Caldera, and C. Ronaghan. 2004. Mindfulness-based stress reduction in women with breast cancer. *Families, Systems, and Health* 22: 193-203.

14. Ramel, W., P. R. Goldin, P. E. Carmona, and J. R. McQuaid. 2004. The effects of mindfulness meditation on cognitive processes and affect in patients with past depression. *Cognitive Therapy and Research* 28: 433-455.

15. Teasdale, J. D., Z. V. Segal, J. M. G. Williams, V. A. Ridgeway, J. M. Soulsby, and M. A. Lau. 2000. Prevention of relapse/recurrence in major depression by mindfulness-based cognitive therapy. *Journal of Consulting and Clinical Psychology* 68: 615-623.

Positive Psychology

1. Peterson, C., and M. E. P. Seligman. 2004. *Character Strengths and Virtues: A Handbook and Classification*. Washington, DC, and New York: American Psychological Association and Oxford University Press.

2. Gable, S. L., and J. Haidt. 2005. What (and why) is positive psychology? *Review of General Psychology* 9: 103-110.

3. Dahlsgaard, K., C. Peterson, and M. E. P. Seligman. 2005. Shared virtue: The convergence of valued human strengths across culture and history. *Review of General Psychology* 9: 203-213.

4. Elliott, T. R., T. E. Witty, S. Herrick, and J. T. Hoffman. 1991. Negotiating reality after physical loss: Hope, depression, and disability. *Journal of Personality and Social Psychology* 61: 608-613.

5. Post, S. G. 2005. Altruism, happiness, and health: It's good to be good. *International Journal of Behavioral Medicine* 12: 66-77.

6. Seligman, M. E. P. 1998. *Learned Optimism*. New York: Simon and Schuster, Inc.

7. Taylor, S. E., M. E. Kemeny, G. M. Reed, J. E. Bower, and T. L. Gruenwald. 2000. Psychological resources, positive illusions, and health. *American Psychologist* 55: 99-109.

8. Pettit, J. W., J. P. Kline, T. Gencoz, F. Gencoz, and T. E. Joiner Jr. 2001. Are happy people healthier? The specific role of positive affect in predicting self-reported health symptoms. *Journal of Research in Personality* 35: 521-536.

9. Argyle, M. 1997. Is happiness a cause of health? *Psychology and Health* 12: 769-781.

10. Harker, L., and D. Keltner. 2001. Expressions of positive emotion in women's college yearbook pictures and their relationship to personality and life outcomes across adulthood. *Journal of Personality and Social Psychology* 80: 112-124.

11. Danner, D. D., D. A. Snowdon, and W. V. Friesen. 2001. Positive emotions in early life and longevity: Findings from the nun study. *Journal of Personality and Social Psychology* 80: 804-813.

12. Seligman, M. E. P., T. A. Steen, N. Park, and C. Peterson. 2005. Positive psychology progress: Empirical validation of interventions. *American Psychologist* 60: 410-421.

Psychoanalysis/Psychodynamic Therapy

1. Freud, S. 1923/1974. The ego and the id. In *Standard Edition of the Complete Psychological Works of Sigmund Freud*, edited by J. Strachey. London: Hogarth Press.

2. Freud, S. 1926/1974. Inhibitions, symptoms and anxiety. In *Standard Edition of the Complete Psychological Works of Sigmund Freud*, edited by J. Strachey. London: Hogarth Press.
3. Freud, S. 1900/1974. The interpretation of dreams. In *Standard Edition of the Complete Psychological Works of Sigmund Freud*, edited by J. Strachey. London: Hogarth Press.
4. Rappoport, A. 2002. How psychotherapy works: The concepts of control-mastery theory. *Bulletin of the American Academy of Clinical Psychology* 8: 10-14.

Rational Emotive Behavior Therapy

1. Ellis, A., and W. Dryden. 1997. *The Practice of Rational-Emotive Behavior Therapy*. New York: Springer.
2. Ellis, A. 2000. Emotional disturbance and its treatment in a nutshell. In *REBT Resource Book for Practitioners*, edited by A. Ellis. New York: Albert Ellis Institute.

Schema-Focused Therapy

1. Young, J. 1999. *Cognitive Therapy for Personality Disorders: A Schema-Focused Approach*. 3rd ed. Sarasota, FL: Professional Resources Press.
2. Bricker, DC, and J. Young. 1991. *A Client's Guide to Schema-Focused Cognitive Therapy*. New York: Cognitive Therapy Center of New York.

Transpersonal Psychology

1. Wilber, K. 1997. *The Eye of the Spirit: An Integral Vision for a World Gone Slightly Mad*. Boston: Shambala.
2. Wilber, K. 1995. *Sex, Ecology, Spirituality: The Spirit of Evolution*. Boston: Shambala.
3. Wilber, K. 1983. *Eye to Eye: The Quest for the New Paradigm*. Garden City, NY: Anchor Press.

INDEX

behavioral activation system, 32

behavioral marital therapy, 139

benzodiazepines, 158-159

binge eating, 52

binge eating disorder, 52

biofeedback: conversion disorder and, 122; pain disorder and, 123

biological factors, 61

bipolar disorder, 44-48; causes of, 46-47; description of, 44-45; problems related to, 45-46; recommended reading on, 200; statistics on, 46; symptoms associated with, 10-11; treatments for, 47-48

black-and-white thinking, 136

body dysmorphic disorder (BDD), 49-51; causes of, 50; description of, 49; problems related to, 49-50; recommended reading on, 200; statistics on, 50; symptoms associated with, 20; treatments for, 51

borderline personality disorder. *See* emotion dysregulation

Braid, James, 152

brain surgery, 93

brief psychodynamic therapy, 135; antisocial personality disorder and, 40; dependent personality disorder and, 57; depression and, 64, 65; PTSD and, 102, 103; recommended reading on, 204; schizoid personality disorder and, 111; self-focused personality disorder and, 118

bulimia, 19, 52-54; causes of, 53; description of, 52; problems related to, 52-53; recommended reading on, 200; statistics on, 53; symptoms

associated with, 19; treatments for, 53-54

bupropion, 160

buspirone, 159

C

Canadian Psychological Association (CPA), 208

cannabinoids, 73

carbamazepine, 162

CBT. *See* cognitive behavioral therapy

checklist of symptoms, 7-26

children: developmental phases of, 168; sexual abuse of, 78, 81, 141

chronic illnesses, 61

cingulotomy, 93

client-centered therapy, 150, 205

cognitive behavioral couples therapy, 139

cognitive behavioral therapy (CBT), 136-138; ADHD and, 43; anger control problems and, 33; anorexia and, 36; antisocial personality disorder and, 40; bipolar disorder and, 48; body dysmorphic disorder and, 51; bulimia and, 53-54; conversion disorder and, 121, 122; dependent personality disorder and, 57; depression and, 64, 65; dissociative disorders and, 67; extreme suspicion of others and, 82; generalized anxiety disorder and, 85; hypochondriasis and, 124; impulse control disorders and, 88, 89; obsessive-compulsive disorder and, 92-93; pain disorder and, 123; panic disorder and, 96; phobias and, 99; PTSD and, 102, 103; recommended reading on,

71; symptoms associated with, 26; treatments for, 67, 69, 70, 71

dissociative fugue, 66, 68-69

dissociative identity disorder, 66, 69-70

divalproex sodium, 162

doctors of osteopathy (DOs), 179

dopamine, 61, 114

double depression, 59

Dr. Phil Show, 4

dreams, 132, 168

drug and alcohol addiction problems, 72-75; causes of, 74; depression and, 62; description of, 72-73; problems related to, 73; PTSD and, 101; recommended reading on, 201; statistics on, 73-74; symptoms associated with, 16; treatments for, 74-75

drugs, prescription. *See* medications

duloxetine, 160

dysthymia, 59, 60, 61

E

eating disorders: anorexia, 18-19, 34-36; bulimia, 19, 52-54

ego, 167

Einstein, Albert, 187

electroconvulsive therapy (ECT), 65

Ellis, Albert, 170

EMDR. *See* eye-movement desensitization and reprocessing

emotion dysregulation, 76-79; causes of, 78-79; description of, 76-77; problems related to, 77; recommended reading on, 201; statistics on, 77; symptoms associated with, 17-18; treatments for, 79, 141

emotional deprivation schema, 104

emotional inhibition schema, 105

emotional reasoning, 136

emotion-focused marital therapy, 140

empathy, 150

empty chair technique, 148

enmeshed family members, 146

enmeshment/undeveloped self schema, 105

entitlement/grandiosity schema, 105

environmental toxins, 62

ethical guidelines, 193-194

exercise: depression and, 65; pain disorder and, 123

existential psychotherapy, 143, 204

exposure and response prevention, 92, 134, 137

exposure therapy, 102

extrapyramidal side effects, 163

extreme suspicion of others, 80-82; causes of, 81; description of, 80; problems related to, 80; recommended reading on, 201; statistics on, 80; symptoms associated with, 23; treatments for, 81-82

eye-movement desensitization and reprocessing (EMDR), 144-145; body dysmorphic disorder and, 51; dissociative disorders and, 67; PTSD and, 102, 103; recommended reading on, 205

eye-movement technique (EMT), 145

F

factitious disorders, 123

failure schema, 105

201; statistics on, 88; symptoms associated with, 23-24; treatments for, 88-89

inhalant abuse, 73

insufficient self-control/self-discipline schema, 105

integrative behavioral couples therapy, 139

intermittent explosive disorder, 87

interpersonal conflicts, 63

interpersonal therapy (IPT), 153-154; antisocial personality disorder and, 40; bipolar disorder and, 48; bulimia and, 54; depression and, 64, 65; extreme suspicion of others and, 82; recommended reading on, 205; schizoid personality disorder and, 111; self-focused personality disorder and, 118; substance abuse problems and, 75

JKL

Jolie, Angelina, 4

Jung, Carl, 7, 131

Jungian psychotherapy, 131-132

kleptomania, 86

libido, 168

life coaches, 184

light therapy, 64-65

lithium, 47, 161-162

loneliness, 63

long-term psychodynamic therapy: schizoid personality disorder and, 111; self- focused personality disorder and, 118

M

magnetic resonance imaging (MRI), 114

malingerers, 123

manic depression. *See* bipolar disorder

manic episodes, 44

marital therapy. *See* couples therapy

marriage and family therapists (MFTs), 181

master's level counselors, 181

McGraw, Phil, 4

meaning, loss of, 63

medical care, 36

medical doctors (MDs), 179

medications, 155-164; ADHD and, 42, 43; anger control problems and, 33; bipolar disorder and, 47, 48; body dysmorphic disorder and, 51; bulimia and, 54; depression and, 61, 63-64, 65; dissociative disorders and, 67; emotion dysregulation and, 79; extreme suspicion of others and, 82; generalized anxiety disorder and, 85; impulse control disorders and, 88, 89; obsessive-compulsive disorder and, 93; pain-relief, 123; panic disorder and, 96; phobias and, 99; psychotherapy and, 2; PTSD and, 102, 103; recommended reading on, 205; schizophrenia and, 114-115; self- focused personality disorder and, 118; somatoform disorders and, 123, 124; substance abuse problems and, 75. *See also specific types of medications*

meditation, 165

melatonin, 61

mental health care professionals, 177-185; advanced practice nurses, 183;

P

pain avoidance, 106

pain disorder, 122-123

pain-relief medications, 123

panic attacks, 94

panic disorder, 94-96; causes of, 95-96; description of, 94; problems related to, 95; recommended reading on, 202; statistics on, 95; symptoms associated with, 12-13; treatments for, 96

paranoid personality disorder. *See* extreme suspicion of others

pathological gambling, 86

Pavlov, Ivan, 133

perfection, obsessions of, 90

Perls, Frederick "Fritz," 148

personality disorders, 76, 80, 116; antisocial personality disorder, 37-40; borderline personality disorder, 76-79; dependent personality disorder, 55-57; obsessive-compulsive personality disorder, 91; paranoid personality disorder, 80-82; schizoid personality disorder, 110-111; self-focused personality disorder, 116-118

person-centered therapy, 150, 205

phobias, 97-99; causes of, 98-99; description of, 97-98; problems related to, 98; recommended reading on, 202; statistics on, 98; symptoms associated with, 11; treatments for, 99

positive psychology, 166, 206

post-traumatic stress disorder (PTSD), 100-103; causes of, 101-102; description of, 100; problems related to, 101; recommended reading on, 202; statistics on, 101; symptoms associated with, 11-12; treatments for, 102-103

premenstrual syndrome (PMS), 61

prescription drugs. *See* medications

primary care provider (PCP), 179

process-oriented psychology, 173

professional help. *See* mental health care professionals

provincial psychological associations, 208-213

psychedelics, 73

psychiatrists, 179

psychoanalysis, 3, 167-169, 206

psychoanalysts, 167

psychoanalytic couples therapy, 139

psychodynamic couples therapy, 139

psychodynamic therapy, 167-169; antisocial personality disorder and, 40; bipolar disorder and, 48; dependent personality disorder and, 57; dissociative disorders and, 67; emotion dysregulation and, 79; extreme suspicion of others and, 82; recommended reading on, 206

psychological associations, 207-214

psychological testing, 180, 196

psychologists, 180

Psychology Today Web site, 214

psychopathic personality traits. *See* antisocial personality disorder

psychopaths, 37-38

psychopharmacologists, 179

psychotherapists. *See* mental health care professionals

psychotherapy: lack of knowledge about, 1-2; medications and, 2; stigma associated with, 3-4. *See also* treatment process psychotropic medications, 155

PTSD. *See* post-traumatic stress disorder

punitiveness schema, 106

pyromania, 86-87

R

rapid cycling bipolar disorder, 45

rational emotive behavior therapy (REBT), 170-171, 206

reassurance behaviors, 90

recommended reading, 199-206

referrals, 188

reframing, 140

registered nurses, 183

relationship problems, 153

relaxation techniques, 124

religious obsessions, 90

repetitious uncertainty, 90

repression, 167

residential treatment centers, 75

resources: contact information, 207-214; recommended reading, 199-206. *See also* Web sites

Ritalin, 42

Rogers, Carl, 150, 177

Rogers, Fred, 27

role-playing, 147

Rolfing, 173

Rosen Method, 173

S

Saint-John's-wort, 65, 121

schema, 104, 138, 172

schema compensation, 106-107

schema maintenance, 106

schema-focused relationship problems, 104-108; causes of, 107; description of, 104-107; problems related to, 107; recommended reading on, 202-203; statistics on, 107; symptoms associated with, 15-16; treatments for, 107-108

schema-focused therapy, 107-108, 172, 206

schizoid personality disorder, 109-111; causes of, 110; description of, 109; problems related to, 109-110; recommended reading on, 203; statistics on, 110; symptoms associated with, 24; treatments for, 110-111

schizophrenia, 112-115; causes of, 114; description of, 112-113; problems related to, 113; recommended reading on, 203; statistics on, 113-114; symptoms associated with, 22-23; treatments for, 114-115

seasonal affective disorder, 61

selective serotonin reuptake inhibitors (SSRIs), 159-160

self-defeating thoughts, 62-63

self-esteem, 116

self-focused personality disorder, 116-118; causes of, 117; description of, 116; problems related to, 117; recommended reading on, 203; statistics on, 117; symptoms associated with, 25; treatments for, 118

self-observational skills, 129-130

self-psychology, 54

self-sacrifice schema, 105

serotonin, 61

serotonin syndrome, 159

somatic psychotherapies, 173;
transpersonal psychology, 174. *See
also* resources

Winfrey, Oprah, 1

withdrawal symptoms, 72-73

World Health Organization, 46, 60

worrying: normal vs. excessive, 83. *See
also* generalized anxiety disorder

XYZ

yoga, 123

Young, Jeffrey, 172

Zen Buddhism, 141

Jeffrey C. Wood, Psy.D., is a psychotherapist, living and working in the San Francisco Bay Area. He specializes in cognitive behavioral treatments for depression, anxiety, and trauma, as well as assertiveness and life-skills coaching. He can be reached at **www.drjeffreywood.com.**

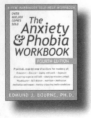
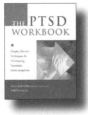
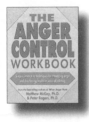